Advances in Urologic Imaging

Editor

SAMIR S. TANEJA

UROLOGIC CLINICS
OF NORTH AMERICA

www.urologic.theclinics.com

Consulting Editor
SAMIR S. TANEJA

August 2018 • Volume 45 • Number 3

ELSEVIER

1600 John F. Kennedy Boulevard • Suite 1800 • Philadelphia, Pennsylvania, 19103-2899

http://www.theclinics.com

UROLOGIC CLINICS OF NORTH AMERICA Volume 45, Number 3
August 2018 ISSN 0094-0143, ISBN-13: 978-0-323-64165-4

Editor: Kerry Holland
Developmental Editor: Sara Watkins

Urologic Clinics of North America (ISSN 0094-0143) is published quarterly by Elsevier Inc., 360 Park Avenue South, New York, NY 10010-1710. Months of issue are February, May, August, and November. Business and Editorial Offices: 1600 John F. Kennedy Blvd., Suite 1800, Philadelphia, PA 19103-2899. Periodicals postage paid at New York, NY and additional mailing offices. Subscription prices are $374.00 per year (US individuals), $721.00 per year (US institutions), $100.00 per year (US students and residents), $431.00 per year (Canadian individuals), $901.00 per year (Canadian institutions), $515.00 per year (foreign individuals), $901.00 per year (foreign institutions), and $240.00 per year (Canadian and foreign students/residents). Foreign air speed delivery is included in all *Clinics* subscription prices. All prices are subject to change without notice. **POSTMASTER:** Send address changes to *Urologic Clinics of North America*, Elsevier Health Sciences Division, Subscription Customer Service, 3251 Riverport Lane, Maryland Heights, MO 63043. **Customer Service: 1-800-654-2452 (US). From outside the United States, call 1-314-447-8871. Fax: 1-314-447-8029. E-mail: JournalsCustomerServiceusa@elsevier.com (for print support)** and **JournalsOnlineSupport-usa@elsevier.com (for online support).**

Reprints. For copies of 100 or more, of articles in this publication, please contact the Commercial Reprints Department, Elsevier Inc., 360 Park Avenue South, New York, New York 10010-1710. Tel.: 212-633-3874; Fax: 212-633-3820; E-mail: reprints@elsevier.com.

Urologic Clinics of North America is covered in MEDLINE/PubMed (*Index Medicus*), *Excerpta Medica, Current Contents/Clinical Medicine, Science Citation Index,* and *ISI/BIOMED.*

Printed in the United States of America.

PROGRAM OBJECTIVE

The goal of *Urologic Clinics of North America* is to keep practicing urologists and urology residents up to date with current clinical practice in urology by providing timely articles reviewing the state of the art in patient care.

TARGET AUDIENCE

Practicing urologists, urology residents and other healthcare professionals practicing in the discipline of urology.

LEARNING OBJECTIVES

Upon completion of this activity, participants will be able to:
- Review the use of dual-energy computed tomography for evaluation of genitourinary diseases
- Discuss image-guided renal interventions
- Recognize imaging of prostate cancer using 11C-Choline PET/Computed Tomography and Fluciclovine

ACCREDITATION

The Elsevier Office of Continuing Medical Education (EOCME) is accredited by the Accreditation Council for Continuing Medical Education (ACCME) to provide continuing medical education for physicians.

The EOCME designates this enduring material for a maximum of 15 *AMA PRA Category 1 Credit*(s)™. Physicians should claim only the credit commensurate with the extent of their participation in the activity.

All other healthcare professionals requesting continuing education credit for this enduring material will be issued a certificate of participation.

DISCLOSURE OF CONFLICTS OF INTEREST

The EOCME assesses conflict of interest with its instructors, faculty, planners, and other individuals who are in a position to control the content of CME activities. All relevant conflicts of interest that are identified are thoroughly vetted by EOCME for fair balance, scientific objectivity, and patient care recommendations. EOCME is committed to providing its learners with CME activities that promote improvements or quality in healthcare and not a specific proprietary business or a commercial interest.

The planning committee, staff, authors and editors listed below have identified no financial relationships or relationships to products or devices they or their spouse/life partner have with commercial interest related to the content of this CME activity:

Sharath K. Bhagavatula, MD; Paolo Castellucci, MD; Francesco Ceci, MD; Petar Duvnjak; Khaled M. Elsayes, MD; Sally Emad-Eldin, MD; Elliot K. Fishman, MD; Sonia Gaur, BS; Kirsi Hannele Härmä, MD; Nicole M. Hindman, MD; Michael Hofman, MBBS, FRACP, FAANMS; Kerry Holland; Jamie N. Holtz, MD; Jiaoti Huang, MD, PhD; Amir Iravani, MD, FRACP; Corey T. Jensen, MD; Fernando U. Kay, MD; Alison Kemp; Martin H. Maurer, MD; Mathias Meyer, MD; Ajaykumar C. Morani, MD; Declan G. Murphy, MBBS, FRACS; Tatenda Nzenza, BMedSci, MBBS, PGDipAnat; Thomas J. Polascik, MD; Andrei S. Purysko, MD; Siva P. Raman, MD; Ariel A. Schulman, MD; Paul B. Shyn, MD; Harriet Thoeny, MD; Baris Turkbey, MD; Federica Vernuccio, MD; Vignesh Viswanathan.

The planning committee, staff, authors and editors listed below have identified financial relationships or relationships to products or devices they or their spouse/life partner have with commercial interest related to the content of this CME activity:

Amir A. Borhani: has acted as a consultant/advisor for Guerbet LLC.
Stefano Fanti, MD: has participated in a speaker's bureau for Astellas Pharma US, Inc., Bayer AG, and Bristol-Myers Squibb Company.
Alessandro Furlan, MD: has received research support and acted as a consultant/advisor for General Electric Company and owns a patent and/or receives royalties and has acted as a consultant/advisor for Elsevier
Rajan T. Gupta, MD: has acted as a consultant/advisor for Bayer AG, Invivo, Halyard Health, Inc. and Siemens AG.
Daniele Marin, MD: receives research support from Siemens Medical Solutions USA, Inc.
Achille Mileto, MD: receives research support from General Electric Company.
Ivan Pedrosa, MD, PhD: has participated in a speaker's bureau for DAVA Oncology
Andrew B. Rosenkrantz, MD: holds a patent and/or receives royalties from Thieme Medical Publishers, Inc.
Bital Savir-Baruch, MD: has received research support from Blue Earth Diagnostics Limited.
David M. Schuster, MD: has participated in a speaker's bureau for PETNET Solutions, Inc. and has been a consultant/advisor for Syncona
Samir S. Taneja, MD: has been a consultant/advisor for Elseiver and INSIGTEC, Ltd, and received research support from MDxHealth. Dr. Taneja has also been a consultant/advisor and received research support from Sophiris Bio Corp.
Antonio C. Westphalen: has acted as an advisor/consultant for 3DBiopsy, Inc.
Lucia Zanoni, MD: has received research support from Blue Earth Diagnostics Limited.

UNAPPROVED/OFF-LABEL USE DISCLOSURE

The EOCME requires CME faculty to disclose to the participants:
1. When products or procedures being discussed are off-label, unlabelled, experimental, and/or investigational (not US Food and Drug Administration [FDA] approved); and

2. Any limitations on the information presented, such as data that are preliminary or that represent ongoing research, interim analyses, and/or unsupported opinions. Faculty may discuss information about pharmaceutical agents that is outside of FDA-approved labelling. This information is intended solely for CME and is not intended to promote off-label use of these medications. If you have any questions, contact the medical affairs department of the manufacturer for the most recent prescribing information.

TO ENROLL
To enroll in the *Urologic Clinics of North America* Continuing Medical Education program, call customer service at 1-800-654-2452 or sign up online at http://www.theclinics.com/home/cme. The CME program is available to subscribers for an additional annual fee of USD $270.

METHOD OF PARTICIPATION
In order to claim credit, participants must complete the following:
1. Complete enrolment as indicated above.
2. Read the activity.
3. Complete the CME Test and Evaluation. Participants must achieve a score of 70% on the test. All CME Tests and Evaluations must be completed online.

CME INQUIRIES/SPECIAL NEEDS
For all CME inquiries or special needs, please contact elsevierCME@elsevier.com.

Contributors

CONSULTING EDITOR

SAMIR S. TANEJA, MD
The James M. Neissa and Janet Riha Neissa
Professor of Urologic Oncology, Professor of
Urology and Radiology, Director, Division of
Urologic Oncology, Department of Urology,
Co-Director, Smilow Comprehensive Prostate
Cancer Center, NYU Langone Health,
New York, New York, USA

EDITOR

SAMIR S. TANEJA, MD
The James M. Neissa and Janet Riha Neissa
Professor of Urologic Oncology, Professor of
Urology and Radiology, Director, Division of
Urologic Oncology, Department of Urology,
Co-Director, Smilow Comprehensive Prostate
Cancer Center, NYU Langone Health, New
York, New York, USA

AUTHORS

SHARATH K. BHAGAVATULA, MD
Resident, Department of Radiology, Harvard
Medical School, Brigham and Women's
Hospital, Boston, Massachusetts,
USA

AMIR A. BORHANI, MD
Department of Radiology, University of
Pittsburgh, Pittsburgh, Pennsylvania, USA

PAOLO CASTELLUCCI, MD
Service of Nuclear Medicine, S. Orsola-Malpighi
University Hospital, University of Bologna,
Bologna, Italy

FRANCESCO CECI, MD
Service of Nuclear Medicine, S. Orsola-
Malpighi University Hospital, University of
Bologna, Bologna, Italy

PETAR DUVNJAK, MD
Assistant Professor, Department of Radiology,
Medical College of Wisconsin, Milwaukee,
Wisconsin, USA (Formerly Fellow in Abdominal
Imaging, Department of Radiology, Duke
University Medical Center, Durham, North
Carolina, USA)

KHALED M. ELSAYES, MD
Professor, Department of Diagnostic
Radiology, The University of Texas MD
Anderson Cancer Center, Houston, Texas,
USA

SALLY EMAD-ELDIN, MD
Assistant Professor, Department of Diagnostic
and Intervention Radiology, Cairo University,
Cairo, Egypt

STEFANO FANTI, MD
Service of Nuclear Medicine, S. Orsola-Malpighi University Hospital, University of Bologna, Bologna, Italy

ELLIOT K. FISHMAN, MD
Department of Radiology, Johns Hopkins University, Baltimore, Maryland, USA

ALESSANDRO FURLAN, MD
Department of Radiology, University of Pittsburgh, Pittsburgh, Pennsylvania, USA

SONIA GAUR, BS
Molecular Imaging Program, National Cancer Institute, National Institutes of Health, Bethesda, Maryland, USA

RAJAN T. GUPTA, MD
Associate Professor, Department of Radiology, Assistant Professor, Department of Surgery, Division of Urologic Surgery, Duke Prostate Center, Duke University Medical Center, Duke Cancer Institute, Durham, North Carolina, USA

KIRSI HANNELE HÄRMÄ, MD
Department of Radiology, Inselspital, Bern University Hospital, University of Bern, Bern, Switzerland

NICOLE M. HINDMAN, MD
Associate Professor, Department of Radiology, NYU School of Medicine, New York, New York, USA

MICHAEL S. HOFMAN, MBBS, FRACP, FAANMS
Professor, Department of Cancer Imaging, Center for Molecular Imaging, Peter MacCallum Cancer Centre, University of Melbourne, Melbourne, Victoria, Australia

JAMIE N. HOLTZ, MD
Department of Radiology, Duke University Medical Center, Durham, North Carolina, USA

JIAOTI HUANG, MD, PhD
Professor and Chair, Department of Pathology, Duke University Medical Center, Duke Cancer Institute, Durham, North Carolina, USA

AMIR IRAVANI, MD, FRACP
Department of Cancer Imaging, Center for Molecular Imaging, Peter MacCallum Cancer Centre, Melbourne, Victoria, Australia

COREY T. JENSEN, MD
Assistant Professor, Department of Diagnostic Radiology, The University of Texas MD Anderson Cancer Center, Houston, Texas, USA

FERNANDO U. KAY, MD
Department of Radiology, The University of Texas Southwestern Medical Center, Dallas, Texas, USA

DANIELE MARIN, MD
Department of Radiology, Duke University Medical Center, Durham, North Carolina, USA

MARTIN H. MAURER, MD
Department of Radiology, Inselspital, Bern University Hospital, University of Bern, Bern, Switzerland

MATHIAS MEYER, MD
Department of Radiology, Duke University Medical Center, Durham, North Carolina, USA

ACHILLE MILETO, MD
Department of Radiology, UW School of Medicine, Seattle, Washington, USA

AJAYKUMAR C. MORANI, MD
Assistant Professor, Department of Diagnostic Radiology, The University of Texas MD Anderson Cancer Center, Houston, Texas, USA

DECLAN G. MURPHY, MBBS, FRACS
Division of Cancer Surgery, Associate Professor, Department of Surgical Oncology, Peter MacCallum Cancer Centre, Melbourne, Victoria, Australia

TATENDA NZENZA, BMedSci, MBBS, PGDipAnat
Division of Cancer Surgery, Department of Surgery, Peter MacCallum Cancer Centre, University of Melbourne, Austin Hospital, Melbourne, Victoria, Australia

IVAN PEDROSA, MD, PhD
Departments of Radiology and Urology, Advanced Imaging Research Center, The University of Texas Southwestern Medical Center, Dallas, Texas, USA

THOMAS J. POLASCIK, MD, FACS
Professor, Department of Surgery, Division of Urologic Surgery, Duke Prostate Center, Duke University Medical Center, Duke Cancer Institute, Durham, North Carolina, USA

ANDREI S. PURYSKO, MD
Section of Abdominal Imaging, Imaging Institute, Cleveland Clinic, Cleveland, Ohio, USA

SIVA P. RAMAN, MD
Department of Radiology, Johns Hopkins University, Baltimore, Maryland, USA

ANDREW B. ROSENKRANTZ, MD
Department of Radiology, NYU Langone Medical Center, New York, New York, USA

BITAL SAVIR-BARUCH, MD
Assistant Professor, Department of Radiology, Loyola University Medical Center, Maywood, Illinois, USA

ARIEL A. SCHULMAN, MD
Fellow in Urologic Oncology, Department of Surgery, Division of Urologic Surgery, Duke Prostate Center, Duke University Medical Center, Durham, North Carolina, USA

DAVID M. SCHUSTER, MD
Associate Professor, Department of Radiology and Imaging Sciences, Emory University Hospital, Emory University, Atlanta, Georgia, USA

PAUL B. SHYN, MD
Associate Professor, Department of Radiology, Harvard Medical School, Brigham and Women's Hospital, Boston, Massachusetts, USA

HARRIET THOENY, MD
Professor, Department of Radiology, Inselspital, Bern University Hospital, University of Bern, Bern, Switzerland

BARIS TURKBEY, MD
Molecular Imaging Program, National Cancer Institute, National Institutes of Health, Bethesda, Maryland, USA

FEDERICA VERNUCCIO, MD
Department of Radiology, Duke University Medical Center, Durham, North Carolina, USA; Section of Radiology -Di.Bi.Med., University Hospital "Paolo Giaccone," University of Palermo, Palermo, Italy

ANTONIO C. WESTPHALEN, MD, PhD
Departments of Radiology and Biomedical Imaging and Urology, University of California, San Francisco, San Francisco, California, USA

LUCIA ZANONI, MD
Department of Nuclear Medicine, Azienda Ospedaliero-Universitaria di Bologna, Policlinico Sant'Orsola-Malpighi, Bologna, Italy

Contents

critical, especially in patients with cancer; the presence of adrenal metastasis changes prognosis and treatment. Characterization of adrenal lesions predominantly relies on morphologic and physiologic features to enable correct diagnosis and management. Key diagnostic features to differentiate benign and malignant adrenal lesions include presence or /absence of intracytoplasmic lipid, fat cells, hemorrhage, calcification, or necrosis and locoregional and distant disease; enhancement pattern and washout values; and lesion size and stability. This article reviews a spectrum of adrenal pathologies.

Computed tomography (CT) urography is the best noninvasive method of evaluating the upper urinary tract for urothelial malignancies. However, the utility of CT urography is heavily contingent on the use of proper image acquisition protocols. This article focuses on the appropriate protocols for optimizing CT urography acquisitions, including contrast administration and the timing of imaging acquisitions, as well as the use of ancillary techniques to increase collecting system distention. In addition, imaging findings are discussed that should raise concern for urothelial carcinoma at each of the 3 segments of the urinary tract: the intrarenal collecting systems, ureters, and bladder.

This review article provides an overview of diffusion-weighted (DW) MR imaging in the urogenital tract. Compared with conventional cross-sectional imaging methods, the additional value of DW-MR imaging in the detection and further characterization of benign and malignant lesions of the kidneys, bladder, prostate, and pelvic lymph nodes is discussed, as well as the role of DW-MR imaging in the evaluation of treatment response.

 Video content accompanies this article at http://www.urologic.theclinics.com.

Multiparametric MR imaging provides detailed anatomic assessment of the prostate as well as information that allows the detection and characterization of prostate cancer. To obtain high-quality MR imaging of the prostate, radiologists must understand sequence optimization to overcome commonly encountered technical challenges. This article discusses the techniques that are used in state-of-the-art MR imaging of the prostate, including imaging protocols, hardware considerations, and important aspects of patient preparation, with an emphasis on the recommendations provided in the prostate imaging reporting and data system version 2 guidelines.

Multiparametric MR imaging of the prostate is a complex study that combines anatomic and functional imaging. The complexity of this technique, along with an increasing demand, has brought new challenges to imaging interpretation. The

Prostate Imaging Reporting and Data System provides radiologists with guidelines to standardize interpretation. This article discusses the interpretation of the pulse sequences recommended in the Prostate Imaging Reporting and Data System version 2 guidelines, reviews advanced quantitative imaging tools, and discusses future directions.

Meaningful changes to the approach of prostate cancer staging and management have been made over the past decade with increasing demand for high-quality multiparametric MR imaging (mpMRI) of the prostate. This article focuses on the evolving paradigm of prostate cancer staging, with emphasis on the role of mpMRI on staging and its integration into clinical decision-making. Current prostate cancer staging systems are defined, and the role of mpMRI in the detection of non–organ-confined disease and how it has an impact on the selection of appropriate next steps are discussed. Several imaging pitfalls, limitations, and future directions of mpMRI also are discussed.

Prostate multiparametric MR imaging (mpMRI) plays an important role in local evaluation after treatment of prostate cancer. After radical prostatectomy, radiation therapy, and focal therapy, mpMRI can be used to visualize normal posttreatment changes and to diagnose locally recurrent disease. An understanding of the various treatments and expected changes is essential for complete and accurate posttreatment mpMRI interpretation.

This article reviews the role of ^{11}C-choline-PET/computed tomography (CT) in patients with prostate cancer for diagnosis, staging, and restaging the disease in case of biochemical recurrence after primary treatment. The main application of this imaging procedure is restaging of the disease in case of biochemical recurrence. ^{11}C-Choline-PET/CT proved its value for metastases-directed salvage therapies and for monitoring therapy response in castration-resistant patients. Prostate-specific antigen (PSA) and PSA kinetics values confirmed their correlation with ^{11}C-choline PET/CT sensitivity. ^{11}C-CholinePET/CT, despite low sensitivity to stage disease or in case of biochemical failure with low PSA levels, has an important impact on the management of patients with prostate cancer.

Prostate cancer is the most common cancer and the second leading cause of cancer death in men in the United States. Despite its high prevalence, diagnosis and surveillance is limited owing to indolent biology. Functional imaging techniques improved the ability to detect disease. Amino acids are building blocks of proteins, and intracellular transport is upregulated in prostate cancer. Normal biodistribution patterns of fluciclovine include uptake in the liver and pancreas with minimal to no urine excretion, a distinct advantage for prostate cancer imaging. This article provides a detailed overview of the use of F-18 fluciclovine PET in prostate cancer imaging.

Radiolabeled prostate-specific membrane antigen (PSMA) PET is emerging as an important modality for imaging prostate cancer (PCa). Promising clinical experience has led to increasing number of studies exploring the role of PSMA PET in different aspects of PCa, including primary detection, risk stratification, targeted biopsy, initial staging, restaging at biochemical recurrence, biologic characterization, treatment response assessment, and prognostication. PSMA PET may prove an important disease biomarker, expand our understanding of the pathogenesis, and pave the way for personalized management of PCa.

UROLOGIC CLINICS OF NORTH AMERICA

THE CLINICS ARE AVAILABLE ONLINE!
Access your subscription at:
www.theclinics.com

Preface
Advances in Urologic Imaging

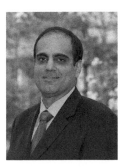

Samir S. Taneja, MD
Editor

Imaging of the urinary tract has long been a fascination of the urologist. We are among the first specialties to introduce imaging into our daily practice in order to enhance our diagnostic capabilities and evolve our treatment paradigms. Since the sequential advent of the intravenous pyelogram, retrograde and antegrade instillation of contrast into urinary lumen, and fluoroscopy, our imaging armamentarium has grown by leaps and bounds. Ultrasonography allowed noninvasive evaluation of stones, bladder emptying, testis masses, and eventually, irreversibly changed the path and trajectory of prostate cancer diagnosis. Cross-sectional imaging has allowed a level of preoperative planning previously thought to be impossible. Through its implementation, our surgical outcomes improved and intraoperative morbidity declined, as we knew the exact location of the stone, the size and extent of the tumor, and the anomalous blood supply of the kidney, before we got there.

With each evolution of imaging has come an evolution of the clinical practice paradigm. Diseases thought to be untreatable have become treatable through better anatomic assessment and, in some cases, earlier detection. Treatment decisions are now often based upon preoperative risk assessment through provision of qualitative parameters of the disease process, rather than just assessment of anatomic detail. In this way, imaging has empowered the urologist to know the intricacies of the individual patient's disease long before tackling the treatment and to assess the likely efficacy of treatment before trial and error.

Imaging continues to rapidly evolve and, in doing so, carries the potential for us to further evolve our practices. Functional imaging sequences not only improve the specificity of disease detection but also provide quantitative metrics by which disease aggressiveness, ideal therapy, or response to therapy might be predicted. In this way, imaging in urologic practice is no longer just a diagnostic tool. It has, instead, become an essential part of the disease management strategy for many urologic diseases. In this unique issue, I have borrowed recently published articles from the *Radiologic Clinics of North America* and the *PET Clinics* that I felt may be of interest to the practicing urologist. Collectively, the articles review the current state-of-the-art in upper and lower genitourinary tract imaging and provide insight into emerging imaging techniques with which urologists may not yet be familiar. It is my belief that these imaging techniques will eventually become a standard tool in the urologist's chest, much like the innovative imaging techniques developed before them. I would like to thank the authors of the articles for allowing us to republish them, and for revising the articles, when needed, to ensure they are up-to-date. It is my hope the issue will be of great value to our readership.

Samir S. Taneja, MD
Division of Urologic Oncology
Smilow Comprehensive Prostate Cancer Center
Department of Urology
NYU Langone Medical Center
150 East 32nd Street, Suite 200
New York, NY 10016, USA

E-mail address:
samir.taneja@nyumc.org

Urol Clin N Am 45 (2018) xv
https://doi.org/10.1016/j.ucl.2018.05.001
0094-0143/18/© 2018 Published by Elsevier Inc.

Use of Dual-Energy Computed Tomography for Evaluation of Genitourinary Diseases

Federica Vernuccio, MD[a,b], Mathias Meyer, MD[a],
Achille Mileto, MD[c], Daniele Marin, MD[a],*

KEYWORDS

- Dual-energy CT • Renal stone • Renal mass • Radiation dose

KEY POINTS

- The elemental physics basis for dual-energy computed tomography imaging is represented by application of 2 different x-ray energies.
- Renal stone mineralization can be noninvasively ascertained using dual-energy computed tomography.
- Dual-energy computed tomography has the potential for ameliorating incidental renal mass and renal cell carcinoma evaluation.
- Potential limitations and pitfalls pertain to dual-energy computed tomography and their knowledge is of utmost importance when dual-energy computed tomography is used for imaging the genitourinary system.
- Dual-energy computed tomography protocols have radiation dose values close to those of traditional computed tomography reference.

INTRODUCTION

Computed tomography (CT) is the most widely used imaging technique in the diagnosis, management, and follow-up of genitourinary diseases.[1] CT scanning can accurately detect and characterize the wide spectrum of genitourinary diseases, such as renal stone or renal parenchymal abnormalities, guiding clinician to the most appropriate treatment.[1] However, many limitations pertain to conventional CT imaging techniques in the evaluation of genitourinary disease.[1]

After its introduction for clinical applications about a decade ago, accumulating evidence has suggested that dual-energy CT scanning may overcome some of the conventional CT limitations and expands CT solution available for assessment of genitourinary system diseases.[2–4]

The aim of this article is 4-fold: to offer a practical synopsis on foundation concepts for dual-energy CT scans, to outline the clinical application of dual-energy CT scans for genitourinary diseases, to critically appraise the strengths and

Portions of this article were previously published in March 2017 *Radiologic Clinics*, Volume 55, Issue 2.

Disclosure: A. Mileto receives research support from GE Healthcare. D. Marin receives research support from Siemens Helthineers. F. Vernuccio and M. Meyer have nothing to disclose.

[a] Department of Radiology, Duke University Medical Center, Box 3808 Erwin Road, Durham, NC 27710, USA; [b] Section of Radiology -Di.Bi.Med., University Hospital "Paolo Giaccone", University of Palermo, Via del Vespro 129, 90127, Palermo, Italy; [c] Department of Radiology, University of Washington School of Medicine, Box 357115, 1959 Northeast Pacific Street, Seattle, WA 98195, USA

* Corresponding author.

E-mail address: danielemarin2@gmail.com

Urol Clin N Am 45 (2018) 297–310
https://doi.org/10.1016/j.ucl.2018.03.012

BASIC PHYSICS PRINCIPLES AND TECHNOLOGY

The differentiation of various materials using conventional single-energy CT scanning is based on their x-ray attenuation expressed as CT numbers in Hounsfield units (HU). CT numbers, however, are arbitrary units of x-ray attenuation, calibrated with reference to water.[5] This inherent limitation of CT numbers results in the potential ambiguity for discriminating different materials owing to considerable overlap in material attenuation. Dual-energy CT scanning may decrease this ambiguity by interrogating the material-specific attenuation properties at different energy levels.[6] Dual-energy CT scanner designs available for clinical use include dual-source, rapid-switching, dual-layer detector, and sequential dual-energy CT scans.

The elemental physical mechanism of dual-energy CT scanning is represented by the photoelectric effect.[7] The photoelectric effect refers to the removal of an electron from the k-shell (the innermost shell) of an atom by an incident photon.[5,7] The photoelectric effect occurs when an incident photon has sufficient energy to overcome the k-shell binding energy of an electron.[5,7] This binding energy is characteristic of each elemental chemical element. The closer the energy level is to the k-edge of a substance such as iodine, the more the substance attenuates. k-edge values (ie, the maximum peak of attenuation for a given material) vary for each element, and they increase as the atomic number increases.[7-10] Indeed, chemical elements with a higher atomic number, such as calcium and iodine, can be characterized from other components of the matter that have a significantly lower k-edge and consequently a different attenuation spectrum.[7-10]

Moreover, dual-energy CT acquisition enables the generation of multiple datasets, having clear advantages in tumor detection, lesion characterization and, possibly, evaluation of treatment response. By interrogating the attenuation characteristics of different materials at different x-ray energies, virtual monochromatic images can generate tissue-specific spectral attenuation curves based on the unique k-edge characteristics of materials with different elemental composition.[10]

Dual-energy CT scanning performs as a single energy CT scan, producing conventional images (ie, blending and monoenergetic images) that can be optimized to improve iodine conspicuity and allow material-specific data analysis. Various material decomposition algorithms can be applied to reconstructed voxels, with some existing differences between dual-source and single-source platforms.[6-10] The 3-materials decomposition algorithm used by dual-source platforms allows for targeting the iodine contrast material: iodine can be either erased from the image thus producing a virtual noncontrast (VNC) image (**Fig. 1**), or selectively portrayed, resulting in a color-coded iodine series (see **Fig. 1**).[6-10] The evaluation of imaged tissues through real-time, computer-based interaction allows for quantitative extraction and measurement of iodine contrast content in milligrams per milliliter (see **Fig. 1**).[7,9] Rapid-switching and spectral detector CT systems use a 2-material decomposition approach targeting companion materials, thus enabling reconstruction of binary sets of images (eg, water-density and iodine-density images). These datasets provide separate material information and, similar to the 3-material

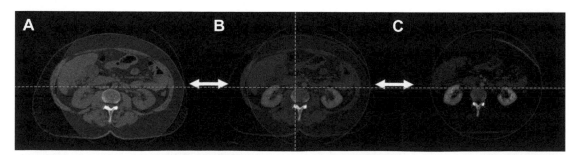

Fig. 1. Three materials decomposition algorithm allows for identifying the iodine contrast material. Iodine can be extracted from reconstructed voxels to obtain a virtual noncontrast image (*A*) or it can be selectively represented in different degrees in the same image dataset, resulting in a color-coded iodine series having varying degrees of representation of the contrast material (*B*) up to an iodine map (*C*). Based on the same principle, iodine can be quantified from a region-of-interest measurement in milligrams per milliliter.

decomposition approach, material can be quantified in milligrams per milliliter.[3,8–11]

APPLICATIONS OF DUAL-ENERGY COMPUTED TOMOGRAPHY FOR THE GENITOURINARY SYSTEM
Dual-Energy Computed Tomography in the Assessment of Urinary Calculi

The mineral composition of urinary calculi is quite variable and comprehends, in the majority of the cases, calcium oxalates (monohydrate or dihydrate) or phosphates (brushite or apatite), uric acid, and cysteine.[12]

The attenuation of different subtypes of calculi overlap on polychromatic CT scanning, limiting the evaluation of calculus composition. Renal calculi protocols with dual-energy CT scans can be used to accurately determine the mineral composition.[13] Mineral composition analysis can play a significant role in stratifying patient treatment as well as, potentially, predicting the likelihood of calculi formation.[14–18]

Dual-energy CT–based material decomposition postprocessing algorithms are able to reliably distinguish between cystine, uric acid, struvite, calcium, and brushite stones.[15–20] These algorithms use basic two-dimensional diagrams plotting out CT attenuation of stones and surrounding urine using data collected at the 2 spectra. The dual-energy CT ratio, which represents the ratio of attenuation delta at low and high energy, can be used to ascertain mineral composition as follows: uric acid stones if the ratio is below 1.13, cystine stones if the ratio is between 1.13 and 1.24, and calcium oxalates/phosphates stones if it is greater than 1.24.[20] By using these cutoffs, dual-energy CT evaluation has shown a sensitivity of 100% and a specificity of 94% in predicting uric acid renal stones composition and an accuracy in differentiating uric acid and nonuric acid stones of 96%.[19] In addition, dual-energy CT ratios combined with volume and morphologic metrics seem to be promising for predicting stone fragility and, these data, if confirmed, may affect surgical management.[21]

Dual-energy CT ratio thresholds for differentiating different stone compositions are highly affected by noise and artifacts occurring in large subjects.[7,22] However, emerging data suggest that discrimination among further subtypes of non–urate-based urinary calculi (ie, cystine, brushite, calcium oxalate, and hydroxyapatite) can be successfully carried out with use of 100/150 Sn kV setting in obese patients as well.[23]

By vendor convention, material decomposition postprocessing algorithms portray different renal calculi subtypes by adopting color-coded maps, where calcium oxalate and uric acid calculi are represented in blue and red, respectively (**Fig. 2**).[7,14]

Dual-Energy Computed Tomography for Renal Mass Evaluation

Single-phase conventional CT scanning can reliably distinguish simple cysts from hyperattenuating lesions when the former display CT attenuation less than 20 Hounsfield units. However, hyperattenuating lesions need further evaluation because often it can be difficult to distinguish benign hyperdense cysts, filled with hemorrhagic or proteinaceous content, from solid renal lesions. Because of this difficulty, the characterization of a renal mass on conventional single-energy CT necessitates both a true unenhanced and a nephrographic phase to determine if there is enhancement of the mass.[3,24] In addition, small benign simple cysts can show a spurious increase in attenuation, or pseudoenhancement, between the unenhanced and enhanced images (**Fig. 3**), which can be a reason for further work-up.

By examining the attenuation changes of various tissues at different x-ray energies, dual-energy quantitative spectral analysis may overcome the confounding effect of energy shift phenomena and can potentially provide a solution to the aforementioned clinical dilemma when encountering pseudoenhancement on conventional multidetector CT scans (see **Fig. 3**).[13,25–28] The mitigation of this phenomenon may be at the root of the improved specificity for characterization of small renal lesions with the use of single-phase contrast-enhanced dual-energy quantitative spectral analysis, compared with conventional single-energy attenuation measurements.[29,30]

Virtual noncontrast and water density images can be used as surrogates of true noncontrast (TNC) images to appreciate baseline characteristics of renal masses.[3,4,9,11,31–34] Indeed, several studies confirmed that VNC images can be comparable with TNC images in terms of renal lesion characterization and detection of contrast enhancement.[34–36] This results in radiation dose decreases of up to 50% in comparison with traditional multiphasic renal CT protocols.[33,34,37]

Moreover, dual-energy CT allows to assess both qualitatively and quantitatively the iodine concentration in a region of interest. Qualitative assessment is performed through dual-energy color-coded iodine overlay images. Iodine overlay images allow the determination of enhancement easier by directly visualizing the presence of iodine within a mass as voxels; iodine is bright or

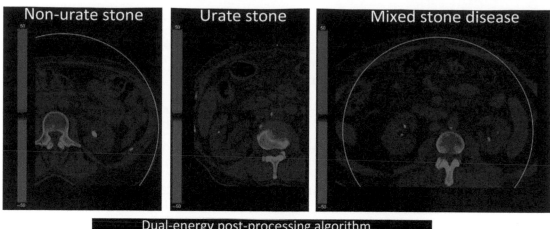

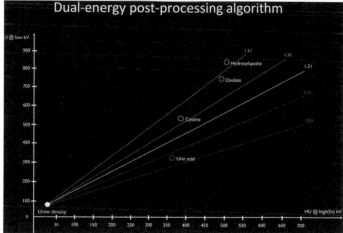

Fig. 2. Dual-energy color-coding representation of mixed stone disease: the 2 nonurate stones are shown in blue, and the urate stone is represented in red. (*Adapted from* Mileto A, Marin D. Dual-energy computed tomography in genitourinary imaging. Radiol Clin North America. 2017;55:375; *with permission* from Siemens Medical Solutions USA, Inc, Malvern, PA.)

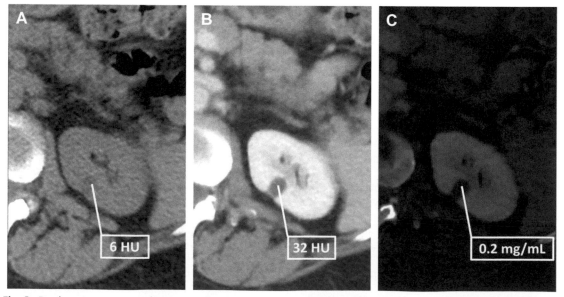

Fig. 3. Dual-energy computed tomography scan in a patient with a renal cyst. Although pseudoenhancement is observed by positioning a region of interest on both (*A*) unenhanced and (*B*) contrast-enhanced images, (*C*) color-coded iodine overlay image provides direct color-coded visualization of iodine content as well as its quantification within the image. Note lack of iodine signal intensity within the cyst, denoting absence of contrast enhancement. HU, Hounsfield unit.

color coded on iodine overlay images.[11] On these datasets, nonenhancing renal cysts can be promptly diagnosed based on the lack of intralesion iodine signal (**Fig. 4**), whereas most enhancing renal masses will demonstrate color within, owing to iodine content (**Fig. 5**).[3,4,9,11,31–33,37–40] As such, the use of dual-energy color-coded iodine overlay images has shown to simplify the workflow of renal CT protocols by decreasing the reader's interpretation time.[34,41–43] The quantitative approach is based on the calculation of iodine concentration, expressed in milligrams per milliliter (see **Fig. 4**).[8] Enhancement of a renal mass is defined by an iodine concentration of greater than 2 and 0.5 mg/mL for rapid kV-switching single-source dual-energy CT scans and dual-source dual-energy CT scans, respectively.[24]

Dual-Energy Computed Tomography in the Assessment of Renal Cell Carcinoma

Dual-energy CT scans can help the radiologist in diagnosing renal cell carcinoma (RCC) and evaluating response to treatment.[44–47] Low-energy virtual monochromatic images reconstructed from the dual-energy dataset can increase the conspicuity of arterially enhancing renal masses, such as RCC, and can allow an accurate preoperative assessment of RCC and renal vasculature.

Iodine quantification with dual-energy CT can also be used to discriminate between clear cell and papillary RCC with high accuracy.[13,48] Optimal imaging thresholds to discriminate between clear cell (**Fig. 6**) and papillary RCC (**Fig. 7**), however, may vary with different dual-energy implementations.[49] This can be due to inherent variation within a broad spectrum in tumor characteristics between these two main RCC subtypes, differences in noise characteristics and spectral separation between the different generations and types of dual-energy implementations.[26–28] This discrepancy in cutoff values may confuse and potentially preclude longitudinal evaluation of the same lesion with different dual-energy platforms.[50–52]

Color-coded iodine overlay images and iodine maps may be useful in the follow-up of patients with RCC after noninvasive locoregional treatment such as percutaneous cryoablation and radiofrequency ablation.[3,4,53,54] Posttreatment changes in these patients include neoangiogenesis and inflammation that result into perinephric stranding, with occurrence of varying-sided hemorrhagic collections in the treatment zone.[53–55] These changes complicate the evaluation of the treatment zone with conventional CT scanning.[53–55] Color-coded iodine overlay images and iodine maps have the potential for resolving these issues, because solid components that uptake iodine contrast are electively displayed, which may streamline the postprocedural follow-up.[3,4,53,54]

The usefulness of dual-energy CT scanning has been also demonstrated for metastatic RCC.[3,56] Metastatic RCC lesions are promptly visualized as highly vascularized masses on color-coded iodine overlay images or iodine maps derived

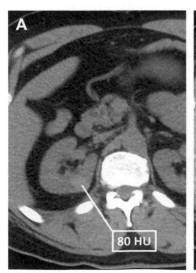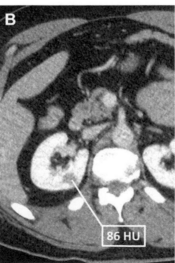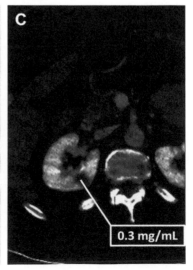

Fig. 4. Dual-energy computed tomography scan in a patient with a high-attenuating cyst. The lesion shows high attenuation values on unenhanced image (*A*) and on nephrographic image (*B*). The iodine map (*C*) allows ruling out any iodine content within lesion, therefore allowing definite diagnosis of high-attenuating cyst. HU, Hounsfield unit.

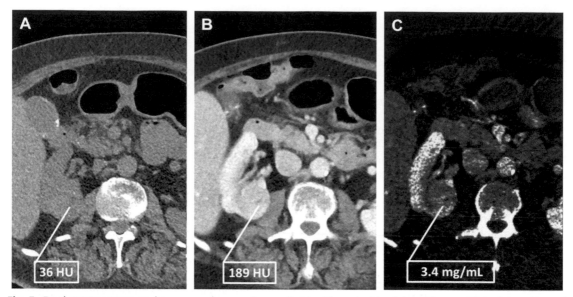

Fig. 5. Dual energy computed tomography scan in a patient with an incidental renal mass. Virtual unenhanced (A) and contrast-enhanced images (B) show an enhancing mass in the right kidney. The color-coded iodine overlay image (C) allows for precisely quantifying iodine content. The patient was operated on and the lesion was diagnosed as oncocytoma, a relatively benign renal tumor. HU, Hounsfield unit.

from dual-energy scan performed in the arterial phase (**Fig. 8**).[3] In addition, the quantitative measurements on iodine maps can be adopted to assess response to treatment rather than commonly used Response Evaluation Criteria in Solid Tumors or Choi criteria.[3,46,57] Measuring pure iodine density or iodine concentration on iodine maps in metastatic RCC proved to show a significantly greater decrease of tumor vascularization owing to antiangiogenic treatment than measuring density alone.[56] It is conceivable that this is due to the effect of this type of therapy, which may induce a disease stability status rather than lesion shrinkage or disappearance.

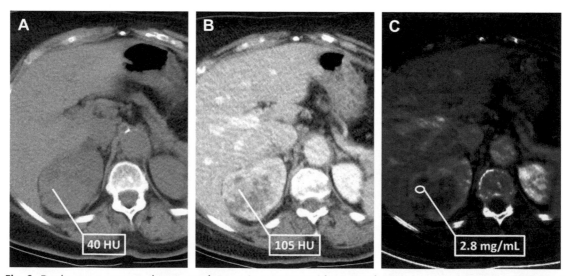

Fig. 6. Dual energy computed tomography scan in a patient with an exophytic renal tumor. Virtual unenhanced (A) and contrast-enhanced images (B) show a heterogeneously enhancing mass in the right kidney. A region-of-interest cursor is drawn in the color-coded iodine overlay image (C) within the viable component of the tumor, which show high iodine content values. The patient was operated on and the lesion was diagnosed as clear cell renal cell carcinoma. HU, Hounsfield unit.

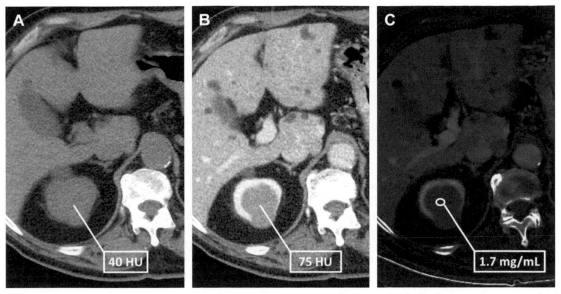

Fig. 7. Dual energy computed tomography (CT) scan in a patient with an exophytic renal tumor. Unenhanced (*A*) and contrast-enhanced images (*B*) show a homogeneously enhancing mass in the upper pole of the right kidney. In the iodine map (*C*) obtained through triangulation, a region of interest is drawn within the tumor, which shows high iodine content values. The patient was operated on and the lesion was diagnosed as papillary renal cell carcinoma. HU, Hounsfield unit.

Dual-Energy Computed Tomography for the Assessment of Incidental Adrenal Nodules

The currently accepted CT protocol for adrenal mass characterization consists of a 3-phase wash-out acquisition protocol, including an unenhanced, a venous, and a delayed phase.[58] The values examined for the workup of an adrenal incidentaloma are the unenhanced attenuation and the absolute washout values of adrenal lesions. An adrenal mass that is 10 HU or less is

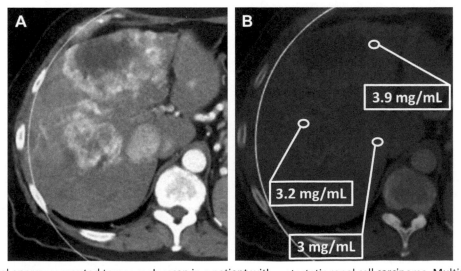

Fig. 8. Dual energy computed tomography scan in a patient with metastatic renal cell carcinoma. Multiple hypervascular liver metastases are appreciated on the linearly blended image (*A*). The 50% iodine overlay images (*B*) are obtained by virtue of a material triangulation-based decomposition approach in which intralesion iodine is observed. Multiple region of interest cursors are drawn within the metastases, which allow for the estimation of iodine content. (*Adapted from* Mileto A, Marin D. Dual-energy computed tomography in genitourinary imaging. Radiol Clin North Am 2017;55:383; with permission.)

classified as a adenoma.[59,60] The venous and delayed phases are essential to differentiate lipid-poor adenomas from other masses to diagnose a lipid-poor adenoma with attenuation of greater than 10 HU on an unenhanced CT image, because adenomas have higher washin and more rapid washout than do masses that are not adenomas, including primary adrenal malignancy (eg, adrenocortical carcinoma) or metastases.[61–63]

Gupta and colleagues[64] reported that the decreased attenuation value of an adrenal lesion at 80-kVp unenhanced CT scan compared with that at 140-kVp unenhanced CT scan is a highly specific sign for adenoma (**Fig. 9**); however, the sensitivity for adenoma was so low that one-half of the adenomas were misclassified on unenhanced dual-energy CT images. Moreover, the clinical use of this strategy was precluded by the need for an additional dual-energy noncontrast series, potentially increasing radiation dose.

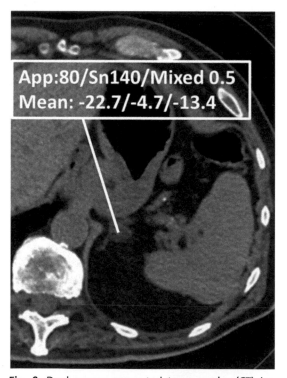

Fig. 9. Dual-energy computed tomography (CT) images obtained with a dual-source CT implementation scan in a patient with adrenal incidentaloma arising from the left adrenal gland. The lesion is seen on the noncontrast image, which was obtained in dual energy mode. A region of interest placed within the adrenal lesion identifies an attenuation shift between the 2 energy spectra, which is suggestive of a fat-containing adrenal adenoma. (*Adapted from* Mileto A, Marin D. Dual-energy computed tomography in genitourinary imaging. Radiol Clin North Am 2017;55:373–91; with permission.)

Dual-energy CT scans can be used to evaluate incidental adrenal nodules with different approaches and options using 2 main dual-energy implementations.[65–67] Using dual-source systems, VNC attenuation values of adrenal lesions could potentially be used to establish the diagnosis of adenoma, thus providing a reasonable surrogate of attenuation measured from TNC series when these are not available. A recent metanalysis including 5 studies performed with dual-source dual-energy CT scans compared the diagnostic accuracy of VNC and TNC for the diagnosis of adrenal adenomas.[68] This metaanalysis showed that there were statistically significant differences reported in measured HU densities between VNC and TNC for the 60-s contrast delays, whereas no significant differences were seen for 150-minute delays.[68] However, the pooled sensitivity of VNC was not significantly different from the pooled sensitivity of TNC.[68] Moreover, calculation of the fat fraction through region of interest measurements from the same spectral series may provide a new quantitative marker facilitating the evaluation of incidental adrenal nodules when the traditional attenuation-based approach is not succesful.[69]

In case of use of rapid-switching dual-energy CT scanning, iodine-subtracted images are generated based on water–iodine 2-material decomposition. The material density images, however, provide density information as opposed to attenuation.[70] Material density based on fat–iodine companion image sets can help in the discrimination of fat-containing adenomas and adrenal metastases.[57,71–73] Another diagnostic possibility for the workup of incidental adrenal lesion with rapid-switching dual-energy CT scans is the interrogation of adrenal nodules across monochromatic curves energy spectrum.[57,73] Indeed, differences in iodine washout between adrenal adenomas and nonadenomatous lesions have been encountered with progressively higher kiloelectronvolts.[73] Datasets at 140 keV (referred to as a pseudovirtual unenhanced series) have been used for evaluating adrenal incidental lesions, because these datasets allow for the maximization of differences in monochromatic attenuation.[73] Recently, a relatively new multimaterial decomposition algorithm has enabled the generation of virtual unenhanced series images with the capability to measure Hounsfield units.[74,75] In this postprocessing technique, the attenuation curve of each voxel is analyzed, and the fraction of different materials can also be calculated. The correlation of attenuation values between VNC and TNC on a population basis proved to be excellent, but intrapatient differences of attenuation values were considerable with attenuation values based on VNC that tend to be higher than TNC attenuation values.[74,75]

LIMITATIONS AND PITFALLS

A certain number of limitations and pitfalls have to be cautiously considered when dual-energy CT scan is adopted routinely for imaging the genitourinary system. First, differences in attenuation between VNC and TNC of more than 10 HU have been reported in some of the measured regions of interest.[74,75] The overestimation or underestimation of attenuation on VNC might potentially lead to an erroneous imaging diagnosis when a threshold of change of 10 HU is used for lesion characterization and further optimization of postprocessing algorithms are necessary before complete replacement of TNC with VNC images. Moreover, an excessive iodine suppression from contrast-enhanced scans may suppress the signal of small stones (usually <3 mm) in the VNC, not allowing their detection (**Fig. 10**).[76]

Second, the degree of enhancement of renal lesions, and hence the measured iodine content within renal lesions, depends on the dual-energy platform used and the acquisition time after contrast administration. The iodine density thresholds are specific for the phase of image acquisition and on the dual-energy CT platform used as well. This limits the routine clinical applicability of iodine density thresholds in follow-up CT examinations.

Third, owing to the inherent shortcomings of the algorithms used to discriminate among materials having similar attenuation coefficient energy dependencies (eg, iodine, iron, and calcium), it happens that lesions containing either a high concentration of hemoglobin or calcium may be misinterpreted as displaying having enhancement or iodine uptake on iodine maps.[34,37]

Fourth, appropriate patient selection is of utmost importance when dual-energy CT scanning is performed. Body sizes may affect the diagnostic performance of dual-energy CT scanning for various clinical applications.[50,77] A larger body size can deteriorate image quality owing to associated increase in noise and the likelihood of lack of x-ray photons not properly reaching the CT detectors.[69,78] This issue is relevant with both dual-source dual-energy CT scanning and rapid kV-switching single-source dual-energy CT scanning.[79] Because of the effect of body size on image quality and diagnostic

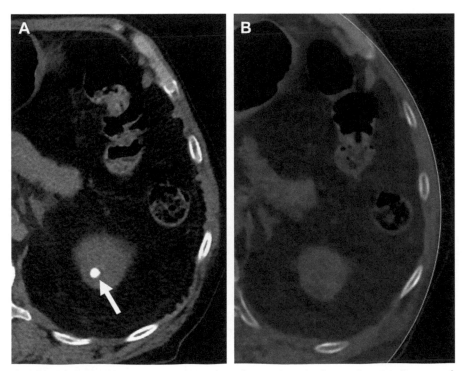

Fig. 10. Dual energy computed tomography scan in a patient with multiple renal stones. True unenhanced scan (A) shows a 4-mm renal stones (*arrow*) in the upper pole of the left kidney. In the corresponding virtual nonenhanced image (B), created subtracting the iodine signal, the 4-mm stone is not identifiable owing to oversubtraction of stone signal.

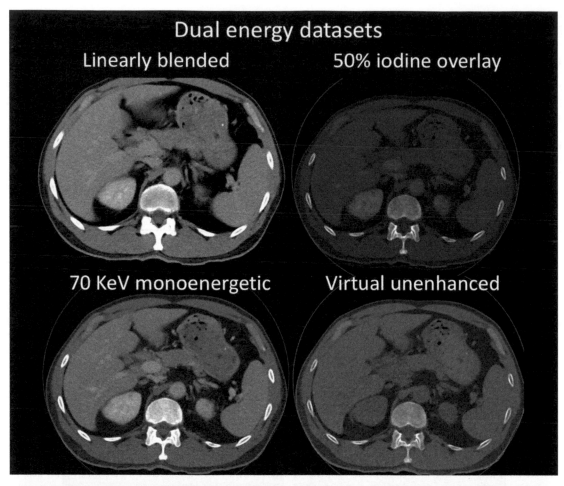

Fig. 11. Collage represents a typical dual energy computed tomography (CT) triple-phase genitourinary protocol: dual energy datasets (*top*), and patient radiation dose protocol showing CT dose index and dose–length product values of all dual energy scans (*bottom*).

performance, many centers use a cutoff to exclude patients from dual-energy CT scanning. The optimal cutoff to generate acceptable image quality with the low tube potential (80-kVp) is reported to be from 34.9 to 35.8 cm for the transverse diameter measured from the initial scout image, depending on the organ of interest being imaged.[80] However, given the paucity of the literature on this topic, the practice patterns vary among different institutions.[79]

Finally, as for other abdominal clinical settings, dual energy raised concerns about possible additional radiation dose because 2 separate datasets are obtained at different tube voltages. However, different technical realizations of dual-energy CT scanning have varying impact on radiation exposure. Initial dual-energy CT hardware implementations were administering substantially higher tube photon outputs limiting the clinical use of early dual-energy CT systems.[6,7,9] Advances in the fabrication of radiation tube and detectors along with development of new software for radiation dose modulation, radiation doses associated with dual-energy CT protocols are identical to those of traditional CT protocols, foremost when a dual-energy CT scan is obtained using a dual-source CT hardware.[78,81,82] Radiation dose neutrality of contemporary dual-energy CT scanners can render opportunities for performing all genitourinary CT protocols in dual-energy mode, thus providing all benefits of dual-energy scanning within the same examination. Moreover, the possibility of substantially reducing radiation dose exposure by decreasing the number of acquired dynamic study phases (omitting the true unenhanced acquisition and replacing it with the virtual unenhanced reconstruction) for some indications leads to further savings in radiation dose while using dual-energy CT techniques (**Fig. 11**).[3,83–87]

SUMMARY

Dual-energy CT scanning has the potential to improve the imaging-based diagnosis of genitourinary diseases. Owing to the information provided by dual-energy CT about how materials behave at different energies, its ability to generate virtual unenhanced datasets, this technology can improve detection and characterization of iodine-containing substances. These capabilities are promising for improved detection and characterization of genitourinary diseases, while the radiation dose exposure to patients is decreased.

REFERENCES

1. Joffe SA, Servaes S, Okon S, et al. Multi-detector row CT urography in the evaluation of hematuria. Radiographics 2003;23:1441–55.
2. Kalender WA, Perman WH, Vetter JR, et al. Evaluation of a prototype dual-energy computed tomographic apparatus. I. Phantom studies. Med Phys 1986;13:334–9.
3. Mileto A, Sofue K, Marin D. Imaging the renal lesion with dual-energy multidetector CT and multi-energy

applications in clinical practice: what can it truly do for you? Eur Radiol 2016;26:3677–90.
4. Mileto A, Marin D, Nelson RC, et al. Dual-energy MDCT assessment of renal lesions: an overview. Eur Radiol 2014;24:353–62.
5. Curry TS III, Dowdey JE, Murry RC. Christensen's physics of diagnostic radiology. 4th edition. Philadelphia: Lea & Febiger; 1990.
6. Johnson TR, Krauss B, Sedlmair M, et al. Material differentiation by dual-energy CT: initial experience. Eur Radiol 2007;17:1510–7.
7. McCollough CH, Leng S, Yu L, et al. Dual- and multi-energy CT: principles, technical approaches, and clinical applications. Radiology 2015;276: 637–53.
8. Coursey CA, Nelson RC, Boll DT, et al. Dual-energy multidetector CT: how does it work, what can it tell us, and when can we use it in abdominopelvic imaging? Radiographics 2010;30:1037–55.
9. Marin D, Boll DT, Mileto A, et al. State of the art: dual-energy CT of the abdomen. Radiology 2014;271: 327–42.
10. Patino M, Prochowski A, Agrawal MD, et al. Material separation using dual-energy CT: current and emerging applications. Radiographics 2016;36: 1087–105.
11. Kaza R, Caoili EM, Cohan RH, et al. Distinguishing enhancing from nonenhancing renal lesions with fast kilovoltage-switching dual-energy CT. AJR Am J Roentgenol 2011;197:1375–81.
12. Saita A, Bonaccorsi A, Motta M. Stone composition: where do we stand? Urol Int 2007;79(Suppl 1):16–9.
13. Mileto A, Marin D. Dual-energy computed tomography in genitourinary imaging. Radiol Clin North Am 2017;55:373–91.
14. Bres-Niewada E, Dybowski B, Radziszewski P. Predicting stone composition before treatment - can it really drive clinical decisions? Cent European J Urol 2014;67:392–6.
15. Graser A, Johnson TR, Bader M, et al. Dual-energy CT characterization of urinary calculi: initial in vitro and clinical experience. Invest Radiol 2008;43: 112–9.
16. Primak AN, Fletcher JG, Vrtiska TJ, et al. Noninvasive differentiation of uric acid versus non-uric acid kidney stones using dual-energy CT. Acad Radiol 2007;14:1441–7.
17. Leng S, Shiung M, Ai S, et al. Feasibility of discriminating uric acid from non-uric acid renal stones using consecutive spatially registered low- and high-energy scans obtained on a conventional CT scanner. AJR Am J Roentgenol 2015;204:92–7.
18. Dale J, Gupta RT, Marin D, et al. Imaging advances in urolithiasis. J Endourol 2017;31:623–9.
19. Bonatti M, Lombardo F, Zamboni GA, et al. Renal stones composition in vivo determination: comparison between 100/Sn140 kV dual-energy CT

and 120 kV single-energy CT. Urolithiasis 2017; 45:255–61.

20. Hidas G, Eliahou R, Duvdevani M, et al. Determination of renal stone composition with dual-energy CT: in vivo analysis and comparison with x-ray diffraction. Radiology 2010;257:394–401.

21. Ferrero A, Montoya JC, Vaughan LE, et al. Quantitative prediction of stone fragility from routine dual-energy CT: ex vivo proof of feasibility. Acad Radiol 2016;23:1545–52.

22. Qu M, Ramirez-Giraldo JC, Leng S, et al. Dual-energy dual-source CT with additional spectral filtration can improve the differentiation of non-uric acid renal stones: an ex vivo phantom study. AJR Am J Roentgenol 2011;196:1279–87.

23. Duan X, Li Z, Yu L, et al. Characterization of urinary stone composition by use of third-generation dual-source dual-energy CT with increased spectral separation. AJR Am J Roentgenol 2015;205:1203–7.

24. Kaza RK, Platt JF. Renal applications of dual-energy CT. Abdom Radiol (NY) 2016;41:1122–32.

25. Jung DC, Oh YT, Kim MD, et al. Usefulness of the virtual monochromatic image in dual-energy spectral CT for decreasing renal cyst pseudoenhancement: a phantom study. AJR Am J Roentgenol 2012;199: 1316–9.

26. Mileto A, Nelson RC, Samei E, et al. Impact of dual-energy multi-detector row CT with virtual monochromatic imaging on renal cyst pseudoenhancement: in vitro and in vivo study. Radiology 2014;272:767–76.

27. Yamada Y, Yamada M, Sugisawa K, et al. Renal cyst pseudoenhancement: intraindividual comparison between virtual monochromatic spectral images and conventional polychromatic 120-kVp images obtained during the same CT examination and comparisons among images reconstructed using filtered back projection, adaptive statistical iterative reconstruction, and model-based iterative reconstruction. Medicine 2015;94:e754.

28. Megibow AJ, Chandarana H, Hindman NM. Increasing the precision of CT measurements with dual-energy scanning. Radiology 2014;272:618–21.

29. Patel BN, Bibbey A, Choudhury KR, et al. Characterization of small (<4 cm) focal renal lesions: diagnostic accuracy of spectral analysis using single-phase contrast-enhanced dual-energy CT. AJR Am J Roentgenol 2017;209:815–25.

30. Marin D, Davis D, Roy Choudhury K, et al. Characterization of small focal renal lesions: diagnostic accuracy with single-phase contrast-enhanced dual-energy CT with material attenuation analysis compared with conventional attenuation measurements. Radiology 2017;284:737–47.

31. Kaza RK, Platt JF, Cohan RH, et al. Dual-energy CT with single- and dual-source scanners: current

applications in evaluating the genitourinary tract. Radiographics 2012;32:353–69.

32. Kaza RK, Platt JF, Megibow AJ. Dual-energy CT of the urinary tract. Abdom Imaging 2013;38:167–79.

33. Ascenti G, Mazziotti S, Mileto A, et al. Dual-source dual-energy CT evaluation of complex cystic renal masses. AJR Am J Roentgenol 2012;199:1026–34.

34. Graser A, Johnson TR, Hecht EM, et al. Dual-energy CT in patients suspected of having renal masses: can virtual nonenhanced images replace true nonenhanced images? Radiology 2009;252: 433–40.

35. Neville AM, Gupta RT, Miller CM, et al. Detection of renal lesion enhancement with dual-energy multidetector CT. Radiology 2011;259:173–83.

36. Song KD, Kim CK, Park BK, et al. Utility of iodine overlay technique and virtual unenhanced images for the characterization of renal masses by dual-energy CT. AJR Am J Roentgenol 2011;197: W1076–82.

37. Graser A, Becker CR, Staehler M, et al. Single-phase dual-energy CT allows for characterisation of renal masses as benign or malignant. Invest Radiol 2010;45:399–405.

38. Mileto A, Nelson RC, Paulson EK, et al. Dual-energy MDCT for imaging the renal mass. AJR Am J Roentgenol 2015;204:W640–7.

39. Mileto A, Allen BC, Pietryga JA, et al. Characterization of incidental renal mass with dual-energy CT: diagnostic accuracy of effective atomic number maps for discriminating nonenhancing cysts from enhancing masses. AJR Am J Roentgenol 2017; 209:W221–30.

40. Mileto A, Marin D, Ramirez-Giraldo JC, et al. Accuracy of contrast-enhanced dual-energy MDCT for the assessment of iodine uptake in renal lesions. AJR Am J Roentgenol 2014;202:W466–74.

41. Ascenti G, Mileto A, Krauss B, et al. Distinguishing enhancing from nonenhancing renal masses with dual-source dual-energy CT: iodine quantification versus standard enhancement measurements. Eur Radiol 2013;23:2288–95.

42. Jayson M, Sanders H. Increased incidence of serendipitously discovered renal cell carcinoma. Urology 1998;51:203–5.

43. Luciani LG, Cestari R, Tallarigo C. Incidental renal cell carcinoma-age and stage characterization and clinical implications: study of 1092 patients (1982-1997). Urology 2000;56:58–62.

44. Goh V, Ganeshan B, Nathan P, et al. Assessment of response to tyrosine kinase inhibitors in metastatic renal cell cancer: CT texture as a predictive biomarker. Radiology 2011;261:165–71.

45. Brufau BP, Cerqueda CS, Villalba LB, et al. Molina CN metastatic renal cell carcinoma: radiologic findings and assessment of response to targeted

antiangiogenic therapy by using multidetector CT. Radiographics 2013;33:1691–716.

46. Smith AD, Shah SN, Rini BI, et al. Morphology, attenuation, size, and structure (MASS) criteria: assessing response and predicting clinical outcome in metastatic renal cell carcinoma on antiangiogenic targeted therapy. AJR Am J Roentgenol 2010;194: 1470–8.

47. Smith AD, Lieber ML, Shah SN. Assessing tumor response and detecting recurrence in metastatic renal cell carcinoma on targeted therapy: importance of size and attenuation on contrast-enhanced CT. AJR Am J Roentgenol 2010;194: 157–65.

48. Mileto A, Marin D, Alfaro-Cordoba M, et al. Iodine quantification to distinguish clear cell from papillary renal cell carcinoma at dual-energy multidetector CT: a multireader diagnostic performance study. Radiology 2014;273:813–20.

49. Zarzour JG, Milner D, Valentin R, et al. Quantitative iodine content threshold for discrimination of renal cell carcinomas using rapid kV-switching dual-energy CT. Abdom Radiol 2017;42:727–34.

50. Marin D, Pratts-Emanuelli JJ, Mileto A, et al. Interdependencies of acquisition, detection, and reconstruction techniques on the accuracy of iodine quantification in varying patient sizes employing dual-energy CT. Eur Radiol 2015;25:679–86.

51. Mileto A, Barina A, Marin D, et al. Virtual monochromatic images from dual-energy multidetector CT: variance in CT numbers from the Same Lesion between single- source projection-based and dual-source image-based implementations. Radiology 2016;279:269–77.

52. Dai C, Cao Y, Jia Y, et al. Differentiation of renal cell carcinoma subtypes with different iodine quantification methods using single-phase contrast-enhanced dual-energy CT: areal vs. volumetric analyses. Abdom Radiol 2017. https://doi.org/10.1007/s00261-017-1253-x.

53. Vandenbroucke F, Van Hedent S, Van Gompel G, et al. Dual-energy CT after radiofrequency ablation of liver, kidney, and lung lesions: a review of features. Insights Imaging 2015;6:363–79.

54. Park SY, Kim CK, Park BK. Dual-energy CT in assessing therapeutic response to radiofrequency ablation of renal cell carcinomas. Eur J Radiol 2014;83:e73–9.

55. Atwell TD, Schmit GD, Boorjian SA, et al. Percutaneous ablation of renal masses measuring 3.0 cm and smaller: comparative local control and complications after radiofrequency ablation and cryoablation. AJR Am J Roentgenol 2013;200:461–6.

56. Hellbach K, Sterzik A, Sommer W, et al. Dual-energy CT allows for improved characterization of response to antiangiogenic treatment in patients with metastatic renal cell cancer. Eur Radiol 2017;27:2532–7.

57. Ju Y, Liu A, Dong Y, et al. The value of nonenhanced single-source dual-energy CT for differentiating metastases from adenoma in adrenal glands. Acad Radiol 2015;22:834–9.

58. Dunnick NR, Korobkin M. Imaging of adrenal incidentalomas: current status. AJR Am J Roentgenol 2002;179:559–68.

59. Lee MJ, Hahn PF, Papanicolaou N, et al. Benign and malignant adrenal masses: CT distinction with attenuation coefficients, size, and observer analysis. Radiology 1991;179:415–8.

60. Boland GW, Lee MJ, Gazelle GS, et al. Characterization of adrenal masses using unenhanced CT: an analysis of the CT literature. AJR Am J Roentgenol 1998;171:201–4.

61. Peña CS, Boland GW, Hahn PF, et al. Characterization of indeterminate (lipid-poor) adrenal masses: use of washout characteristics at contrast-enhanced CT. Radiology 2000;217:798–802.

62. Park BK, Kim CK, Kim B, et al. Comparison of delayed enhanced CT and chemical shift MR for evaluating hyperattenuating incidental adrenal masses. Radiology 2007;243:760–5.

63. Caoili EM, Korobkin M, Francis IR, et al. Adrenal masses: characterization with combined unenhanced and delayed enhanced CT. Radiology 2002;222:629–33.

64. Gupta RT, Ho LM, Marin D, et al. Dual-energy CT for characterization of adrenal nodules: initial experience. AJR Am J Roentgenol 2010;194:1479–83.

65. Gnannt R, Fischer M, Goetti R, et al. Dual-energy CT for characterization of the incidental adrenal mass: preliminary observations. AJR Am J Roentgenol 2012;198:138–44.

66. Ho LM, Marin D, Neville AM, et al. Characterization of adrenal nodules with dual- energy CT: can virtual unenhanced attenuation values replace true unenhanced attenuation values? AJR Am J Roentgenol 2012;198:840–5.

67. Kim YK, Park BK, Kim CK, et al. Adenoma characterization: adrenal protocol with dual-energy CT. Radiology 2013;267:155–63.

68. Connolly MJ, McInnes MDF, El-Khodary M, et al. Diagnostic accuracy of virtual non-contrast enhanced dual-energy CT for diagnosis of adrenal adenoma: a systematic review and meta-analysis. Eur Radiol 2017;27:4324–35.

69. Sodickson A. Dual-energy CT fat fraction for characterizing adrenal nodules. 18th Annual International Symposium on Multidetector-row CT. International Society of Computed Tomography. San Francisco, CA, June 20–23, 2016.

70. Morgan DE. Dual-energy CT of the abdomen. Abdom Imaging 2014;39:108–34.

71. Morgan DE, Weber AC, Lockhart ME, et al. Differentiation of high lipid content from low lipid content adrenal lesions using single-source rapid kilovolt

(peak)-switching dual-energy multidetector CT. J Comput Assist Tomogr 2013;37:937–43.

72. Mileto A, Nelson RC, Marin D, et al. Dual-energy multidetector CT for the characterization of incidental adrenal nodules: diagnostic performance of contrast-enhanced material density analysis. Radiology 2015;274:445–54.

73. Glazer DI, Maturen KE, Kaza RK, et al. Adrenal Incidentaloma triage with single- source (fast-kilovoltage switch) dual-energy CT. AJR Am J Roentgenol 2014;203:329–35.

74. Kaza RK, Raff EA, Davenport MS, et al. Variability of CT attenuation measurements in virtual unenhanced images generated using multimaterial decomposition from fast kilovoltage-switching dual-energy CT. Acad Radiol 2017;24:365–72.

75. Borhani AA, Kulzer M, Iranpour N, et al. Comparison of true unenhanced and virtual unenhanced (VUE) attenuation values in abdominopelvic single-source rapid kilovoltage-switching spectral CT. Abdom Radiol 2017;42:710–7.

76. Takahashi N, Vrtiska TJ, Kawashima A, et al. Detectability of urinary stones on virtual nonenhanced images generated at pyelographic-phase dual-energy CT. Radiology 2010;256:184–90.

77. Mileto A, Nelson RC, Samei E, et al. Dual-energy MDCT in hypervascular liver tumors: effect of body size on selection of the optimal monochromatic energy level. AJR Am J Roentgenol 2014;203:1257–64.

78. Yu L, Christner JA, Leng S, et al. Virtual monochromatic imaging in dual-source dual-energy CT: radiation dose and image quality. Med Phys 2011;38: 6371–9.

79. Patel BN, Alexander L, Allen B, et al. Dual-energy CT workflow: multi-institutional consensus on standardization of abdominopelvic MDCT protocols. Abdom Radiol 2017;42:676–87.

80. Guimarães LS, Fletcher JG, Harmsen WS, et al. Appropriate patient selection at abdominal dual-energy CT using 80 kV: relationship between patient size, image noise, and image quality. Radiology 2010;257:732–42.

81. Yu L, Primak AN, Liu X, et al. Image quality optimization and evaluation of linearly mixed images in dual-source, dual-energy CT. Med Phys 2009;36: 1019–24.

82. McCollough CH, Primak AN, Saba O, et al. Dose performance of a 64-channel dual- source CT scanner. Radiology 2007;243:775–84.

83. Ascenti G, Mileto A, Gaeta M, et al. Single-phase dual-energy CT urography in the evaluation of haematuria. Clin Radiol 2013;68:87–94.

84. Karlo CA, Gnannt R, Winklehner A, et al. Split-bolus dual-energy CT urography: protocol optimization and diagnostic performance for the detection of urinary stones. Abdom Imaging 2013;38:1136–43.

85. Chen CY, Hsu JS, Jaw TS, et al. Split-bolus portal venous phase dual-energy CT urography: protocol design, image quality, and dose reduction. AJR Am J Roentgenol 2015;205:W492–501.

86. Hansen C, Becker CD, Montet X, et al. Diagnosis of urothelial tumors with a dedicated dual-source dual-energy MDCT protocol: preliminary results. AJR Am J Roentgenol 2014;202:W357–64.

87. Takeuchi M, Kawai T, Ito M, et al. Split-bolus CT-urography using dual-energy CT: feasibility, image quality and dose reduction. Eur J Radiol 2012; 81:3160–5.

Imaging of Solid Renal Masses

Fernando U. Kay, MD, Ivan Pedrosa, MD, PhD*

KEYWORDS

- Renal cell carcinoma • Lymphoma • Angiomyolipoma • Renal oncocytoma • Ultrasonography
- X-ray computed tomography • MR imaging • Image-guided biopsy

KEY POINTS

- Solid renal masses include various types of malignant and benign histologic diagnoses.
- Noninvasive lesion characterization is achievable in a substantial number of cases, with the use of state-of-the-art imaging techniques and evidence-based interpretation criteria.
- Cross-sectional imaging has the potential to improve patients' outcomes by reducing the number of unnecessary biopsies and/or surgical procedures.

INTRODUCTION

The incidence of renal cancer increased from 7.1 to 10.8 cases per 100,000 patients between 1983 and 2002, with most primary tumors initially diagnosed as incidental small renal masses (ie, measuring ≤4 cm) on imaging studies performed for other clinical reasons.[1] Paradoxically, this increase in diagnosis has not been associated with better clinical outcomes, with a reported increase in mortality from 1.5 to 6.5 deaths per 100,000 patients within the same time interval.[1] Furthermore, most incidentally detected tumors either grow slowly[2] or do not show detectable growth over time.[3,4] Therefore, cost-effective strategies are necessary to identify clinically significant renal masses that could evolve into life-threatening disease, while avoiding the unnecessary morbidity and financial costs associated with overtreatment of benign or more indolent malignant conditions.

The first step in the workup of incidentally found renal lesions is to differentiate benign cysts from solid masses.[5,6] Solid renal masses contain little or no fluid and are composed predominantly of vascularized tissue (ie, elements enhancing with the administration of exogenous contrast agents).[6] Despite their lower prevalence compared with cystic lesions, up to 90% of solid masses are malignant.[7–9] The risk of malignancy is influenced by size, occurring in approximately 50% for lesions smaller than 1 cm and more than 90% for masses greater than or equal to 7 cm.[7]

Solid malignant masses most frequently encountered in clinical practice are renal cell carcinoma (RCC), urothelial carcinoma, lymphoma, and metastasis, whereas the most frequently encountered benign solid renal masses are angiomyolipoma (AML), oncocytoma, and inflammatory pseudotumors or pseudolesions. This article provides a comprehensive imaging approach to common malignant and benign solid renal masses on state-of-the-art ultrasonography (US), computed tomography (CT), and multiparametric magnetic resonance (MR) imaging, proposing strategies to

Portions of this article were previously published in March 2017 *Radiologic Clinics*, Volume 55, Issue 2.
Disclosure: This article was supported by the National Institutes of Health (grants P50CA196516, awarded to I. Pedrosa; and R01 5RO1CA154475, awarded to I. Pedrosa).
Department of Radiology; UT Southwestern Medical Center, 2201 Inwood Road, Suite 210, Dallas, TX 75390, USA
* Corresponding author.
E-mail address: ivan.pedrosa@utsouthwestern.edu

Urol Clin N Am 45 (2018) 311–330
https://doi.org/10.1016/j.ucl.2018.03.013
0094-0143/18/

differentiate benign from malignant lesions and to distinguish RCC subtypes.

Malignant Lesions

Cancer arising in the kidney and renal pelvis accounts for 5% of all malignancies in men and 3% of malignancies in women.[10] RCC is more common among men (1.6:1, M:F). Patients with localized disease have a reported 93% 5-year survival, whereas this rate decreases to 66% and 12% for those with regional and distant metastasis, respectively.[10]

Renal cell carcinoma

The World Health Organization classification subdivides RCC into different histologic groups,[11] with clear cell RCC (ccRCC) accounting for 70% to 75%, papillary RCC (pRCC) accounting for 10% to 21%, and chromophobe RCC (chrRCC) accounting for 5% of all RCC cases.[11,12] Survival heavily depends on staging, histologic grade (ie, Furhman/International Society of Urological Pathology), presence of sarcomatoid features, and necrosis. In addition, ccRCC is associated with worse prognosis than pRCC and chrRCC.[11,13] Different histopathologic subtypes have distinct features on imaging studies, and these are discussed later.

Urothelial carcinoma

Urothelial carcinoma originates from the epithelium of calyces and renal pelvis and may comprise up to 15% of all renal tumors.[14] Median age at diagnosis is more than 60 years, with an approximately 2:1 M/F ratio, and hematuria is the most frequent symptom at presentation.[14,15] Synchronous and metachronous involvement of the urinary tract may occur in 24% and 11% of patients with renal urothelial carcinoma, respectively.[15] Differentiation of upper-tract urothelial carcinoma from RCC and other solid renal masses is simpler during earlier stages, when the presentation is characterized by wall thickening of the urothelial tract or filling defects in the collecting system. Infiltrative masses in the renal sinus or parenchyma are features of advanced disease, in which distinction from aggressive forms of RCC is difficult.[16]

Lymphoma

Lymphomatous involvement of the kidneys is most frequently the result of secondary spread of non-Hodgkin disease, with prevalence at autopsy reaching 50% in this population.[17] Renal lymphoma may present as multiple masses, solitary lesions simulating RCC, retroperitoneal/perirenal disease, and infiltrative renal disease. A pattern of multiple renal masses is encountered in up to 60% of the patients, typically ranging from 1 to 3 cm, with homogeneous attenuation (CT) or signal intensity (MR imaging), and low-level postcontrast enhancement compared with background parenchyma (**Fig. 1**).[18] Contiguous involvement of the kidneys by bulky retroperitoneal disease is another common presentation of lymphoma on imaging.[18] Solitary lesions occur in 10% to 20% of the patients, and although differentiation from ccRCC may be possible because of the characteristic homogeneous signal/attenuation and low-grade enhancement of lymphoma, biopsy may be needed to discriminate from non-ccRCC subtypes, especially papillary tumors.

Metastases

The reported prevalence of metastatic disease to the kidneys in oncologic patients differs depending on the method of assessment, varying from 20% on autopsy studies to less than 1% in clinicopathologic studies.[19] Commonly, the primary tumor is already known or diagnosed at the same time as the renal lesion, with more than half of the cases occurring in patients older than 60 years.[19] The most common primary sites are lung, breast, female genital tract, head and neck, colon, and prostate. Bilateral or multiple masses are found in 23% and 30% of the patients, respectively.[19] Renal metastases occur more commonly at the junction of the renal cortex and medulla, often showing ill-defined borders and low-level enhancement, except in the case of hypervascular primary tumors (eg, RCC, thyroid, choriocarcinoma). These features may help to suggest the diagnosis and differ from the most common well-defined appearance of cortical-based RCCs, although a definitive diagnosis may require a biopsy.

Benign Lesions

The reported prevalence of benign histology is 13% to 16% of all surgically resected renal masses.[7,9] The likelihood of benign histology in small solid renal masses is influenced by size, with a prevalence of up to 40% in lesions less than 1 cm in diameter.[20] AMLs and oncocytomas comprise most of the benign solid masses, representing 44% and 35%, respectively.[9]

Angiomyolipoma

AMLs are benign neoplasms, consisting of aberrant blood vessels, smooth muscle, and mature adipose tissue,[21] representing 2% to 6% of all resected tumors in surgical series.[22,23] Most of these neoplasms are found incidentally on imaging (eg, 0.1%–0.2% of US examinations), with a female preponderance (1:2, M/F).[24] AMLs can

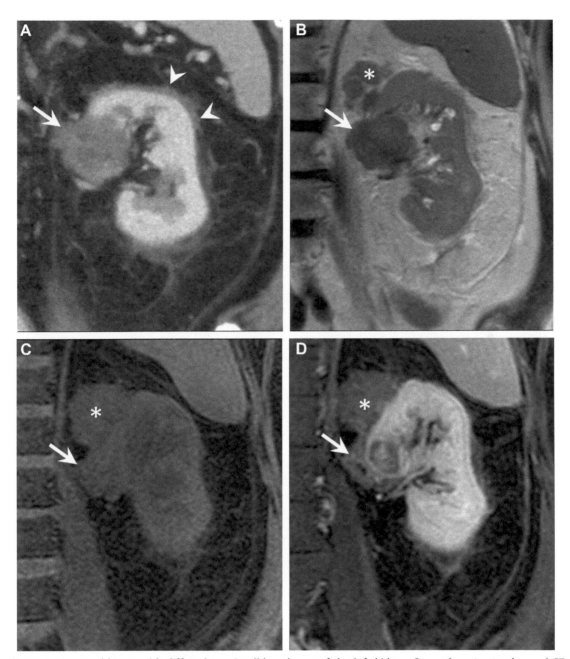

Fig. 1. A 69-year-old man with diffuse large B cell lymphoma of the left kidney. Coronal contrast-enhanced CT image (*A*) showing a solid infiltrative lesion in the perihilar region of the left kidney (*arrow*). Note the perinephric soft tissue component surrounding the renal capsule (*arrowheads*). Coronal single-shot fast spin-echo T2-weighted MR image (*B*) shows low-intermediate signal intensity in the mass (*arrow*), with interval development of new perinephric nodules (*asterisk*) compared with the prior CT (*A*). Coronal 3-dimensional (3D) fat-saturated Dixon T1-weighted MR images before (*C*) and after (*D*) administration of contrast agent show low-level enhancement of the lesion (*arrows*) in comparison with the renal cortex. Also note low-level homogeneous enhancement of the perirenal component (*asterisks*). (*From* Kay FU, Pedrosa I. Imaging of solid renal masses. Radiol Clin North Am 2017;55(2):245; with permission.)

occur sporadically or in association with genetic syndromes. AML prevalence in patients with tuberous sclerosis varies from 55% to 90%, and in patients with lymphangioleiomyomatosis from 30% to 50%.[21] Larger AMLs may cause symptoms and spontaneous hemorrhage (Wunderlich syndrome), a life-threatening complication in larger tumors.[25]

The detection of fatty tissue (ie, adipocytes) by CT or MR imaging is regarded as the most specific feature for this diagnosis, although many pathologically proven AMLs do not show fatty tissue on imaging, causing a diagnostic challenge.[26] The diagnosis of classic and AML with minimal or absent fat is discussed later.

Oncocytoma

Oncocytomas are relatively uncommon cortical tumors (approximately 7% of renal masses in surgical series) composed of oncocytes (polygonal or round cells, with moderate to abundant granular cytoplasm) surrounded by thin capillaries and stroma.[27] Patients are usually asymptomatic, being more frequently men (1.2:1, M/F), with a mean age of 65 years at diagnosis. Intratumoral hemorrhage and central scars are present in 20% and 33% of all oncocytomas, respectively, and multifocality may occur in 13% of the patients.[27] Although oncocytomas are classified as benign tumors,[11] case reports have described malignant potential.[28] Similarly, aggressive local behavior may manifest with intravascular extension into branches of the renal vein[29] and invasion of the perinephric fat, the latter occurring in up to 7% of all oncocytomas (**Fig. 2**).[30]

Inflammatory conditions and pseudotumors

A variety of nonneoplastic conditions may mimic solid renal masses. Developmental renal pseudotumors (eg, prominent columns of Bertin, dromedary humps, persistent fetal lobulations) are easily differentiated from true renal masses by the delineation of normal renal parenchyma imaging features in the suspicious region (eg, on multiphasic dynamic contrast-enhanced imaging). However, other conditions, such as infectious, inflammatory, and granulomatous diseases (eg, pyelonephritis/abscess, xanthogranulomatous pyelonephritis), may pose a significant diagnostic challenge.[31] Interpretation of the imaging findings in the appropriate clinical context is crucial, because focal or multifocal pyelonephritis is usually accompanied by characteristic symptoms, such as chills, fever, flank pain, and pyuria. US-Doppler and contrast-enhanced CT or MR may show single or multiple hypoperfused wedge-shaped areas, extending from the papilla to the cortex. Perirenal inflammatory changes are common.[32] Xanthogranulomatous pyelonephritis can also present as renal masses in patients with flank pain and fever and is more commonly observed in middle-aged women with urinary stones, infection (most common by *Escherichia coli* and *Proteus*), and/or congenital anomalies.[33,34] This disease is characterized by destruction of the normal renal architecture, enlarged kidney, contracted pelvis, staghorn calculus, and perinephric inflammatory changes.[32]

Imaging Techniques

Ultrasonography

US is generally the first-line imaging modality for patients with suspected renal disease given its lower cost, wide availability, and lack of ionizing radiation. There is no current role for RCC screening with US in the general population. The prevalence of incidental renal masses in asymptomatic individuals undergoing US is about 0.4%, with half of the cases resulting in RCC.[35] US is indicated in the evaluation of upper urinary tract symptoms and in the workup of indeterminate renal masses (American College of Radiology [ACR] Appropriateness Criteria rating 8).[36] It has been favored over nonenhanced MR imaging and CT in patients with contraindications to intravenous contrast, with lower sensitivity in the detection of small lesions compared with contrast-enhanced CT.[37–39] US is not indicated to stage renal cancer (ACR Appropriateness Criteria rating 3).[40]

Characterization of cystic renal lesions is most frequently straightforward on US, although the appearance of complex cystic masses and solid lesions may overlap. Simple renal cysts are anechoic structures with positive through-transmission and refraction along the sidewalls, showing sharp and smooth walls.[41] Cysts with hemorrhagic or protein contents may harbor internal echoes or debris. Harmonic imaging can minimize reverberation artifacts related to so-called dirty echoes, facilitating the distinction of cysts from solid masses.[42,43] As with other imaging techniques, the detection of blood flow on Doppler, or lesion enhancement after intravenous contrast injection, represents unequivocal evidence of a solid mass.[44]

Computed tomography

The most commonly used method to evaluate indeterminate renal masses is contrast-enhanced CT (ACR Appropriateness Criteria rating 9).[36] It is also considered the method of choice to stage RCC (ACR Appropriateness Criteria rating 9),[40] with high accuracies in both early and advanced stages.[45] A CT protocol for evaluation of renal masses is proposed in **Table 1**.

The sensitivity of CT for small renal masses is higher than 90%,[37] approaching 100% for lesions larger than 2 cm.[38] An advantage of CT compared with US and MR imaging is the ability to characterize lesions in Hounsfield units (HU), a quantitative standardized x-ray attenuation scale. Differences of at least 10 HU between precontrast and postcontrast CT images have been historically proposed as cutoff values to differentiate

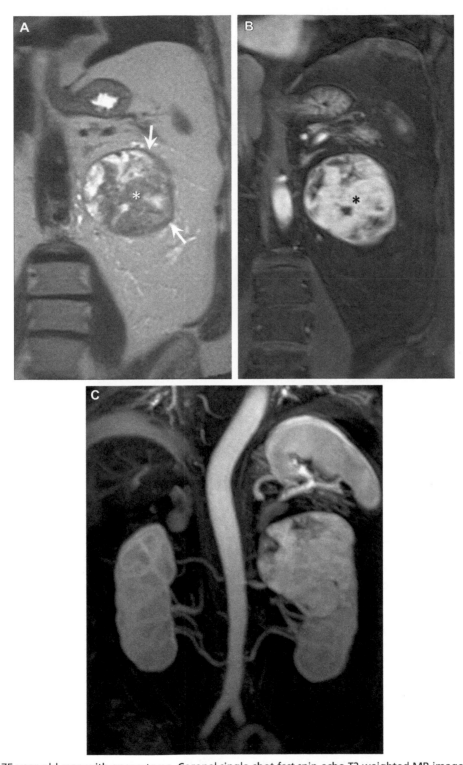

Fig. 2. A 75-year-old man with oncocytoma. Coronal single-shot fast spin-echo T2-weighted MR image (*A*) shows a large mass in the left kidney (*arrows*) with foci of high signal intensity in the periphery and central areas of intermediate signal intensity. Note that the central component (*asterisk in A*) shows avid postcontrast enhancement on the fat-saturated Dixon-based T1-weighted gradient echo acquisition during the corticomedullary phase (*asterisk in B*). Maximum intensity projection of postcontrast T1-weighted Dixon-based acquisition (*C*) shows invasion of the renal hilum fat, which was confirmed after nephrectomy. (*From* Kay FU, Pedrosa I. Imaging of solid renal masses. Radiol Clin North Am 2017;55(2):245; with permission.)

Table 1
Multidetector contrast-enhanced computed tomography protocol for renal mass characterization

Renal Mass Multidetector CT Protocol				
Phases	Noncontrast	Corticomedullary[a]	Nephrographic	Delayed
Phase timing	—	40 s	100–120 s	5–7 min
Coverage	Kidneys	Diaphragm through kidneys	Diaphragm through kidneys	Kidneys
FOV	Whole body	Whole body	Whole body	Whole body
Reconstructions	Axial: 3 mm	Axial: 3 mm Coronal: 2 mm Sagittal: 2 mm	Axial: 3 mm Coronal: 2 mm Sagittal: 2 mm	Axial: 3 mm Coronal: 2 mm Sagittal: 2 mm

Intravenous contrast: 100 to 150 mL of low-osmolar iodinated contrast at 5 mL/s.
Abbreviation: FOV, field of view.
[a] Optional.
From Kay FU, Pedrosa I. Imaging of solid renal masses. Radiol Clin North Am 2017;55(2):247; with permission.

solid masses from renal cysts.[46,47] More conservative values, such as 15 to 20 HU, have been used in clinical practice to account for volume averaging artifacts and misregistration among acquisitions.[48] Similarly, enhancement of adjacent renal parenchyma may cause pseudoenhancement (ie, increased HU on contrast-enhanced images) in renal cysts due to x-ray beam hardening.[49] A practical approach is to consider a 20-HU difference between precontrast and postcontrast CT images as unequivocal evidence of enhancement, and a difference between 10 and 20 HU is equivocal for enhancement. The average attenuation of renal lesions larger than 1 cm on nonenhanced CT scans is also useful in their characterization: homogeneously distributed values than 20 HU or more than 70 HU are associated with simple and hemorrhagic cysts, respectively.[50]

The last decade witnessed the emergence of multienergy CT as a promising technique to evaluate renal masses, with increased specificity in the detection of postcontrast enhancement (ie, reducing the effect of pseudoenhancement), and the potential role to reduce reduce radiation dose by minimizing multiphase scanning.[51]

MR imaging

MR imaging is indicated in the evaluation of indeterminate renal masses and staging of renal cancer (ACR Appropriateness Criteria rating 8).[36] The specificity of MRI for benign lesions may be superior to that of CT.[52] MR is particularly helpful to distinguish solid from cystic lesions when enhancement of renal masses is equivocal on CT (ie, between 10 and 20 HU).[5] However, more recent evidence with multienergy CT technology has shown comparable performance of both methods for differentiation of pRCC from hemorrhagic cysts.[53] MR is more accurate than conventional venography and CT in delineating vena caval tumor thrombus.[54]

Current state-of-the-art MR protocols for imaging renal masses include multiple parameters that allow a more comprehensive and systematic analysis of tumor phenotypes.[55,56] For instance, diffusion-weighted imaging (DWI) and dynamic contrast-enhanced MR imaging can provide specific information about tumor histology.[57] As discussed later, the use of those parameters may help to differentiate benign from malignant renal masses, differentiate the RCC subtype, and predict tumor grade.

Shortcomings of MR imaging include a longer scan time, cost, and potential concerns related to the use of gadolinium-based contrast agents (GBCA). Group I GBCA (gadodiamide, gadopentate dimeglumine, and gadoversetamide) are currently contraindicated in dialysis, acute kidney injury, and severe or end-stage chronic kidney disease (CKD 4 or 5; ie, estimated glomerular filtration [eGFR], <30 mL/min/1.73 m^2).[58] These GBCA have been associated with nephrogenic systemic fibrosis, which is a rare and potentially fatal fibrosing disease caused by accumulation of free gadolinium.[59] Group II GBCA (gadobenate dimeglumine, gadoteridol, gadoteric acid, and gadobutrol) are considered safe agents with few, if any, unconfounded cases of nephrogenic systemic fibrosis,[60,61] and can be used in patients with CKD stages 4 and 5 (estimated glomerular filtration rate [eGFR] <30 mL/min/1.73 m^2). Accordingly, the most recent recommendations from the ACR indicate that the need to screen for renal function is optional when using class II GBCAs. More recently, the use of GBCA has also been associated with gadolinium deposition in the basal ganglia, but no harmful effects have been reported to date.[62,63] Alternatively, nonenhanced sequences, such as arterial spin labeling (ASL), may aid in the evaluation of vascularity in renal masses without the necessity of exogenous contrast agents.[64] Perfusion levels estimated by ASL are correlated with those obtained by dynamic contrast-enhanced MR imaging as well as with microvessel density at histology in renal tumors.[65] However, currently ASL sequences are used primarily in research protocols.

An MR imaging protocol for evaluation of renal masses is provided in **Table 2**. Images are acquired in end expiration to improve the consistency of kidney position between scans, with the patient's arms located above the head, when possible, to avoid phase-wrap artifacts.[66]

Impact of Imaging on Patient Management

Increased detection rates and lower intrinsic prevalence of malignancy in small renal masses challenge patient management. Mainstream treatment of renal cancer is still surgical. Nephron-sparing techniques achieve similar oncologic results to radical nephrectomy in small RCC.[67,68] However, subgroups of patients, such as the elderly, those with multiple comorbidities, and those with favorable tumor histology, may benefit from conservative approaches such as active surveillance.[2,69] Current strategies propose the use of size, histologic subtype, nuclear grade, and clinical criteria as parameters for the decision between active surveillance or surgical treatment.[70] Therefore, the role of imaging is to facilitate management by offering a noninvasive diagnosis of benign disease and, ideally, distinguish indolent from aggressive renal malignancies.

Diagnosis of benign disease
The ability to distinguish benign from malignant solid renal masses by US is limited.[71] Even the classic appearance of AML on US as hyperechoic masses is not specific, overlapping with RCC features.[72–74] However, contrast-enhanced US (CEUS) is a promising modality that can potentially add value in the characterization of renal masses. In a large cohort of patients, CEUS performed with a sensitivity of 100% and specificity of 95% in the diagnosis of malignancy among cystic and solid indeterminate renal masses.[75]

Unequivocal demonstration of bulk fat (ie, adipocytes) by CT or MR imaging in a renal lesion is a specific finding for the diagnosis of AML.[76,77] On unenhanced CT, determination of macroscopic fat is achieved when values less than −10 HU are present within the mass (**Fig. 3**).[78] On MR imaging, bulk fat follows the signal intensity of subcutaneous and intra-abdominal fat on all sequences, characterized by (a) hyperintense signal on T1-weighted or T2-weighted images, with signal saturation after application of a frequency-selective fat-saturation technique; (b) high signal intensity on T1-weighted in-phase (IP) and opposed-phased (OP) imaging, with signal dropout on OP imaging at the interface of the

---

Table 2
Contrast-enhanced MR imaging protocol for renal mass characterization

Acquisition	Renal Mass MR Protocol (3T)						
	TR (ms)	TE (ms)	Flip Angle (degrees)	Bandwidth (Hz/pixel)	Slice Thickness/Gap	FOV (cm)	Matrix
Coronal T2-weighted SSFSE	960	80	90	652	5/1	40 × 45	312 × 279
Axial T2-weighted fat-saturated SSFSE	920	80	90	543	5/1	40 × 30	304 × 168
Axial 2D T1-weighted GRE IP/OP	120	2.3/1.15	55	1215	5/1	40 × 38	400 × 269
Axial DWI	1060	53	90	36.5	7/1	44 × 35	144 × 115
Sagittal oblique 3D Dixon (kidneys)[a]	3.7	1.32/2.3	10	1568	3/−1.5	30 × 30	248 × 230
Coronal 3D Dixon[b]	3.8	1.7/2.1	10	1923	3/−1.5	39 × 40	260 × 223
Axial 3D Dixon	2.2	1.16/2.1	10	1852	3/−1.5	38 × 33	252 × 218

Intravenous contrast: 0.1 mmol/kg gadolinium chelate at 2 mL/s, followed by 20-mL saline flush.

Abbreviations: 2D, 2-dimensional; GRE, gradient recalled echo; SSFSE, single-shot fast spin echo; TE, echo time; TR, repetition time.

[a] Precontrast and postcontrast (3 min).

[b] Before, bolus-tracking (breathing instructions start at left ventricle enhancement), early arterial (ask for 2 breaths in/breaths out, then hold), corticomedullary (40 s), nephrographic (90 s).

From Kay FU, Pedrosa I. Imaging of solid renal masses. Radiol Clin North Am 2017;55(2):248; with permission.

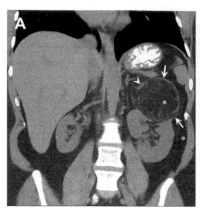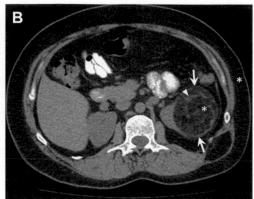

Fig. 3. A 47-year-old woman with AML in the left kidney. Coronal (*A*) and axial (*B*) non–contrast-enhanced CT images show an 8-cm circumscribed mass in the left upper pole (*arrows*), predominantly composed of low-attenuation elements (bulk fat), similar to that of retroperitoneal and subcutaneous fat (*asterisks*). Also note some streaks of soft tissue within the lesion, corresponding with vascular and smooth muscle components (*arrowheads*). (*From* Kay FU, Pedrosa I. Imaging of solid renal masses. Radiol Clin North Am 2017;55(2):249; with permission.)

lesion with the kidney (India-ink artifact); (c) high signal intensity on fat-only reconstructions from Dixon-based acquisitions (**Fig. 4**).[79] Coexistence of areas of both bulk and intravoxel fat (scant amounts of fat mixed with smooth muscle and vessels), the latter manifested as intratumoral areas of decreased signal on OP images compared with IP images, is common in AML.[80]

Some AMLs may not show bulk fat on imaging (AML with minimal fat [mfAML]),[81] whereas signal loss on OP images is also commonly present in ccRCC given the presence of intracytoplasmic lipid-containing vacuoles.[55,82] Therefore, in the authors' experience, the isolated presence of decreased signal on OP imaging relative to IP imaging is not useful in the differentiation of ccRCC from mfAML in small renal masses.[83] The diagnosis of mfAML should be considered for renal masses with homogeneous low signal intensity relative to renal cortex on T2-weighted images, particularly for smaller lesions found in women, in the absence of bulk fat, plus or minus intravoxel fat (ie, decreased signal intensity on OP imaging).[83] In contrast, the presence of intratumoral necrosis and cystic changes favors ccRCC over mfAML.[83] In addition, a simplified vascular parameter, known as arterial-to-delayed enhancement ratio, and defined as the difference in signal intensity between arterial and precontrast phase divided by the difference between delayed and precontrast phase, has been proposed to distinguish mfAML from RCC, with values greater than 1.5 favoring the first.[84] Ultimately, the combination of multiple MR imaging parameters may provide better diagnostic performances, with up to 100% sensitivity and 89% specificity for the diagnosis of mfAML (**Fig. 5**).[85]

DWI can provide surrogate information about cellular density and can potentially assist in the differentiation of benign and malignant lesions. A meta-analysis reported significantly lower apparent diffusion coefficients (ADCs) in RCC, with 95% confidence intervals ranging from 1.45×10^{-3} to 1.77×10^{-3} mm²/s, whereas values obtained from benign lesions ranged between 1.92×10^{-3} and 2.28×10^{-3} mm²/s. Particularly, oncocytomas had significantly higher ADC values than malignant lesions, ranging from 1.84×10^{-3} to 2.17×10^{-3} mm²/s, whereas this was not observed for AML, with values between 1.25×10^{-3} and 1.83×10^{-3} mm²/s.[86]

The presence of a heterogeneous pattern of postcontrast enhancement known as segmental enhancement inversion (ie, intratumor hyperenhancing areas on the corticomedullary phase that become hypoenhancing on the early excretory phase with other areas in the same tumor exhibiting the opposite enhancement pattern) was initially reported to have 80% sensitivity and 99% specificity to distinguish oncocytomas from RCC on CT.[87] However, a study comparing oncocytomas and chrRCC did not show significant differences in the prevalence of the segmental enhancement inversion sign on MRI between these 2 entities.[88] A recent study by the authors confirmed segmental inversion enhancement as an independent predictor of oncocytoma. However, interreader agreement for this finding was only moderate (κ = 0.49), leading to large variability in the sensitivity (17%–83%) and specificity (91%–99%) for this diagnosis.[89] Higher ASL perfusion levels were reported in oncocytomas compared with clear

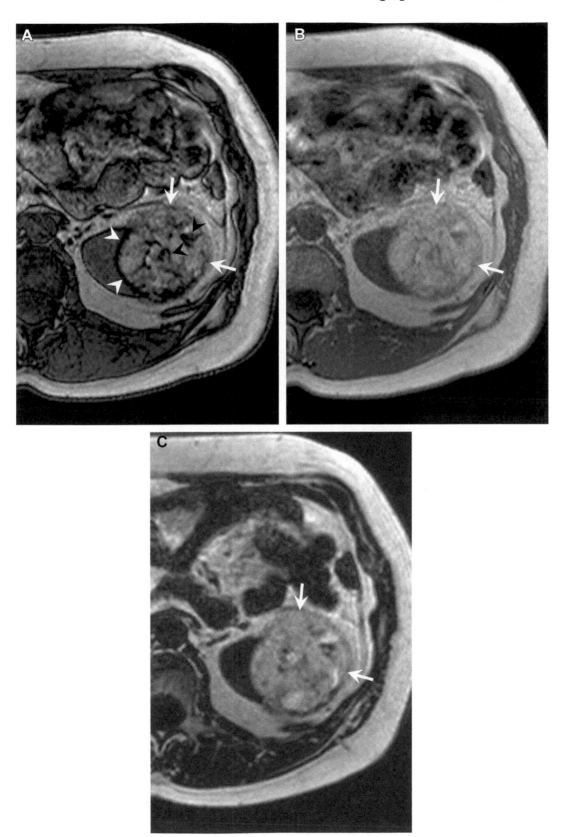

Fig. 4. A 47-year-old woman with AML in the left kidney (same patient from **Fig. 3**). OP (*A*), IP (*B*), and fat-only (*C*) reconstructions from an axial T1-weighted Dixon acquisition. The circumscribed mass (*arrows*) shows high signal

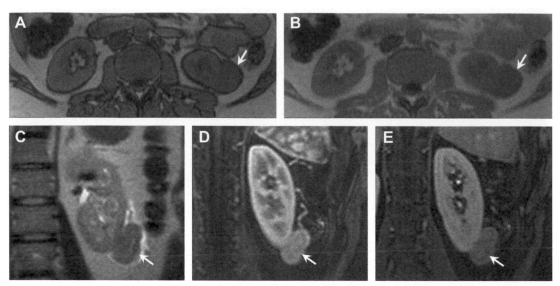

Fig. 5. A 40-year-old woman with minimal-fat AML in the left kidney. Axial GRE T1-weighted OP (*A*) and IP (*B*) MR images show a slightly hypointense circumscribed lesion in the lower pole of the left kidney (*arrows*), without significant signal dropout to suggest intravoxel fat. Coronal non–fat-saturated single-shot fast spin-echo T2-weighted MR image (*C*) shows homogeneous hypointense signal in the lesion (*arrow*). Dynamic contrast-enhanced fat-saturated spoiled gradient recalled (SPGR) T1-weighted MR images during corticomedullary (*D*) and excretory (*E*) phases show avid early enhancement of the lesion and subsequent washout (*arrows*). (*From* Kay FU, Pedrosa I. Imaging of solid renal masses. Radiol Clin North Am 2017;55(2):251; with permission.)

cell and non–clear cell subtypes of RCC,[90] although some overlap exists. A recent study reported promising results in a prospective trial using [^{99}Tc]-Technetium Sestamibi single-proton emission computed tomography (SPECT) for the diagnosis of oncocytoma and mixed oncocytic/chromophobe tumors, which exhibit intense uptake ("hot tumors"), compared with RCC and AML not showing uptake ("cold" tumors).[91]

Characterization of renal cell carcinoma subtypes

Attempts to characterize RCCs on Doppler or CEUS have been inconsistent so far.[92] On CT, differentiation of RCC subtypes generally relies on analyses of postcontrast time-attenuation curves and lesion homogeneity. Postcontrast enhancement of ccRCC is significantly higher than that observed for pRCC and chrRCC, whereas heterogeneity is also more frequently seen in ccRCCs (**Fig. 6**).[93–95]

Relative ratios of renal mass enhancement to enhancement of the aorta are significantly lower for pRCC than for nonpapillary histology on CT, with sensitivity and specificity of 86% and 85%, respectively, using a cutoff of 0.25.[96] Relative enhancement ratios in the renal mass compared with the renal parenchyma are also significantly higher for ccRCC than for pRCC (**Fig. 7**).[97]

The MR imaging phenotype of papillary neoplasms is variable because these tumors evolve from solid hypoenhancing homogeneous masses with low signal intensity on T2-weighted images to more heterogeneous tumors after intratumoral hemorrhage. pRCC often presents as hemorrhagic cystic masses with peripheral enhancing components, contained by a well-developed tumor capsule.[55] Regardless of the MR imaging phenotype, the viable, vascularized portions of the tumor usually show homogeneous low signal intensity on T2-weighted images and low-level progressive enhancement (**Fig. 8**).[98,99]

Papillary tumors are further subdivided into type 1 (basophilic, usually low-grade) and type 2 (eosinophilic, usually high-grade) groups, the latter with worse prognosis.[100] Distinction between these

intensity on all images, following the same pattern of retroperitoneal and subcutaneous fat. On OP images, note the signal dropout at the interface between the mass and the kidney (*white arrowheads*), also known as India-ink artifact. Signal dropout in areas within the mass (*black arrowheads*) indicates coexistence of fat and nonfat elements (ie, intravoxel fat). (*From* Kay FU, Pedrosa I. Imaging of solid renal masses. Radiol Clin North Am 2017;55(2):243–58; with permission.)

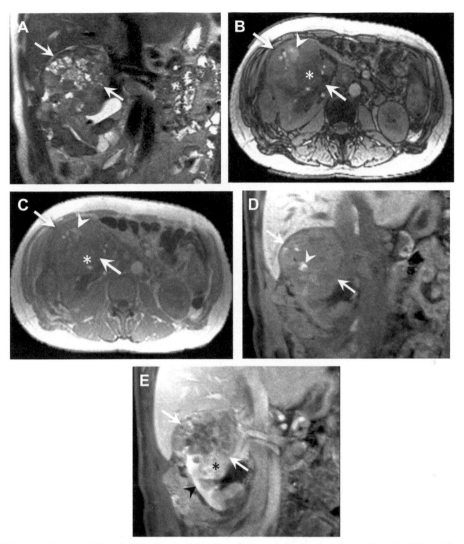

Fig. 6. A 55-year-old man with ccRCC in the right kidney. Coronal single-shot fast spin-echo T2-weighted MR image (*A*) shows an infiltrative mass (*arrows*) with heterogeneous and predominantly high signal intensity in the right upper pole. Area of signal dropout (*asterisk*) is identified in the T1-weighted OP image (*B*) compared with the IP image (*C*), consistent with intravoxel fat. There are also foci of high signal intensity (*white arrowheads*), related to hemorrhage, better seen on the precontrast fat-saturated T1-weighted SPGR acquisition (*D*). Postcontrast image using the same acquisition as in (*D*), during the corticomedullary (*E*) phase, shows heterogeneous enhancement in the mass (*arrows*) with areas of avid enhancement (*asterisk*), similar to that of normal renal cortex (*black arrowhead*). (*From* Kay FU, Pedrosa I. Imaging of solid renal masses. Radiol Clin North Am 2017;55(2):252; with permission.)

2 types by imaging is in general not possible for those tumors presenting as localized renal masses, albeit type 2 tumors tend to be larger.[101] A subgroup of type 2 pRCC can present as ill-defined, invasive tumors, commonly with centripetal growth and renal vein invasion, complicated by pulmonary embolism.[102] This infiltrative phenotype is associated with worse prognosis than well-defined pRCC, independent of histology type (ie. type 1 vs 2).[101]

Three-point time-intensity curve analyses have also shown value in RCC subtyping. ccRCC has significantly greater signal intensity change (difference between postcontrast and precontrast, divided by precontrast signal intensity) on both corticomedullary and nephrographic phases (205.6% and 247.1%, respectively) compared with pRCC (32.1% and 96.6%), whereas chrRCC has intermediate enhancement values (109.9% and 192.5%) (**Fig. 9**). Distinction of ccRCC from pRCC was achieved with near perfect sensitivity and specificity using 84% signal intensity change as the threshold on corticomedullary

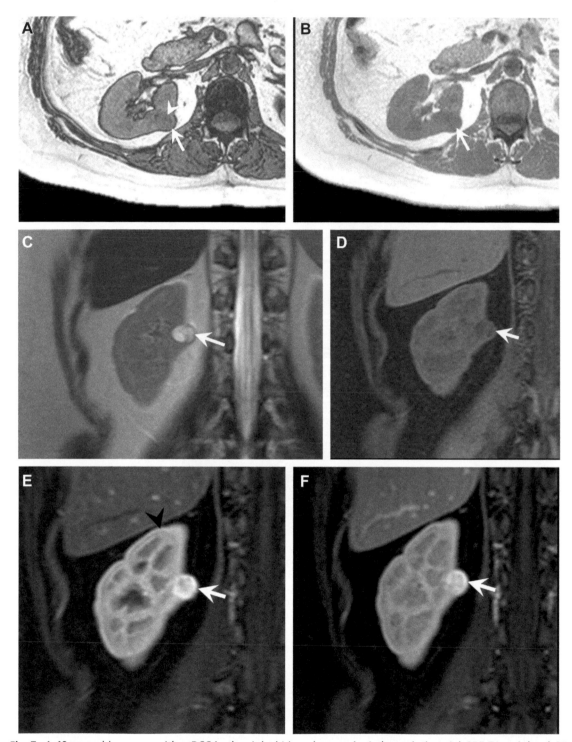

Fig. 7. A 40-year-old woman with ccRCC in the right kidney (*arrows in A through F*). Axial GRE T1-weighted OP (*A*) and IP (*B*) MR images show mild signal dropout within the mass (*arrowhead*), consistent with intravoxel fat. There is marked hyperintense signal on coronal single-shot fast spin-echo T2-weighted MR images (*C*). Note the early and avid enhancement on dynamic postcontrast images (*E–F*; precontrast, *D*), higher than that of normal renal cortex (*arrowhead in E*). (*From* Kay FU, Pedrosa I. Imaging of solid renal masses. Radiol Clin North Am 2017;55(2):253; with permission.)

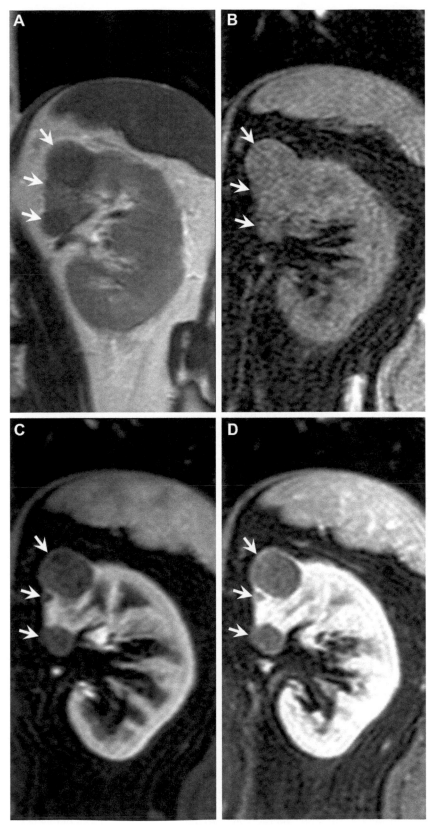

Fig. 8. A 65-year-old man with multifocal pRCC. Coronal single-shot fast spin-echo T2-weighted MR image (*A*) shows 3 circumscribed lesions (*arrows*) with homogeneous hypointense signal in the perihilar and upper pole

acquisitions.[103] Perfusion in pRCC by ASL is also lower than perfusion levels observed for ccRCC, chrRCC, unclassified RCC, and oncocytoma.[90]

Imaging-Guided Biopsy

Percutaneous renal biopsy has been shown to help avoid surgery in up to 33% of the cases initially considered to be malignant on imaging.[104] Renal biopsy shows high sensitivity and specificity in identifying malignancy,[70,104,105] although the number of nondiagnostic samples may vary between 9%[70] and 29%.[104,106] Considering only diagnostic samples, biopsy of small renal masses has shown up to 94% accuracy in defining histology,[70] with lower accuracies for determining Fuhrman grade (46%–85%).[81] Severe complications are rare, occurring in less than 1%,[107] leading some clinicians/urologists to advocate the incorporation of imaging-guided biopsy into management algorithms of small renal masses.[70]

Standardized Diagnostic Algorithms

Recent attempts have been made to standardize the interpretation criteria for multiparametric MR imaging in the characterization of solid renal masses.[108–110] T2-weighted images and dynamic postcontrast series are key features of most proposed algorithms. Although DWI may aid in the differentiation of oncocytomas from RCC, its usefulness in subtyping RCCs has not been proven.[111] Exploration of quantitative capabilities of multiparametric MR could aid increasing diagnostic reproducibility.[56]

Fig. 10 summarizes a diagnostic algorithm used by the authors for the characterization of solid renal masses on MR imaging. Note that in those columns with more than one diagnosis, the MR imaging findings of different histologic subtypes can overlap, and even with the use of ancillary findings (eg, homogeneity, necrosis, scar), a specific diagnosis may not be possible. In a recent study using multiparametric MRI, the authors assessed the performance of a 5-scale clear cell likelihood score (ccLS) based on this algorithm.[108] As the ccLS increased from 1 to 5, the likelihood of ccRCC also increased. The overall diagnostic accuracy, sensitivity, specificity, and positive and negative predictive values for clear cell histology across 7 different radiologists using ccLS of 4 and 5 were approximately 80%. Conversely, the specificity of ccLS 1 and 2 to exclude clear cell histology was 95% with a positive predictive value for other histologies of 93%.

The described algorithm could support a change in the management of small renal masses in which patients with a ccLS 4 to 5 would be encouraged to undergo curative intervention; patients with a ccLS 1 to 2 could be placed on active surveillance, especially if lesions are less than 3 cm, and patients with a ccLS of 3 would undergo a renal mass biopsy. In the authors' experience, this approach would result in a biopsy rate of only 20%, with unnecessary treatment of oncocytoma and lipid-poor AML in 4.5% and 1.7% of the surgical cohort, respectively, and 4.4% of patients with ccRCC placed on active surveillance.[108] Further refinements in the algorithm may improve these results. Furthermore, additional noninvasive tests such as [99Tc]-Technetium Sestamibi SPECT could be contemplated in patients with ccLS 3 for the diagnosis of oncocytoma and mixed oncocytic/chromophobe tumors.[91] Ultimately, the diagnostic performance of different imaging tests and/or the morbidity/complication rate associated with percutaneous biopsies will not be the only factors to be considered in the workup of small renal masses, a careful cost-benefit analysis of any proposed algorithm will be necessary.

Prediction of Histologic Grade

Tumor histologic grade has prognostic implications and therefore may affect patient management. However, the accuracy in presurgical grade prediction has been limited for imaging methods and even percutaneous biopsy. On MR imaging, multivariate models taking into consideration morphologic features of RCC showed that renal vein thrombosis and retroperitoneal collaterals were predictive of high-grade ccRCC, whereas peripheral location and homogeneous enhancement were associated with low-grade pRCC.[55] DWI may aid in the differentiation of low-grade from high-grade ccRCC, with sensitivities between 65% and 90%, specificities between 71% and 83%, and overall accuracy of 83%.[111] Focal areas of marked restricted diffusion increase the likelihood of high-grade clear cell histology.[111]

Radiomics

A novel field in medical imaging commonly named "Radiomics" explores the ability of advanced

of the left kidney. Coronal 3D fat-saturated Dixon T1-weighted MR images before (*B*) and after contrast injection, during the corticomedullary (*C*) and nephrographic (*D*) phases show low-level homogeneous progressive enhancement (*arrows*). (*From* Kay FU, Pedrosa I. Imaging of solid renal masses. Radiol Clin North Am 2017;55(2):253; with permission.)

325

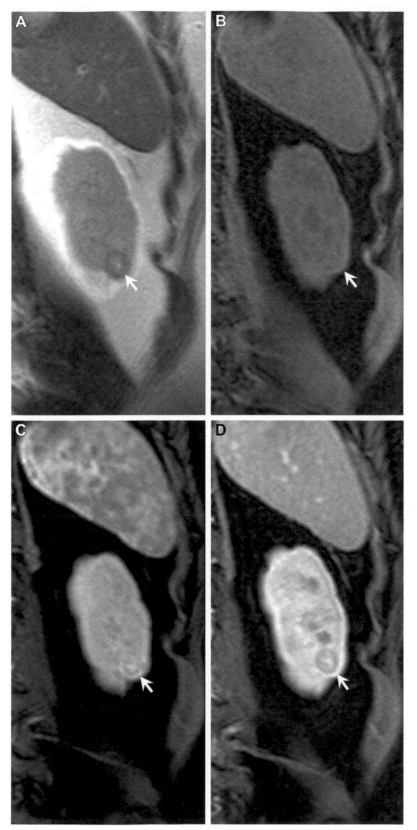

Fig. 9. A 42-year-old woman with chrRCC in the left kidney (*arrows*). Coronal single-shot fast spin-echo T2-weighted MR image (*A*) shows a 1.3-cm, slightly heterogeneous, predominantly hypointense lesion in the left lower pole. Fat-saturated 3D Dixon T1-weighted MR image shows moderate enhancement of the lesion on the corticomedullary (*C*) and nephrographic (*D*) phases compared with precontrast image (*B*). (*From* Kay FU, Pedrosa I. Imaging of solid renal masses. Radiol Clin North Am 2017;55(2):254; with permission.)

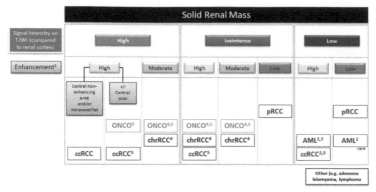

Fig. 10. Diagnostic algorithm for characterization of solid renal masses. 1) Enhancement during corticomedullary phase: Intense, greater than or equal to renal cortex; moderate, approximately 50% of renal cortex; mild, approximately 25% to 30% of renal cortex. 2) Arterial-to-delayed enhancement ratio (ADER), which is the difference in signal intensity between arterial and precontrast phase divided by the difference between delayed and precontrast phase. ADER greater than 1.5 favors minimal-fat AML, whereas less than 1.5 favors ccRCC. 3) ccRCC is typically heterogeneous; minimal-fat AML is typically homogeneous (i.e. except if intratumor bleed). 4) Oncocytoma (ONCO) is more commonly hypervascular (enhances similarly to renal cortex), whereas chrRCC shows more commonly homogeneous moderate enhancement (approximately 50% of renal cortex). 5) Oncocytoma if segmental enhancement inversion (i.e. hyperenhancing tumor areas on corticomedullary phase with relative hypoenhancement on delayed phases and hypoenhancing areas of corticomedullary phase that enhance avidly during delay phases) and/or central scar (ie, central initial nonenhancing area with delayed enhancement), whereas ccRCC is more likely if necrosis (ie, nonenhancing central area) is present or if tumor is heterogeneous. T2WI, T2-weighted imaging. (*Adapted from* Kay FU, Pedrosa I. Imaging of solid renal masses. Radiol Clin North Am 2017;55(2):255; with permission.)

image analysis to extract textural and morphologic features beyond the human perception that could reflect histologic, genomic, and proteomic patterns, resulting in better diagnosis and risk stratification.[112] It has been shown that some phenotypical features of ccRCC could be associated with genomic mutations.[113] Textural features of ADC and intravoxel incoherent motion imaging can identify tumors with metastatic potential[114] and some subtypes of renal masses.[115] Texture analysis applied to CT has also shown promising results in differentiation of renal tumors.[116,117] The incorporation of quantitative imaging techniques such as Dixon MRI in multiparametric MRI protocols may provide additional information about the metabolism and aggressiveness of ccRCC.[118]

SUMMARY

The continued evolution of imaging methods and evolving management options has bolstered the noninvasive assessment of solid renal masses. The combination of multiple parameters obtained from imaging studies offers an opportunity for evaluating the biology and ultimately the clinical significance of solid renal masses. As a result, patient management may be positively affected with the use of cutting-edge imaging protocols, along with the development of evidence-based diagnostic algorithms that integrate these novel imaging criteria and percutaneous biopsies.

ACKNOWLEDGMENTS

The authors thank Dr Jeffrey A. Caddedu, MD for reviewing this article.

REFERENCES

1. Hollingsworth JM, Miller DC, Daignault S, et al. Rising incidence of small renal masses: a need to reassess treatment effect. J Natl Cancer Inst 2006;98(18):1331–4.
2. Chawla SN, Crispen PL, Hanlon AL, et al. The natural history of observed enhancing renal masses: meta-analysis and review of the world literature. J Urol 2006;175(2):425–31.
3. Kassouf W, Aprikian AG, Laplante M, et al. Natural history of renal masses followed expectantly. J Urol 2004;171(1):111–3 [discussion: 3].
4. Volpe A, Panzarella T, Rendon RA, et al. The natural history of incidentally detected small renal masses. Cancer 2004;100(4):738–45.
5. Israel GM, Bosniak MA. How I do it: evaluating renal masses. Radiology 2005;236(2):441–50.
6. Silverman SG, Israel GM, Herts BR, et al. Management of the incidental renal mass. Radiology 2008;249(1):16–31.
7. Frank I, Blute ML, Cheville JC, et al. Solid renal tumors: an analysis of pathological features related to tumor size. J Urol 2003;170(6 Pt 1):2217–20.
8. Li G, Cuilleron M, Gentil-Perret A, et al. Characteristics of image-detected solid renal masses:

implication for optimal treatment. Int J Urol 2004; 11(2):63–7.

9. Kutikov A, Fossett LK, Ramchandani P, et al. Incidence of benign pathologic findings at partial nephrectomy for solitary renal mass presumed to be renal cell carcinoma on preoperative imaging. Urology 2006;68(4):737–40.

10. Siegel RL, Miller KD, Jemal A. Cancer statistics, 2017. CA Cancer J Clin 2017;67(1):7–30.

11. Lopez-Beltran A, Carrasco JC, Cheng L, et al. 2009 update on the classification of renal epithelial tumors in adults. Int J Urol 2009;16(5):432–43.

12. Remzi M, Ozsoy M, Klingler HC, et al. Are small renal tumors harmless? Analysis of histopathological features according to tumors 4 cm or less in diameter. J Urol 2006;176(3):896–9.

13. Amin MB, Amin MB, Tamboli P, et al. Prognostic impact of histologic subtyping of adult renal epithelial neoplasms: an experience of 405 cases. Am J Surg Pathol 2002;26(3):281–91.

14. Guinan P, Vogelzang NJ, Randazzo R, et al. Renal pelvic cancer: a review of 611 patients treated in Illinois 1975-1985. Cancer Incidence and End Results Committee. Urology 1992;40(5):393–9.

15. Hall MC, Womack S, Sagalowsky AI, et al. Prognostic factors, recurrence, and survival in transitional cell carcinoma of the upper urinary tract: a 30-year experience in 252 patients. Urology 1998;52(4):594–601.

16. Caoili EM, Cohan RH, Inampudi P, et al. MDCT urography of upper tract urothelial neoplasms. AJR Am J Roentgenol 2005;184(6):1873–81.

17. Xiao JC, Walz-Mattmuller R, Ruck P, et al. Renal involvement in myeloproliferative and lymphoproliferative disorders. A study of autopsy cases. Gen Diagn Pathol 1997;142(3–4):147–53.

18. Urban BA, Fishman EK. Renal lymphoma: CT patterns with emphasis on helical CT. Radiographics 2000;20(1):197–212.

19. Wu AJ, Mehra R, Hafez K, et al. Metastases to the kidney: a clinicopathological study of 43 cases with an emphasis on deceptive features. Histopathology 2015;66(4):587–97.

20. Johnson DC, Vukina J, Smith AB, et al. Preoperatively misclassified, surgically removed benign renal masses: a systematic review of surgical series and United States population level burden estimate. J Urol 2015;193(1):30–5.

21. Flum AS, Hamoui N, Said MA, et al. Update on the diagnosis and management of renal angiomyolipoma. J Urol 2016;195(4 Pt 1):834–46.

22. Fujii Y, Komai Y, Saito K, et al. Incidence of benign pathologic lesions at partial nephrectomy for presumed RCC renal masses: Japanese dual-center experience with 176 consecutive patients. Urology 2008;72(3):598–602.

23. Milner J, McNeil B, Alioto J, et al. Fat poor renal angiomyolipoma: patient, computerized tomography and histological findings. J Urol 2006;176(3):905–9.

24. Fujii Y, Ajima J, Oka K, et al. Benign renal tumors detected among healthy adults by abdominal ultrasonography. Eur Urol 1995;27(2):124–7.

25. Chronopoulos PN, Kaisidis GN, Vaiopoulos CK, et al. Spontaneous rupture of a giant renal angiomyolipoma-Wunderlich's syndrome: report of a case. Int J Surg Case Rep 2016;19:140–3.

26. Lane BR, Aydin H, Danforth TL, et al. Clinical correlates of renal angiomyolipoma subtypes in 209 patients: classic, fat poor, tuberous sclerosis associated and epithelioid. J Urol 2008;180(3):836–43.

27. Perez-Ordonez B, Hamed G, Campbell S, et al. Renal oncocytoma: a clinicopathologic study of 70 cases. Am J Surg Pathol 1997;21(8):871–83.

28. Oxley JD, Sullivan J, Mitchelmore A, et al. Metastatic renal oncocytoma. J Clin Pathol 2007;60(6):720–2.

29. Hes O, Michal M, Sima R, et al. Renal oncocytoma with and without intravascular extension into the branches of renal vein have the same morphological, immunohistochemical and genetic features. Virchows Arch 2008;452(3):285–93.

30. Gudbjartsson T, Hardarson S, Petursdottir V, et al. Renal oncocytoma: a clinicopathological analysis of 45 consecutive cases. BJU Int 2005;96(9): 1275–9.

31. Bhatt S, MacLennan G, Dogra V. Renal pseudotumors. AJR Am J Roentgenol 2007;188(5):1380–7.

32. Craig WD, Wagner BJ, Travis MD. Pyelonephritis: radiologic-pathologic review. Radiographics 2008; 28(1):255–77 [quiz: 327–8].

33. Chuang CK, Lai MK, Chang PL, et al. Xanthogranulomatous pyelonephritis: experience in 36 cases. J Urol 1992;147(2):333–6.

34. Osca JM, Peiro MJ, Rodrigo M, et al. Focal xanthogranulomatous pyelonephritis: partial nephrectomy as definitive treatment. Eur Urol 1997;32(3): 375–9.

35. Haliloglu AH, Gulpinar O, Ozden E, et al. Urinary ultrasonography in screening incidental renal cell carcinoma: is it obligatory? Int Urol Nephrol 2011; 43(3):687–90.

36. Heilbrun ME, Remer EM, Casalino DD, et al. ACR appropriateness criteria indeterminate renal mass. J Am Coll Radiol 2015;12(4):333–41.

37. Warshauer DM, McCarthy SM, Street L, et al. Detection of renal masses: sensitivities and specificities of excretory urography/linear tomography, US, and CT. Radiology 1988;169(2):363–5.

38. Jamis-Dow CA, Choyke PL, Jennings SB, et al. Small (≤ 3-cm) renal masses: detection with CT versus US and pathologic correlation. Radiology 1996;198(3):785–8.

39. Kang SK, Kim D, Chandarana H. Contemporary imaging of the renal mass. Curr Urol Rep 2011;12(1): 11–7.

40. Vikram R, Beland MD, Blaufox MD, et al. ACR appropriateness criteria renal cell carcinoma staging. J Am Coll Radiol 2016;13(5):518–25.

41. Hartman DS, Choyke PL, Hartman MS. From the RSNA refresher courses: a practical approach to the cystic renal mass. Radiographics 2004;24(Suppl 1):S101–15.

42. Desser TS, Jeffrey RB. Tissue harmonic imaging techniques: physical principles and clinical applications. Semin Ultrasound CT MR 2001;22(1):1–10.

43. Schmidt T, Hohl C, Haage P, et al. Diagnostic accuracy of phase-inversion tissue harmonic imaging versus fundamental B-mode sonography in the evaluation of focal lesions of the kidney. AJR Am J Roentgenol 2003;180(6):1639–47.

44. Quaia E. Microbubble ultrasound contrast agents: an update. Eur Radiol 2007;17(8):1995–2008.

45. Catalano C, Fraioli F, Laghi A, et al. High-resolution multidetector CT in the preoperative evaluation of patients with renal cell carcinoma. AJR Am J Roentgenol 2003;180(5):1271–7.

46. Bosniak MA. The small (less than or equal to 3.0 cm) renal parenchymal tumor: detection, diagnosis, and controversies. Radiology 1991;179(2):307–17.

47. Silverman SG, Lee BY, Seltzer SE, et al. Small (≤ 3 cm) renal masses: correlation of spiral CT features and pathologic findings. AJR Am J Roentgenol 1994;163(3):597–605.

48. Maki DD, Birnbaum BA, Chakraborty DP, et al. Renal cyst pseudoenhancement: beam-hardening effects on CT numbers. Radiology 1999;213(2):468–72.

49. Birnbaum BA, Hindman N, Lee J, et al. Renal cyst pseudoenhancement: influence of multidetector CT reconstruction algorithm and scanner type in phantom model. Radiology 2007;244(3):767–75.

50. Pooler BD, Pickhardt PJ, O'Connor SD, et al. Renal cell carcinoma: attenuation values on unenhanced CT. AJR Am J Roentgenol 2012;198(5):1115–20.

51. Mileto A, Nelson RC, Paulson EK, et al. Dual-energy MDCT for imaging the renal mass. AJR Am J Roentgenol 2015;204(6):W640–7.

52. Kreft BP, Muller-Miny H, Sommer T, et al. Diagnostic value of MR imaging in comparison to CT in the detection and differential diagnosis of renal masses: ROC analysis. Eur Radiol 1997;7(4):542–7.

53. Dilauro M, Quon M, McInnes MD, et al. Comparison of contrast-enhanced multiphase renal protocol CT versus MRI for diagnosis of papillary renal cell carcinoma. AJR Am J Roentgenol 2016;206(2):319–25.

54. Goldfarb DA, Novick AC, Lorig R, et al. Magnetic resonance imaging for assessment of vena caval tumor thrombi: a comparative study with venacavography and computerized tomography

scanning. J Urol 1990;144(5):1100–3 [discussion: 1103–4].

55. Pedrosa I, Chou MT, Ngo L, et al. MR classification of renal masses with pathologic correlation. Eur Radiol 2008;18(2):365–75.

56. Cornelis F, Tricaud E, Lasserre AS, et al. Routinely performed multiparametric magnetic resonance imaging helps to differentiate common subtypes of renal tumours. Eur Radiol 2014;24(5):1068–80.

57. Pedrosa I, Alsop DC, Rofsky NM. Magnetic resonance imaging as a biomarker in renal cell carcinoma. Cancer 2009;115(10 Suppl):2334–45.

58. ACR Committee on Drugs and Contrast Media. Manual on Contrast Media v10.3 2017. Available at: https://www.acr.org/Quality-Safety/Resources/Contrast-Manual. Accessed November 30,2017.

59. Zhang B, Liang L, Chen W, et al. An updated study to determine association between gadolinium-based contrast agents and nephrogenic systemic fibrosis. PLoS One 2015;10(6):e0129720.

60. Nandwana SB, Moreno CC, Osipow MT, et al. Gadobenate dimeglumine administration and nephrogenic systemic fibrosis: is there a real risk in patients with impaired renal function? Radiology 2015;276(3):741–7.

61. Soulez G, Bloomgarden DC, Rofsky NM, et al. Prospective cohort study of nephrogenic systemic fibrosis in patients with stage 3-5 chronic kidney disease undergoing MRI with injected gadobenate dimeglumine or gadoteridol. AJR Am J Roentgenol 2015;205(3):469–78.

62. Kanda T, Nakai Y, Hagiwara A, et al. Distribution and chemical forms of gadolinium in the brain: a review. Br J Radiol 2017;90(1079):20170115.

63. FDA. FDA Drug Safety Communication: FDA identifies no harmful effects to date with brain retention of gadolinium-based contrast agents for MRIs; Available at: https://www.fda.gov/Drugs/DrugSafety/ucm559007.htm. Accessed November 30, 2017

64. Pedrosa I, Rafatzand K, Robson P, et al. Arterial spin labeling MR imaging for characterisation of renal masses in patients with impaired renal function: initial experience. Eur Radiol 2012;22(2):484–92.

65. Zhang Y, Kapur P, Yuan Q, et al. Tumor vascularity in renal masses: correlation of arterial spin-labeled and dynamic contrast-enhanced magnetic resonance imaging assessments. Clin Genitourin Cancer 2016;14(1):e25–36.

66. Khatri G, Pedrosa I. 3T MR imaging protocol for characterization of renal masses. Appl Radiol 2012;41(Suppl):22–6.

67. Butler BP, Novick AC, Miller DP, et al. Management of small unilateral renal cell carcinomas: radical versus nephron-sparing surgery. Urology 1995;45(1):34–40 [discussion: 40–1].

68. Lerner SE, Hawkins CA, Blute ML, et al. Disease outcome in patients with low stage renal cell carcinoma treated with nephron sparing or radical surgery. 1996. J Urol 2002;167(2 Pt 2):884–9 [discussion: 889–90].

69. Rosales JC, Haramis G, Moreno J, et al. Active surveillance for renal cortical neoplasms. J Urol 2010; 183(5):1698–702.

70. Halverson SJ, Kunju LP, Bhalla R, et al. Accuracy of determining small renal mass management with risk stratified biopsies: confirmation by final pathology. J Urol 2013;189(2):441–6.

71. Harvey CJ, Alsafi A, Kuzmich S, et al. Role of US contrast agents in the assessment of indeterminate solid and cystic lesions in native and transplant kidneys. Radiographics 2015;35(5):1419–30.

72. Yamashita Y, Takahashi M, Watanabe O, et al. Small renal cell carcinoma: pathologic and radiologic correlation. Radiology 1992;184(2):493–8.

73. Forman HP, Middleton WD, Melson GL, et al. Hyperechoic renal cell carcinomas: increase in detection at US. Radiology 1993;188(2):431–4.

74. Sidhar K, McGahan JP, Early HM, et al. Renal cell carcinomas: sonographic appearance depending on size and histologic type. J Ultrasound Med 2016;35(2):311–20.

75. Barr RG, Peterson C, Hindi A. Evaluation of indeterminate renal masses with contrast-enhanced US: a diagnostic performance study. Radiology 2014; 271(1):133–42.

76. Bosniak MA, Megibow AJ, Hulnick DH, et al. CT diagnosis of renal angiomyolipoma: the importance of detecting small amounts of fat. AJR Am J Roentgenol 1988;151(3):497–501.

77. Simpson E, Patel U. Diagnosis of angiomyolipoma using computed tomography-region of interest < or = -10 HU or 4 adjacent pixels < or = -10 HU are recommended as the diagnostic thresholds. Clin Radiol 2006;61(5):410–6.

78. Davenport MS, Neville AM, Ellis JH, et al. Diagnosis of renal angiomyolipoma with Hounsfield unit thresholds: effect of size of region of interest and nephrographic phase imaging. Radiology 2011; 260(1):158–65.

79. Wang Y, Li D, Haacke EM, et al. A three-point Dixon method for water and fat separation using 2D and 3D gradient-echo techniques. J Magn Reson Imaging 1998;8(3):703–10.

80. Israel GM, Hindman N, Hecht E, et al. The use of opposed-phase chemical shift MRI in the diagnosis of renal angiomyolipomas. AJR Am J Roentgenol 2005;184(6):1868–72.

81. Jinzaki M, Tanimoto A, Narimatsu Y, et al. Angiomyolipoma: imaging findings in lesions with minimal fat. Radiology 1997;205(2):497–502.

82. Outwater EK, Bhatia M, Siegelman ES, et al. Lipid in renal clear cell carcinoma: detection on opposed-phase gradient-echo MR images. Radiology 1997;205(1):103–7.

83. Hindman N, Ngo L, Genega EM, et al. Angiomyolipoma with minimal fat: can it be differentiated from clear cell renal cell carcinoma by using standard MR techniques? Radiology 2012;265(2):468–77.

84. Sasiwimonphan K, Takahashi N, Leibovich BC, et al. Small (<4 cm) renal mass: differentiation of angiomyolipoma without visible fat from renal cell carcinoma utilizing MR imaging. Radiology 2016; 280(2):653.

85. Schieda N, Dilauro M, Moosavi B, et al. MRI evaluation of small (<4 cm) solid renal masses: multivariate modeling improves diagnostic accuracy for angiomyolipoma without visible fat compared to univariate analysis. Eur Radiol 2016;26(7): 2242–51.

86. Lassel EA, Rao R, Schwenke C, et al. Diffusion-weighted imaging of focal renal lesions: a meta-analysis. Eur Radiol 2014;24(1):241–9.

87. Kim JI, Cho JY, Moon KC, et al. Segmental enhancement inversion at biphasic multidetector CT: characteristic finding of small renal oncocytoma. Radiology 2009;252(2):441–8.

88. Rosenkrantz AB, Hindman N, Fitzgerald EF, et al. MRI features of renal oncocytoma and chromophobe renal cell carcinoma. AJR Am J Roentgenol 2010;195(6):W421–7.

89. Kay FU, Canvasser NE, Xi Y, et al. Diagnostic performance and interreader agreement of a standardized MR imaging approach in the prediction of small renal mass histology. Radiology 2018; 287(2):543–53.

90. Lanzman RS, Robson PM, Sun MR, et al. Arterial spin-labeling MR imaging of renal masses: correlation with histopathologic findings. Radiology 2012; 265(3):799–808.

91. Gorin MA, Rowe SP, Baras AS, et al. Prospective evaluation of (99m)Tc-sestamibi SPECT/CT for the diagnosis of renal oncocytomas and hybrid oncocytic/chromophobe tumors. Eur Urol 2016;69(3): 413–6.

92. Tamai H, Takiguchi Y, Oka M, et al. Contrast-enhanced ultrasonography in the diagnosis of solid renal tumors. J Ultrasound Med 2005; 24(12):1635–40.

93. Sheir KZ, El-Azab M, Mosbah A, et al. Differentiation of renal cell carcinoma subtypes by multislice computerized tomography. J Urol 2005;174(2): 451–5 [discussion: 455].

94. Kim JK, Kim TK, Ahn HJ, et al. Differentiation of subtypes of renal cell carcinoma on helical CT scans. AJR Am J Roentgenol 2002;178(6): 1499–506.

95. Sureka B, Lal A, Khandelwal N, et al. Dynamic computed tomography and Doppler findings in different subtypes of renal cell carcinoma with their

histopathological correlation. J Cancer Res Ther 2014;10(3):552–7.

96. Herts BR, Coll DM, Novick AC, et al. Enhancement characteristics of papillary renal neoplasms revealed on triphasic helical CT of the kidneys. AJR Am J Roentgenol 2002;178(2):367–72.

97. Bata P, Gyebnar J, Tarnoki DL, et al. Clear cell renal cell carcinoma and papillary renal cell carcinoma: differentiation of distinct histological types with multiphase CT. Diagn Interv Radiol 2013;19(5): 387–92.

98. Oliva MR, Glickman JN, Zou KH, et al. Renal cell carcinoma: t1 and t2 signal intensity characteristics of papillary and clear cell types correlated with pathology. AJR Am J Roentgenol 2009;192(6): 1524–30.

99. Roy C, Sauer B, Lindner V, et al. MR imaging of papillary renal neoplasms: potential application for characterization of small renal masses. Eur Radiol 2007;17(1):193–200.

100. Pignot G, Elie C, Conquy S, et al. Survival analysis of 130 patients with papillary renal cell carcinoma: prognostic utility of type 1 and type 2 subclassification. Urology 2007;69(2):230–5.

101. Rosenkrantz AB, Sekhar A, Genega EM, et al. Prognostic implications of the magnetic resonance imaging appearance in papillary renal cell carcinoma. Eur Radiol 2013;23(2):579–87.

102. Yamada T, Endo M, Tsuboi M, et al. Differentiation of pathologic subtypes of papillary renal cell carcinoma on CT. AJR Am J Roentgenol 2008;191(5): 1559–63.

103. Sun MR, Ngo L, Genega EM, et al. Renal cell carcinoma: dynamic contrast-enhanced MR imaging for differentiation of tumor subtypes–correlation with pathologic findings. Radiology 2009;250(3):793–802.

104. Vasudevan A, Davies RJ, Shannon BA, et al. Incidental renal tumours: the frequency of benign lesions and the role of preoperative core biopsy. BJU Int 2006;97(5):946–9.

105. Caoili EM, Bude RO, Higgins EJ, et al. Evaluation of sonographically guided percutaneous core biopsy of renal masses. AJR Am J Roentgenol 2002; 179(2):373–8.

106. Leveridge MJ, Finelli A, Kachura JR, et al. Outcomes of small renal mass needle core biopsy, nondiagnostic percutaneous biopsy, and the role of repeat biopsy. Eur Urol 2011;60(3):578–84.

107. Wang R, Wolf JS, Wood DP, et al. Accuracy of percutaneous core biopsy in management of small renal masses. Urology 2009;73(3):586–90 [discussion: 90–1].

108. Canvasser NE, Kay FU, Xi Y, et al. Diagnostic accuracy of multiparametric magnetic resonance imaging to identify clear cell renal cell carcinoma in cT1a renal masses. J Urol 2017;198(4):780–6.

109. Lopes Vendrami C, Parada Villavicencio C, DeJulio TJ, et al. Differentiation of solid renal tumors with multiparametric MR imaging. Radiographics 2017;37(7):2026–42.

110. Cornelis F, Grenier N. Multiparametric magnetic resonance imaging of solid renal tumors: a practical algorithm. Semin Ultrasound CT MR 2017; 38(1):47–58.

111. Kang SK, Zhang A, Pandharipande PV, et al. DWI for renal mass characterization: systematic review and meta-analysis of diagnostic test performance. AJR Am J Roentgenol 2015;205(2):317–24.

112. Lambin P, Rios-Velazquez E, Leijenaar R, et al. Radiomics: extracting more information from medical images using advanced feature analysis. Eur J Cancer 2012;48(4):441–6.

113. Karlo CA, Di Paolo PL, Chaim J, et al. Radiogenomics of clear cell renal cell carcinoma: associations between CT imaging features and mutations. Radiology 2014;270(2):464–71.

114. Kierans AS, Rusinek H, Lee A, et al. Textural differences in apparent diffusion coefficient between low- and high-stage clear cell renal cell carcinoma. AJR Am J Roentgenol 2014;203(6):W637–44.

115. Gaing B, Sigmund EE, Huang WC, et al. Subtype differentiation of renal tumors using voxel-based histogram analysis of intravoxel incoherent motion parameters. Invest Radiol 2015;50(3):144–52.

116. Raman SP, Chen Y, Schroeder JL, et al. CT texture analysis of renal masses: pilot study using random forest classification for prediction of pathology. Acad Radiol 2014;21(12):1587–96.

117. Yu H, Scalera J, Khalid M, et al. Texture analysis as a radiomic marker for differentiating renal tumors. Abdom Radiol (NY) 2017;42(10): 2470–8.

118. Zhang Y, Udayakumar D, Cai L, et al. Addressing metabolic heterogeneity in clear cell renal cell carcinoma with quantitative Dixon MRI. JCI Insight 2017;2(15) [pii:94278].

Imaging of Cystic Renal Masses

Nicole M. Hindman, MD

KEYWORDS

• Renal • Kidney • Bosniak • Classification • Cystic • Complex • Indeterminate

KEY POINTS

- Cystic renal lesions are generally more indolent than solid renal lesions.
- The Bosniak classification system is an imaging framework for differentiating benign and malignant cystic renal masses.
- The key feature that separates malignant from benign Bosniak cystic lesions is that Bosniak 3 and 4 lesions demonstrate enhancement of solid components. Benign lesions do not demonstrate internal solid enhancement.
- Although gray-scale ultrasound is useful for definitive characterization of simple renal cysts, it tends to erroneously upgrade benign renal cysts, which have internal debris, given its high sensitivity to morphology and lack of sensitivity to internal vascularity.
- The Bosniak classification system is a contrast-enhanced CT-defined classification system; however, it has been shown to be equally accurate when applied to contrast-enhanced MR imaging.

INTRODUCTION: DISCUSSION OF PROBLEM/CLINICAL PRESENTATION

Cystic renal masses are a common diagnostic challenge in daily imaging. These lesions are frequently detected incidentally in patients imaged for other reasons, and the optimal management of these lesions can be challenging. Both benign and malignant renal lesions may have a cystic imaging appearance. The imaging definition of "cystic" is a lesion that, on imaging, has a mostly fluid-filled growth pattern with a solid portion occupying a maximum of one-fourth of the tumor volume[1–3] or a mass that is mostly composed of fluid-filled spaces.[4] Cystic renal mass lesions represent only 15% of all renal mass lesions (the other 85% are solid renal masses)[5,6] and malignant cystic renal lesions are associated with a much lower morbidity and mortality rate than malignant solid renal mass lesions.[1,7–11] This more indolent behavior of malignant cystic renal masses than malignant solid renal masses allows greater leeway in surveillance imaging of cystic renal masses, prior to definitive surgical intervention.

The most common benign cystic renal mass is a simple renal cyst, which is estimated to be seen incidentally in up to 17% to 41% of patients imaged for other reasons.[12,13] Typically, these simple renal cysts can be readily diagnosed as benign on the initial imaging study that detected them[14] and appropriately ignored. The diagnostic challenge with cystic renal masses is distinguishing between benign and malignant complex cystic renal masses. The Bosniak classification system, introduced in 1986 by Dr Morton Bosniak, provides a robust imaging approach for the differentiation of benign and malignant cystic renal masses and is widely used in the international urologic and radiologic communities for its utility in assisting with management of these lesions.[15–21]

This article reviews the imaging evaluation of cystic renal masses (through the Bosniak classification), discusses the CT and MR imaging

This article was previously published in March 2017 *Radiologic Clinics*, Volume 55, Issue 2.
Disclosure Statement: The author has nothing to disclose.
Department of Radiology, NYU School of Medicine, 660 First Avenue, New York, NY 10016, USA
E-mail address: Nicole.Hindman@nyumc.org

Urol Clin N Am 45 (2018) 331–349
https://doi.org/10.1016/j.ucl.2018.03.006

techniques for evaluation of the cystic renal mass, provides an image-rich differential diagnosis of cystic renal mass lesions (benign and malignant), and reviews current approaches to management of these lesions.

NORMAL ANATOMY AND IMAGING TECHNIQUE: DISCUSSION OF IMPORTANT ANATOMIC CONSIDERATIONS

Most renal masses, including cystic renal masses, are found incidentally at the time of cross-sectional imaging for another reason.[4,16,22,23] Most of these incidental masses are simple renal cysts that can be diagnosed at the time of the initial scan without additional work-up or treatment.[4,22] Incidental solid and complex cystic masses may also be found, however, which need characterization, because some are malignant and need to be surgically excised, and others are benign. Careful attention to proper technique in evaluating these masses is essential to guide appropriate management. If the initial examination that detects the cystic renal mass is inadequate for characterization, then a dedicated renal mass CT or MR imaging can be performed, with gray-scale sonography reserved for the characterization of suspected simple cysts or some proteinaceous cysts. The CT and MR imaging protocols and recommended technique for the analysis of renal masses are presented, with the acknowledgment that these protocols are not extensive (for example, the presurgical work-up of a known malignant renal mass, including arterial, nephrographic, and urographic phases, is not included, for the sake of brevity).

CT TECHNIQUE

For evaluation of a known renal mass, a CT scan must include a noncontrast examination prior to the contrast-enhanced examination, because a noncontrast baseline is essential to determine true enhancement on the postcontrast scan. Nonionic intravenous contrast is given at a weight-based dose (1.5 mL/kg), using a power injector for a rate of 3 mL/s to 4 mL/s to guarantee that a high concentration of intravenous contrast is delivered for uniform opacification of the kidneys postcontrast. By using a multidetector row CT scanner, contrast material–enhanced imaging is routinely performed using a scan delay of 80 seconds to 90 seconds; this should ensure that there is opacification of the renal arteries and that there is a uniform nephrogram in the kidneys. In select cases, a corticomedullary phase at a 40-second delay also is added to the evaluation

of the renal mass, particularly if a vascular lesion (pseudoaneurysm) or if a renal pseudotumor (column of Bertin) is suspected. Renal mass lesion should not be characterized on the corticomedullary phase of contrast enhancement, because renal masses may have attenuation similar to that of the renal medulla and are invisible on this phase of contrast. Additionally, hypoenhancing renal lesions, such as papillary neoplasms, may not demonstrate internal enhancement on this phase.

Typically, the data sets are acquired at 0.6 mm and are reconstructed to 4-mm sections, which are sent to a picture archiving and communication system (PACS). If smaller slices are required for analysis of a small renal tumor, then these thinner slices (various multiples of 0.6 mm) are evaluated on the scanner or workstation, without need to rescan the patient (**Table 1**). This data set can then be analyzed on a 3-D workstation to create volume-rendered and 3-D images, for improved analysis of the renal tumor and its relationship to renal vasculature and the hilum.

The Bosniak classification is a CT-defined classification system,[14,24] and imaging performed on a multidetector CT scanner, using the previously described renal mass technique,[25] characterizes most renal cystic lesions. Known challenges in using CT for lesion characterization include the phenomenon of pseudoenhancement (the artifactual increase in attenuation on contrast-enhanced CT images by 10 Hounsfield units [HU] or more, thought to be secondary to beam hardening artifact) and the pitfall of partial volume averaging in small lesions (which occurs when the size of the lesion is less than twice the slice thickness used to scan).[26] Virtual monochromatic imaging in dual-energy multidetector CT may completely eliminate renal cyst pseudoenhancement in cysts larger than 1.5 cm.[27]

MR IMAGING TECHNIQUE

The average renal mass MR exam lasts approximately 30 minutes on the magnet, which can be a long time for a patient who is not adequately prepared for the examination. Therefore, discussion with patients about the length of a scan, the breath-holds required, the placement of phased array coils in contact with the body, and the noises (from gradient coil switching) should be explained; this helps decrease anxiety. At the author's institution, all breath-hold sequences are held during end expiration (because this has been shown to have improved diaphragmatic level reproducibility and thus allows for improved registration on subtraction images).[28]

Table 1
Renal mass characterization CT protocol: Siemens single-source 128-slice multidetector CT

	Noncontrast	Contrast
kV	100–120[a]	100–120[a]
mA	150[b]	150[b]
Detector collimation	0.6 mm	0.6 mm
Display field of view	Skin to skin	Skin to skin
Thin-slice reconstruction	0.6 mm q 0.6 mm	0.6 mm q 0.6 mm
Networking	0.6-mm slices ONLY to workstation	0.6 mm slices ONLY to workstation
Axial slice thickness (display)	4 mm	4 mm
Reconstruction interval	4 mm	4 mm
Coronal slice thickness	3 mm	3 mm
Coronal slice interval	3 mm	3 mm
Networking	Thick slices to PACS	Thick slices to PACS
Scan delay	Not applicable	90 s
Pitch	0.9	0.9
Gantry rotation time	0.5 s	0.5 s
Strength iterative Reconstruction	SAFIRE 3	SAFIRE 3
Reconstruction algorithm	I 40	I 40
Phase of respiration	Inspiration	Inspiration

Contrast type/volume/rate: nonionic contrast, weight based (1.5 mL/kg), 3 mL/s to 4 mL/s.
Abbreviation: SAFIRE, sinogram affirmed iterative reconstruction.
[a] Care kV determines optimal value.
[b] Based on high-kW tube power and most efficient detector.

Prior to contrast material administration, a transverse dual-echo 2-D T1-weighted gradient-echo sequence (**Table 2**), a transverse and coronal T2-weighted half-Fourier single-shot turbo spin-echo sequence, and an axial diffusion-weighted sequence are performed.

In all patients referred for evaluation of a renal mass, corticomedullary, nephrographic, and early excretory phases are acquired by using an axial breath-hold 3-D fat-suppressed T1-weighted spoiled gradient-echo sequence before and at multiple time points after administration of 0.1 mL/kg body weight (0.1 mmol/kg) of a gadolinium-based contrast material (gadobutrol is the multicyclic agent of choice at the author's institution). The 3-D imaging slab is collimated to the area of interest to maximize spatial resolution. Similarly, the matrix size is adjusted to maximize in-plane spatial resolution, balancing the need to keep the sequences less than the typical breath-hold capacity of a patient (approximately 15 seconds is the typical breath-hold capacity). The slice thickness is ideally kept between 1.5 mm and 2 mm, not to exceed 3 mm (even in poor breath-holders). The imaging delay for the arterial phase is based on a timing run with a power injector

and 1 mL of gadolinium-based contrast material followed by a 20-mL saline flush.[29] Nephrographic and early excretory phases are obtained at 70 seconds and 180 seconds postinjection, respectively. A delayed coronal acquisition is obtained after approximately 4 to 5 minutes postinjection. These sequences are useful for depicting the renal vasculature and the relationship of the tumor to the collecting system, for presurgical planning, which can help in planning for nephron preservation surgery (eg, partial nephrectomies). Finally, in-between the early excretory and coronal acquisitions, an axial 3-D image through the liver is included, because typically the dome of the liver is cut off from the field of view for renal examinations, and this helps characterize any incidental hepatic lesions, without requiring additional imaging.

Although the Bosniak classification is a CT-defined classification system, several articles have shown that renal mass MR imaging is equivalent to renal mass CT for the accurate classification of cystic renal masses in the Bosniak classification system.[30–32] MR imaging is superior to CT for the detection of internal enhancement in hemorrhagic or calcified lesions, by the use of

Table 2
Renal mass MR imaging protocol at 3T. Example given is for Siemens Prisma 3T magnet

	Sequence	Plane	Slice Thickness	Field of View	Matrix	Repetition Time (ms)	Echo Time (ms)	B Value (s/mm²)	Contrast Delay
Scout	T2WI	Cor/Sag/Ax	7–8 mm	40 cm	192 × 144	700	1.13	—	—
HASTE	T2WI	Cor	5 mm	35 cm (adjust to pt habitus)	320 × 288	Infinite	91	—	—
In/out	T1WI	Ax	5 mm	35 cm (adjust to pt habitus)	256 × 232	168	1.1/2.2 (3T)	—	—
Diffusion	T2WI	Ax	5 mm	35 cm (adjust to pt habitus)	192 × 113	5600 (minimize)	61 (minimize)	0, 400, 800	—
HASTE	T2WI	Ax	5 mm	35 cm (adjust to pt habitus)	320 × 240	Infinite	92	—	—
Precontrast VIBE	T1WI	Ax	1.5–2 mm (max 3 mm)	35 cm (adjust to pt habitus)	256 × 179	3 (minimize)	1.4 (minimize)	—	—
Postcontrast VIBE	T1WI	Ax	1.5–2 mm (max 3 mm)	35 cm (adjust to pt habitus)	256 × 179	3 (minimize)	1.4 (minimize)	—	30, 70, 180 s
VIBE cover liver	T1WI	Ax	1.5–2 mm (max 3 mm)	35 cm (adjust to pt habitus)	256 × 179	3 (minimize)	1.4 (minimize)	—	Between 70 and 180 s
VIBE	T1WI	Cor	1.5–2 mm	35 cm (adjust to pt habitus)	256 × 179	3 (minimize)	1.5 (minimize)	—	After 180 s
Subtraction VIBEs sent to PACS	T1 sub	Ax	1.5–2 mm	—	256 × 179	3	1.4	—	—

Contrast type/volume/rate: gadolinium contrast/weight based (0.1 mL/kg body weight [0.1 mmol/kg]): typically for gadobutrol (Gadavist), this is 6 mL for a 60-kg patient with a 2 mL/s flow rate.

Abbreviations: Ax, axial; Cor, coronal; HASTE, half fourier acquisition single shot turbo spin Echo; max, maximum; pt, patient; Sag, sagittal; Sub, subtraction; T1WI, T1 weighted image; T2WI, T2 weighted image; VIBE, volume interpolated breath hold examination.

subtraction imaging.[23,33,34] Known pitfalls with subtraction imaging in MR imaging include problems with image alignment (misregistration) and with discriminating signal from true internal enhancement from signal resulting from the additive noise on subtraction images.[35] An additional pitfall with MR imaging is its increased sensitivity for depiction of subtle internal septations and wall thickening[31] as well as its superior contrast resolution (but inferior spatial resolution) compared with CT, both of which may cause less experienced readers of MR imaging to erroneously upgrade cystic renal lesions.[30,31,36] Morphology alone (increased depiction of septations or apparent wall thickening), however, without associated enhancement does not upgrade a lesion in the Bosniak classification system; the morphologic change must be associated with enhancement. New advances in MR imaging with evolving motion-robust sequences, using high-resolution free-breathing radial 3-D fat-suppressed T1 gradient echo,[37] allow improved detection and clarification of internal enhancement in small cystic renal masses, with superior spatial resolution, approaching that of the spatial resolution of CT. Diffusion-weighted imaging techniques cannot yet accurately differentiate a cystic renal mass from a simple renal cyst; however, preliminary studies have shown promising results.[38–40] Characterization of cystic renal masses is frequently challenging; for indeterminate CT scans; the author's institution tends to use contrast-enhanced MR imaging.

GRAY-SCALE ULTRASOUND

Gray-scale ultrasound without contrast is limited in the diagnosis of complex renal masses, with specific exceptions. It is not sensitive for the detection of small renal lesions.[41] The poor sensitivity to vascular flow using color Doppler techniques limits the technique to only describing morphology, which in the absence of contrast enhancement/associated vascularity is inadequate for the accurate characterization of renal mass lesions. Morphology alone cannot upgrade a lesion in the Bosniak classification system; enhancement of that morphologic finding is the key.[14,24] Pitfalls in gray-scale ultrasound without contrast include the erroneous upgrading of cystic renal masses that appear solid or contain internal debris.[42] Gray-scale ultrasound, however, has utility for the following cases. If a cystic lesion is seen on ultrasound and meets sonographic criteria for a simple cyst (is anechoic, has a well-defined border, and demonstrates increased posterior through-transmission), then no further follow-up is

necessary.[43] Ultrasound is also useful in characterizing cystic renal masses that measure between 20 HU and 40 HU on CT, because these lesions typically contain internal proteinaceous material and appear simple on ultrasound, allowing for definitive characterization. Renal cystic masses with an attenuation higher than 40 HU on CT, however, are more likely to be hemorrhagic cysts and therefore appear complex (and thus indeterminate) on ultrasound.[4] Multiple recent articles have evaluated the accuracy of contrast-enhanced ultrasound in evaluating cystic renal masses using the Bosniak classification, and the results have shown promise.[44–47]

IMAGING FINDINGS/PATHOLOGY
The Bosniak Classification

Renal cystic lesions can be accurately classified with the Bosniak classification into 1 of 5 categories (1, 2, 2F, 3, and 4) on the basis of imaging features (**Fig. 1**, **Tables 3** and **4**).

Category 1 (simple) cysts
Category 1 (simple) cysts are fluid attenuation cysts, which measure less than 20 HU and are homogeneous in attenuation on noncontrast or post-contrast CT. On MR imaging, they are uniform in signal intensity on T1-weighted and T2-weighted images. These cysts have a pencil-thin wall without internal solid component and no enhancement postcontrast. These are benign and require no follow-up.

Category 2 (mildly complicated) cysts
Cysts in category 2 (mildly complicated) may contain a few pencil-thin septations with a thin wall. Minimal enhancement of the pencil-thin septations may be visually appreciated/suggested (called *perceived enhancement*), but cannot be measured with a region-of-interest measurement (ie, there is no measureable enhancement). Non-enhancing cysts smaller than 3 cm with high attenuation on noncontrast CT or uniformly high signal on precontrast T1-weighted MR imaging sequences are in this category. These cysts are benign and require no follow-up.

Category 2F (complicated) cystic lesions
Category 2F (complicated) cysts are most likely benign but may have minimal thickening of the wall or septae and have an increased number of thin internal septations. There may be perceived enhancement of the sepate or wall, but no measureable enhancement is seen. These cysts require follow-up studies, typically at 6-month intervals for the first year, then annually thereafter. Some studies have suggested that follow-up cease after

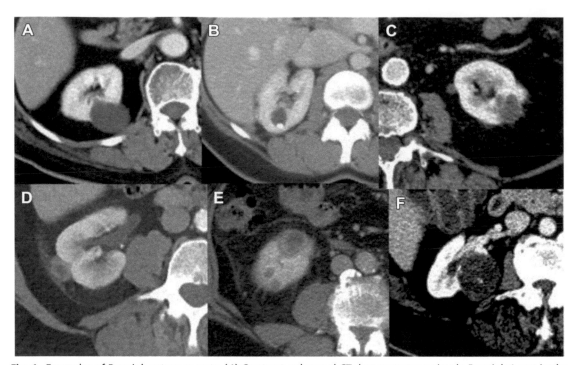

Fig. 1. Examples of Bosniak category cysts. (*A*) Contrast-enhanced CT demonstrates a simple Bosniak 1 cyst in the right posterior upper pole. (*B*) Contrast-enhanced CT demonstrates dependent layering calcification, with a well-defined wall and no internal enhancement consistent with a Bosniak 2 cyst. (*C*) There is a cyst with a mildly thickened internal smooth septation consistent with a Bosniak 2F (*F* indicates follow-up) cyst; this grew into a simple cyst on follow-up. (*D*) There is a cyst with a diffusely thickened peripheral wall with adjacent fluid along the right perirenal space, consistent with a Bosniak 3 cystic lesion (this was a collapsing renal cyst, a benign entity that disappeared on follow-up studies). (*E*) There is a thickened right lower pole intrarenal mass with a thickened wall consistent with a Bosniak 3 lesion; this was a clear cell cystic RCC on follow-up. (*F*) There is a cystic mass with irregular thickened internal septations with nodular enhancement consistent with a Bosniak 4 lesion (this was resected and was an MLCRCC).

Table 3 Diagnostic criteria: Bosniak classification	
1	A benign simple cyst with fluid attenuation with a pencil-thin wall. This cyst does not contain soft tissue, septa, or calcifications. There is no enhancement.
2	A benign cyst with a pencil-thin wall that may contain a few pencil-thin septa where faint minimal enhancement may be perceived in the septa. Thin calcifications or short segments of thickened calcification may be present. Homogeneous high-attenuation nonenhancing lesions less than 3 cm with a well-defined wall are in this category. No further evaluation is needed for these cysts.
2F (*F* indicates follow-up)	Cysts in this category may have multiple thin septa or minimal smooth thickening of the septa or wall. Faint minimal enhancement and calcifications of the septa or wall may be present; however, no associated measurable contrast enhancement is seen. These lesions are well circumscribed. Endophytic, intrarenal nonenhancing high-attenuation renal lesions greater than 3 cm are in this category. All lesions in this category require follow-up imaging to prove benignity.
3	These cystic lesions have a thickened wall or septa (smooth or irregular) with measureable (ie, via region of interest placement) enhancement. These are surgical lesions, typically with 50% of these lesions malignant (eg, cystic RCC and MLCRCC) and 50% benign (eg, complex hemorrhagic cysts, abscesses, N, and MEST).
4	These cystic lesions have the features described in category 3 as well as a solid enhancing soft tissue component separate from the wall or septum. These are surgical lesions.

Table 4	
Differential diagnosis: Bosniak renal lesions by category	
Bosniak Category	**Differential Diagnosis**
Category 1	Benign causes: simple renal cyst
Category 2	Benign causes: hemorrhagic, proteinaceous or posttraumatic cyst
Category 2F	Benign causes (common): hemorrhagic, proteinaceous, posttraumatic cysts, infected cyst/abscess, localized cystic disease of the kidney, pyelocalyceal diverticula, milk of calcium cysts, CN/MEST Malignant causes (uncommon): MLCRCC, cystic clear cell carcinoma, tubulocystic carcinoma, clear cell tubulopapillary RCC
Category 3	Benign causes (estimated 50% of Bosniak 3 lesions): hemorrhagic, proteinaceous, posttraumatic cysts, infected cyst/abscess, localized cystic disease of the kidney, pyelocalyceal diverticula, milk of calcium cysts, CN/MEST Malignant causes (estimated 50% of Bosniak 3 lesions): MLCRCC, cystic clear cell carcinoma, tubulocystic carcinoma, clear cell tubulopapillary RCC
Category 4	Malignant causes (common): MLCRCC, cystic clear cell carcinoma, tubulocystic carcinoma, clear cell tubulopapillary RCC Benign causes (uncommon): CN/MEST

stability is demonstrated for 4 to 5 years. If these lesions progress on follow-up imaging (ie, demonstrate increased soft tissue components [septal thickening/wall thickening with associated enhancement]), then this becomes a surgical lesion. Conversely, if this lesion becomes simple on follow-up imaging (loses the internal septations or wall thickening), then this becomes a nonsurgical lesion. Malignancy rates for Bosniak 2F cysts are on average considered approximately 11% (range 5%–38%), so that cysts in this category have an 11% chance of being malignant.[16,30,48–51]

Category 3 (indeterminate) cystic lesions

Category 2 (indeterminate) cystic lesions may have thickened internal septations or walls with associated measureable enhancement but do not contain frankly nodular enhancing soft tissue in association with the wall or septations, which distinguishes these lesions from category 4 lesions. The malignancy rate of a cyst in this category is approximately 50% (range 25%–100%).[16,30,48–51] For this reason, cysts in this category are considered surgical lesions. It is well recognized, however, that benign hemorrhagic cysts, infected cysts/abscesses, scarred cysts from trauma, multiloculated cysts, and cystic nephromas (CNs) may have features that are indistinguishable from malignant cysts (such as the multilocular cystic renal cell carcinoma [MLCRCC] and cystic renal cell carcinoma [RCC]) in this category. If there is additional history to suggest an infected cyst or a posttraumatic cyst, then management may include surveillance after treatment (for a suspected abscess) or an attempt to obtain

prior films (if a traumatic collapsed cyst is suspected).

Category 4 (malignant) cystic lesions

Cystic lesions in category 4 (malignant) demonstrate measureable enhancement of internal soft tissue components and are unequivocally malignant. Malignancy rates for cystic lesions in this category are approximately 80% (range 67%–100%).[16,30,48–51] These are considered surgical lesions. Imaging surveillance has been considered an acceptable alternative management approach in patients with a short life expectancy or comorbidities.

Malignant cystic renal mass lesions, which represent 15% of all renal mass lesions,[5,6] are associated with a much lower morbidity and mortality rate than malignant solid renal mass lesions.[1,7–11] The definitive treatment of Bosniak 3 and 4 renal lesions is surgical excision. Resection of renal masses, however, is not without risk. This is particularly true because the greatest incidence of renal masses (cystic and solid) occur in patients 70 years old and older, in whom medical comorbidities (cardiovascular disease, pulmonary disease, renal disease, and so forth) may increase the risks of radical or partial nephrectomy. Several articles have demonstrated increased cardiovascular morbidity, secondary to worsening/development of chronic kidney disease, in patients who have a radical nephrectomy as opposed to a partial nephrectomy.[52–55] For these reasons, when the tumor is amenable to partial nephrectomy, this technique is becoming the gold standard for treatment of renal lesions.

The ongoing clinical challenge lies in the ability to definitively differentiate the benign (or benign-behaving) Bosniak 2F, 3, and 4 lesions from the malignant Bosniak 2F, 3, and 4 lesions and to further evaluate which patient (young/old; healthy/ill) and lesion level (eg, a Bosniak 3 lesion but with clinical/imaging features of a benign abscess) factors will help inform the suggested management.

Size

Size is not considered a separate component of the Bosniak classification system, because small cystic renal masses can be malignant and large cystic masses can be benign. Small size, however, should arguably be considered an important consideration in the management of cystic renal lesions, because small renal lesions are more indolent than large renal lesions.[7,11,56–61] Small renal lesions (smaller than 1.5 cm) are overwhelmingly likely to be benign (excluding patients with a demographic/genetic predisposition to cancer).[62] Incidental detection of a benign-appearing very small renal cystic mass in a patient with no risk factors for malignancy can be presumed benign and does not warrant further characterization.[4]

Biopsy

Some studies have suggested that biopsy of cystic renal masses is helpful in distinguishing benign from malignant etiologies[48]; however, in general it is not a high-yield technique. This is secondary to the paucity of cells within cystic renal masses that limits a definitive sample and, therefore, limits the likelihood of a definitive diagnosis from pathology. Biopsy and/or drainage is useful for cystic renal masses that are suspected to be renal abscesses. Additionally, biopsy may be useful in patients who are poor surgical candidates, with the caveat that unless at an institution with experienced cytopathologists and interventional proceduralists, frequently the sample may be insufficient to give a definitive diagnosis.[63]

BENIGN/BENIGN-BEHAVING BOSNIAK 2F, 3, AND 4 LESIONS

Benign/benign-behaving lesions may have the imaging appearance of a Bosniak 2F, 3, or 4 category cyst but have imaging features that may allow for the accurate suggestion of benignity. The benign lesions that can be diagnosed as benign based on distinct imaging features include localized cystic disease of the kidney, pyelocalyceal diverticula, milk of calcium cysts, and vascular partially thrombosed pseudoaneurysms (which can occasionally mimic a cystic mass). Also included in this category are benign lesions where imaging may heavily suggest a benign diagnosis; however, tissue is ultimately needed to confirm the diagnosis. These lesions include the renal abscess, CN, and mixed epithelial stromal tumor (MEST).

Localized cystic disease is a benign process that is always unilateral. This disease is characterized by a cluster of multiple cysts of various sizes separated by normal or atrophic renal tissue, which presents as a conglomerate mass.[64] This can be suggestive of a cystic neoplasm. The key to confidently diagnosing this entity as benign is the ability to find, within the conglomerate mass, a slightly separate renal cyst, which is surrounded by normal renal parenchyma (**Fig. 2**).

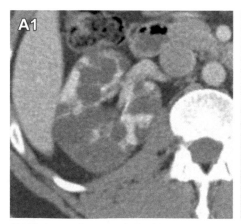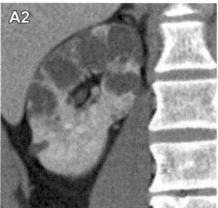

Fig. 2. Localized cystic disease. A 54-year-old man with contrast-enhanced CT images demonstrating multiple cysts, with a posterior cystic lesion in the right midpole (*A1, A2*). A single cyst can be separated from the conglomeration of cysts, which enables the diagnosis of localized cystic disease. This was followed for many years and was stable on follow-up.

Pyelocalyceal diverticula are outpouchings of the intrarenal collecting system that project into the renal cortex. These diverticula may contain stones and typically communicate with the collecting system (best depicted on the excretory phase) (**Fig. 3**).

Milk of calcium cysts are thought to arise from pyelocalyceal diverticula, which have internal precipitations of calcium salts; these cysts have lost communication with the adjacent collecting system. On imaging, the internal precipitation layer and often have a horizontal sharp upper border. No enhancement in these cysts is seen postcontrast (**Fig. 4**).

Although not a cystic renal mass, vascular causes (arteriovenous malformations and pseudoaneurysms) should be considered in the diagnosis of a cystic renal masses. When a patient has had a prior intervention (biopsy or surgery) and a new or growing cystic lesion is seen, either Doppler ultrasound imaging or arterial-phase CT or MR imaging should be performed to demonstrate internal signal/attenuation that follows the aortic signal/attenuation (**Fig. 5**).

Renal abscesses have a thickened homogeneous peripheral rim with perilesional edema. There is frequently mild stranding in the perirenal fat adjacent to the renal abscess (**Fig. 6**). In the setting of a lesion with this appearance, correlation with a patient's clinical symptoms (flank pain, urine analysis, and urine cultures) and imaging follow-up and/or tissue aspiration should be considered.

BENIGN/BENIGN-BEHAVING RENAL NEOPLASMS THAT CANNOT BE CONFIDENTLY DIAGNOSED ON PREOPERATIVE IMAGING STUDIES AND, THEREFORE, MAY REQUIRE SURGICAL EXCISION

CN, previously termed the multilocular CN, is a rare, nonfamilial tumor, which has a bimodal age and gender distribution. In the pediatric population, it has a male predilection; however, it affects middle-aged women in the adult population. CN herniates into the sinus and occasionally protrudes into the collecting system (**Fig. 7**).

MEST is currently thought, by pathologists, to be a lesion on the same spectrum as the CN, with the vast majority of these lesions in middle-aged women, also occasionally demonstrating herniation into the collecting system.[65,66] On pathology, CNs have more fluid and cysts within them, whereas MESTs have a greater solid ovarian stromal component (**Fig. 8**).[67] Some pathologists have recommended use of the term, *renal epithelial and stromal tumor*, to refer to both CN and MEST.[68]

The multilocular cystic RCC (MLCRCC) is a low-grade neoplasm of excellent prognosis.

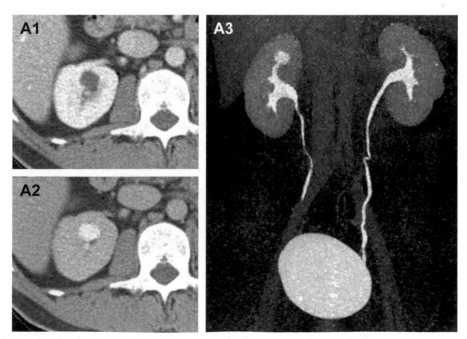

Fig. 3. Calyceal diverticulum. A 49-year-old women with a low attenuation cyst in the upper pole (*A1*), which fills uniformly with contrast on delayed excretory imaging (*A2*). Volume-rendered imaging through both kidneys demonstrates the communication of the calyceal diverticulum with the right upper pole collecting system (*A3*).

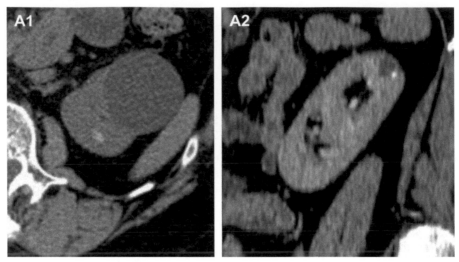

Fig. 4. Milk of calcium cysts. A 59-year-old man with layering calcium seen in a small posterior left upper pole cyst (*A1*) on noncontrast CT. In a different patient, a 52-year-old woman, there is an upper pole cyst with layering calcium (*A2*) consistent with a milk of calcium cyst.

This lesion has a male predominance, with a male-to-female ratio of 3:1.[69] Some pathologists suspect it is essentially benign because there are no cases of progression or metastases in reported series.[8] This lesion can range in appearance from a Bosniak 2F to a Bosniak 4 lesion, and it resembles a CN on gross pathology. It lacks solid nodules of carcinoma histologically.[8]

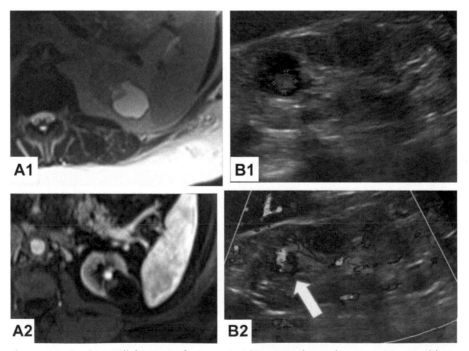

Fig. 5. Renal aneurysm in the medial aspect of a cyst mimicking a cystic renal mass. A 60-year-old woman with a cystic lesion that developed after a renal biopsy. Axial T2-weighted single-shot fast spin-echo images (*A1*) demonstrate a thick-walled cyst, which demonstrates a focus of central enhancement on arterial T1 gradient-recalled echo images (*A2*), which is as bright as the aorta, consistent with a small aneurysm. Corresponding ultrasound shows a cystic lesion with a focus of internal soft tissue (*B1*) with a yin-yang turbulent signal on color Doppler images (*B2*), consistent with an aneurysm.

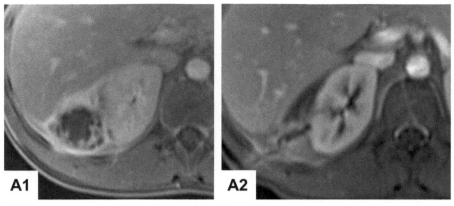

Fig. 6. Renal abscess. An 11-year-old boy with right costovertebral tenderness and fever after an appendectomy. In the right posterior upper pole, contrast-enhanced MR imaging T1 gradient-recalled echo images demonstrate a thick-walled renal cystic mass with shaggy internal peripheral enhancement and hyperemia in the perinephric fat (*A1*). This was drained percutaneously and subsequently (*A2*) resolved.

It is important to emphasize that there is no imaging feature that can suggest the diagnosis of this benign-behaving neoplasm prior to surgical excision, and other malignant lesions (such as the cystic clear cell RCC) can have an identical appearance; therefore, it is considered a surgical lesion (**Fig. 9**).

Malignant Bosniak 2F, 3, and 4 Lesions

Malignant cystic RCCs are all rare relative to the incidence of solid RCCs. These malignant cystic lesions include the cystic clear cell carcinoma, the clear cell tubulopapillary RCC, tubulocystic carcinomas, and the benign-behaving MLCRCC.

Cystic clear cell carcinoma is a cystic lesion with an irregularly thickened wall with large areas of solid nodularity within the wall. This lesion demonstrates a male predominance (male-to-female ratio of 2:1), mostly occurring in the sixth to seventh decades.[70] These cancers show extensive cystic change, not resulting from necrosis and are usually multiloculated. When there is no necrosis (based on histopathology), these neoplasms are typically cured with resection (**Fig. 10**).[71]

The clear cell tubulopapillary RCC is a neoplasm that is composed of clear cells of low nuclear grade, with variable papillary tubular/acinar and cystic architecture. This tumor has no gender predilection, occurs at a mean age of 61 years, and

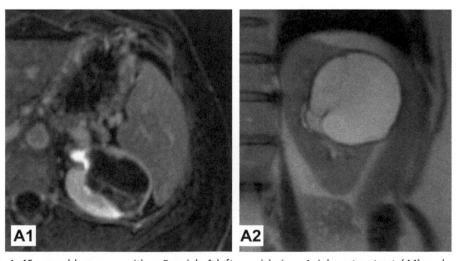

Fig. 7. CN. A 46-year-old woman with a Bosniak 4 left renal lesion. Axial postcontrast (*A1*) and coronal T2-weighted images (*A2*) through the left kidney demonstrate a complex cystic lesion with thickened internal septations and soft tissue nodularity. There is herniation into the collecting system, a feature that can be seen in CN or MESTs. Even herniation into the collecting system, however, can be seen in malignant lesions; therefore, this lesion was surgically resected and was a cystic nephroma on surgical pathology.

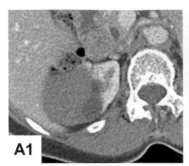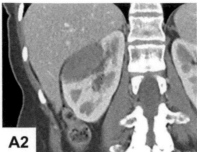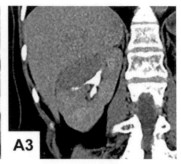

Fig. 8. MEST. A 47-year-old woman with a solid-appearing mass in the right upper pole seen on axial (*A1*) and coronal (*A2*) contrast-enhanced CT images with delayed urographic-phase images (*A3*), showing herniation into the collecting system. This lesion was resected and was a MEST on surgical pathology.

presents at a low stage with indolent behavior and no metastases reported.[72,73]

Tubulocystic carcinoma is a neoplasm, which histologically contains a mixture of tubules with microcysts and macrocysts with low-grade nuclear features lined by a single layer of cuboidal or columnar cells with distinct nuclei that have a hobnail appearance. This lesion is also termed *low-grade collecting duct carcinoma* and *Bellini duct carcinoma*; this occurs mostly in men (85% men and 15% women), with a mean age of 54 years. The prognosis is excellent, with rare metastases.[73,74]

Multilocular Cystic Renal Cell Carcinoma

MLCRCC is a benign-behaving neoplasm (also termed, *neoplasm of low malignant potential*), which is almost entirely fluid-filled, with the septa between the cystic components containing small clusters of clear cells without solid expansile nodules of clear cell carcinoma.[75] This lesion has a variable imaging appearance, ranging from a Bosniak 2F lesion to a Bosniak 4 lesion, with the higher

Bosniak categories corresponding to an increased degree of vascularized fibrosis within the lesion (see **Fig. 9**).[8]

Solid Renal Neoplasms Mimicking Cystic Renal Cell Carcinomas

Solid RCCs may mimic a cystic RCC on imaging. This is partly due to variance in the definition of a true cystic lesion on imaging. An accepted imaging definition for *cystic* is a lesion that, on imaging, has a mostly fluid-filled growth pattern with a solid portion occupying a maximum of one-fourth of the tumor volume[1–3] or a mass that is mostly composed of fluid-filled spaces.[4] Histologically, a solid renal mass may present erroneously as mostly fluid either secondary to nearly absent internal enhancement (which can occur in a hypovascular solid papillary RCC) or secondary to extensive necrosis in a solid RCC with a thickened rind of residual non-necrotic tumor.[76] Necrosis in a solid lesion can be, and has been, mistaken for an intrinsically cystic lesion (**Fig. 11**); however, attention to detailed imaging features should prevent

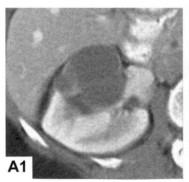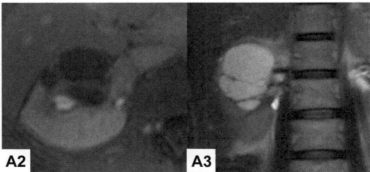

Fig. 9. MLCRCC. A 56-year-old woman with a Bosniak 4 lesion in the right upper pole. Contrast-enhanced axial CT (*A1*) and corresponding contrast-enhanced T1 gradient-recalled echo (*A2*) and coronal T2 single shot fast spin echo (SSFSE) images (*A3*) demonstrate a cystic mass with thickened enhancing internal septations. This was resected and was an MLCRCC on surgical pathology.

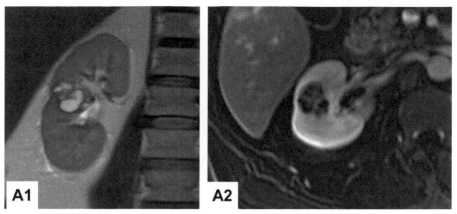

Fig. 10. Cystic clear cell RCC. A 52-year-old man with a Bosniak 4 lesion in the right kidney. Coronal T2 SSFSE (*A1*) and axial postcontrast T1 gradient-recalled echo (*A2*) images show a cystic renal mass with multiple thickened internal septations (*A1*) with associated irregular enhancement postcontrast (*A2*) consistent with a Bosniak 4 lesion. This was a cystic clear cell RCC on final surgical pathology.

this mistake. In the Smith and colleagues[50] article evaluating the outcomes of cystic renal masses, 1 of the lesions prospectively read as a Bosniak 3 lesion (of 113 total Bosniak 3 lesions) was a sarcomatoid RCC (presumably extensively necrotic), and, although the patient had a history of a surgically resected solid papillary tumor, presumably the subsequent rapid tumor progression of the category 3 lesion and associated pulmonary metastases were secondary to this sarcomatoid tumor. Similarly, a lesion prospectively classified as a Bosniak 4 lesion, in the same article, was a necrotic solid papillary RCC on histopathology, and the patient eventually died of metastases from this lesion. The problem is, therefore, that solid necrotic tumors can be mistaken for cystic

benign-behaving renal neoplasms on imaging. A solid, hypovascular papillary RCC without any internal necrosis has also been mistaken for a cystic lesion on imaging. This is because, histopathologically, papillary carcinomas may have a partially cystic arrangement with papillae that variably fill a cystic space. For solid papillary renal lesions with low density of papillae within the lesion, it appears more cystic on pathology. Additionally, the solid variant of papillary RCC, composed of cells in tightly packed tubules, can also mimic a cystic lesion on imaging, depending on the density of internal tissue.[8,77,78] Finally, papillary RCCs are commonly hypovascular on imaging. This means that they may not demonstrate internal contrast uptake to reach the threshold needed to suggest

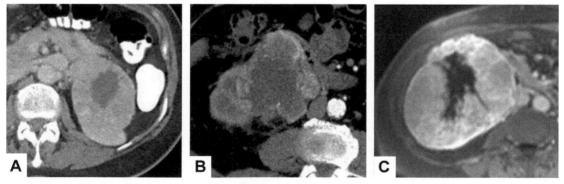

Fig. 11. Necrotic solid RCCs should not be confused with Bosniak 4 lesions. Three separate patients with solid RCCs. (*A*) Axial CT images demonstrate a solid clear cell RCC with central necrosis; this should not be confused with a cystic renal mass, because the lesion is predominantly solid. (*B*) Contrast-enhanced CT images demonstrate a thickened peripheral solid rind of tissue (measuring up to 15 mm in thickness) with central nonenhancement; this is an aggressive solid necrotic clear cell RCC and should not be classified as a Bosniak 4 lesion; this should be read as a necrotic solid mass. Contrast-enhanced T1 gradient-recalled echo (*C*) similarly shows a large solid mass with central nonenhancement, which was a scar in a pathology-proved chromophobe RCC; this is not a cystic renal mass.

true enhancement within a lesion. (Typically, on CT, true enhancement is considered an increase by 20 HU between precontrast and postcontrast CT. On MR imaging, internal enhancement is suggested by internal signal in a lesion on subtraction MR images.) Therefore, these lesions may mimic a nonenhancing renal lesion on imaging and be falsely categorized as a cystic lesion.[79,80] It is, therefore, known that an overlap exists in the imaging appearance between truly cystic lesions on histopathology (eg, cystic clear cell RCC, MLCRCC, complicated hemorrhagic cysts, infected cysts, and posttraumatic cysts) and solid papillary hypovascular tumors. A study by Huber and colleagues[2] suggested that, regardless of the final histopathology, a cystic appearance on imaging is associated with a lower malignant potential in these lesions. This article by Huber and colleagues assumes that a necrotic solid aggressive tumor is not placed into the imaging category of cystic renal mass. Several articles offer guides to accurately diagnosing necrosis in a solid tumor and in better predicting true cystic benign-behaving pathology accurately based on imaging appearance.[2,81] For example, necrosis is typically centrally located in larger renal mass lesions. If a lesion with a thickened solid peripheral rind is seen, with nonenhancement centrally (see **Fig. 11**), then necrosis in a solid tumor should be favored, and this lesion should not be categorized with the Bosniak classification as a Bosniak 4 lesion but instead described as a solid necrotic mass.

PEARLS, PITFALLS, AND VARIANTS

- Evaluation of cystic renal masses requires careful attention to technique.
- Renal pseudotumors (benign lesions that appear malignant) can be seen, when an unusual appearance of normal renal parenchyma protrudes adjacent to a simple cyst. Arterial-phase imaging in the corticomedullary phase shows corticomedullary differentiation in the nodule, which allows for it to be diagnosed as benign.
- True enhancement on CT imaging is considered an increase from precontrast to postcontrast imaging by 20 HU or more.
- Pseudoenhancement on CT imaging is a phenomenon when a benign renal cyst appears falsely to enhance on postcontrast images by 10 HU or more. This phenomenon is thought secondary to beam hardening artifact.
- Pseudoenhancement on CT imaging can be suspected in a benign renal cyst that is small

(<2 cm), completely intrarenal, and surrounded by very bright hyperattenuating renal parenchyma. If pseudoenhancement is suspected in a cyst that otherwise seems completely benign, contrast-enhanced MR imaging or ultrasound can be useful to confirm the diagnosis of a cyst.
- Pitfalls in MR imaging enhancement include subtraction misregistration, which is when there is poor alignment of the precontrast and postcontrast images, falsely suggesting enhancement in a nonenhancing renal lesion. This can be suspected by the presence of a thick rind of signal surrounding the organs on subtraction images. If this rind is seen, another method should be used to determine MR imaging enhancement.
- If the subtraction sequences are not reliable, the percentage enhancement can be determined with signal intensity units.[82]

DEMOGRAPHICS WITH INCREASED RISK

Several recent studies have described demographic features that are associated with an increased risk for malignancy in cystic renal lesions.[83] In an article by Smith and colleagues,[51] there was an increased risk of malignancy in Bosniak category 2F and 3 lesions in patients with a history of a primary renal malignancy, with a coexisting Bosniak category 4 cystic renal lesion or a solid renal mass, or with multiple Bosniak category 3 renal lesions. Similarly, in a study of Bosniak 2F cystic lesions, the author and colleagues reported a trend toward increased risk for malignancy in Bosniak category 2F cysts in men more than 50 years old with a prior solid RCC.[30] Therefore, on the basis of these studies, in men more than 50 years old with a history of a prior RCC (cystic or solid), the risk of malignancy in a cystic renal lesion seems increased relative to that of the general population. Larger studies of this subgroup of patients need to be performed to confirm this suspected association.

MANAGEMENT RECOMMENDATIONS

Several recent review articles have described reasonable approaches to the management of both solid and cystic renal masses.[4,59] For cystic renal lesions, the Bosniak categorization is followed, with surgery recommended for Bosniak 3 and 4 lesions and follow-up surveillance for Bosniak 2F lesions (Bosniak 1 and 2 cysts require no follow-up). Malignant cystic renal lesions are traditionally managed surgically (with partial nephrectomy as opposed to radical nephrectomy now considered the standard of care).[55] There is a growing interest in conservative management (eg, surveillance) for these cystic lesions in selected cases. Malignancy rates in Bosniak 2F, 3, and 4 lesions range from approximately 5% for Bosniak 2F lesions (lowest reported percentage in the literature) up to 100% for Bosniak 4 lesions. Some investigators are challenging whether, even in the case of true malignancy, cystic renal mass lesions are optimally treated by surgical removal, based on multiple studies showing that cystic RCCs have lower malignant potential than solid RCCs.[16,17,20,21] This surveillance approach, for a selected population, is safe as long as necrotic solid RCCs are not mistaken for cystic renal lesions.[22,50] The reports that show that cystic renal lesions are benign-behaving rely on the accurate diagnosis of these lesions as cystic on both imaging and on pathology (eg, Bosniak 3 and 4 lesions that on surgical resection prove to be MLCRCC, cystic clear cell RCC, or cystic papillary RCC).

Size is becoming a factor in management, with some recommendations more liberally allowing for the incidentally detected very small cystic renal lesion (less than 2 cm or 1.5 cm in size, depending on the article) that is benign appearing to be definitively called a simple cyst and ignored.[21,62] Surveillance imaging is cautiously used even for solid tumors (mean size 7.1 cm in the Mues and colleagues[21,84,85] series) in selected patient populations (elderly patients with comorbidities), with most patients not progressing to metastases even with these high-risk large tumors (in this article, progression to metastatic disease was seen in 2 of 36 patients (5.6%)). If extrapolated to cystic renal masses, which are more indolent than solid tumors, then selected patients with Bosniak 3 and 4 lesions are candidates for surveillance imaging. Almost all series to date report the absence of recurrent or metastatic disease after surgical resection of Bosniak 2F and 3 lesions, with favorable outcomes after surgical resection of Bosniak 4 lesions.[30,51,86–88] Further investigations are needed to evaluate the safety of surveillance in cystic renal masses.

The role of ablation in the treatment of cystic renal masses is an area of current investigation. Smith and colleagues[50] suggested that there are less complications and lower cost associated with cystic renal mass ablation, as opposed to surgery. Ablation is only selectively used for cystic renal masses, however, depending on the size and location of the cystic lesion,[89,90] with long-term data and analysis of complications still preliminary.

WHAT THE REFERRING PHYSICIAN NEEDS TO KNOW

- To characterize a cystic renal lesion on imaging, both precontrast and a postcontrast images are needed.
- Enhancement within a lesion cannot be assumed on a postcontrast image only; a noncontrast baseline is necessary to determine enhancement.
- Enhancement is a key component of cystic renal lesion characterization. Enhancement of a solid component (thickened wall, internal septation, nodule) allows for accurate imaging categorization of a cystic renal lesion as a malignant lesion (and, therefore, a surgical lesion) using the Bosniak classification system.
- There can be internal nonenhancing soft tissue within benign cystic renal lesions, such as clumped blood in a hemorrhagic cyst. This does not enhance and allows this lesion to be accurately characterized as benign. This prevents unnecessary upgrading of a lesion and prevents unnecessary surgery.
- True enhancement in a lesion is when a region of interest can be placed on a morphologically visible structure (thickened wall, septation, nodule) and an increase from precontrast to postcontrast images of 20 HU or more is noted.
- Contrast-enhanced CT and MR imaging are both acceptable modalities for Bosniak cystic lesion classification.
- Contrast-enhanced ultrasound shows promise in Bosniak cystic lesion classification, because it uses contrast bubbles to show enhancement in renal lesions, with preliminary studies demonstrating good accuracy.
- Gray-scale ultrasound without contrast has select applications for Bosniak cystic lesion characterization. It is good for characterizing a simple renal cyst and can characterize some hemorrhagic cysts as benign. It misses small renal lesions (less than 1 cm in size), however, and it erroneously upgrades many benign cystic lesions to malignant Bosniak 3 or 4 lesions, due to its reliance on morphology and its lack of sensitivity/specificity for internal blood flow within the lesion. Because of this, gray-scale ultrasound is not an accurate modality for characterizing Bosniak 2F, 3, or 4 cystic lesions. If a Bosniak 2F, 3, or 4 lesion is suspected on gray-scale ultrasound, a contrast-enhanced CT or MR image should be obtained

SUMMARY

In conclusion, cystic renal masses are common in daily practice. The Bosniak classification is an established method for the imaging classification and management of these lesions. Careful attention to excellent CT and MR imaging technique is important to accurately apply the Bosniak classification system and, therefore, to guide the appropriate management of these lesions. Knowledge of the pathognomonic features of certain benign Bosniak 2F/3 lesions is important to avoid surgery on these lesions (eg, localized cystic disease, calyceal diverticula, and renal abscesses).

REFERENCES

1. Corica FA, Iczkowski KA, Cheng L, et al. Cystic renal cell carcinoma is cured by resection: a study of 24 cases with long-term followup. J Urol 1999;161(2):408–11.
2. Huber J, Winkler A, Jakobi H, et al. Preoperative decision making for renal cell carcinoma: cystic morphology in cross-sectional imaging might predict lower malignant potential. Urol Oncol 2014;32(1):37.e1-6.
3. Park HS, Lee K, Moon KC. Determination of the cutoff value of the proportion of cystic change for prognostic stratification of clear cell renal cell carcinoma. J Urol 2011;186(2):423–9.
4. Silverman SG, Israel GM, Herts BR, et al. Management of the incidental renal mass. Radiology 2008;249(1):16–31.
5. Hartman DS, Davis CJ Jr, Johns T, et al. Cystic renal cell carcinoma. Urology 1986;28(2):145–53.
6. Moch H. Cystic renal tumors: new entities and novel concepts. Adv Anat Pathol 2010;17(3):209–14.
7. Han KR, Janzen NK, McWhorter VC, et al. Cystic renal cell carcinoma: biology and clinical behavior. Urol Oncol 2004;22(5):410–4.
8. Hindman NM, Bosniak MA, Rosenkrantz AB, et al. Multilocular cystic renal cell carcinoma: comparison of imaging and pathologic findings. AJR Am J Roentgenol 2012;198(1):W20–6.
9. Koga S, Nishikido M, Hayashi T, et al. Outcome of surgery in cystic renal cell carcinoma. Urology 2000;56(1):67–70.
10. Winters BR, Gore JL, Holt SK, et al. Cystic renal cell carcinoma carries an excellent prognosis regardless of tumor size. Urol Oncol 2015;33(12):505.e9-13.
11. Hollingsworth JM, Miller DC, Daignault S, et al. Rising incidence of small renal masses: a need to reassess treatment effect. J Natl Cancer Inst 2006;98(18):1331–4.
12. Carrim ZI, Murchison JT. The prevalence of simple renal and hepatic cysts detected by spiral computed tomography. Clin Radiol 2003;58(8):626–9.
13. O'Connor SD, Silverman SG, Ip IK, et al. Simple cyst-appearing renal masses at unenhanced CT: can they be presumed to be benign? Radiology 2013;269(3):793–800.
14. Bosniak MA. The current radiological approach to renal cysts. Radiology 1986;158(1):1–10.
15. Cloix P, Martin X, Pangaud C, et al. Surgical management of complex renal cysts: a series of 32 cases. J Urol 1996;156(1):28–30.
16. Curry NS, Cochran ST, Bissada NK. Cystic renal masses: accurate Bosniak classification requires adequate renal CT. AJR Am J Roentgenol 2000;175(2):339–42.
17. Levy P, Helenon O, Merran S, et al. Cystic tumors of the kidney in adults: radio-histopathologic correlations. J Radiol 1999;80(2):121–33 [in French].
18. Graumann O, Osther SS, Karstoft J, et al. Bosniak classification system: a prospective comparison of CT, contrast-enhanced US, and MR for categorizing complex renal cystic masses. Acta Radiol 2016;57(11):1409–17.
19. Warren KS, McFarlane J. The Bosniak classification of renal cystic masses. BJU Int 2005;95(7):939–42.
20. Koga S, Nishikido M, Inuzuka S, et al. An evaluation of Bosniak's radiological classification of cystic renal masses. BJU Int 2000;86(6):607–9.
21. Silverman SG, Israel GM, Trinh QD. Incompletely characterized incidental renal masses: emerging data support conservative management. Radiology 2015;275(1):28–42.
22. Israel GM, Bosniak MA. How I do it: evaluating renal masses. Radiology 2005;236(2):441–50.
23. Israel GM, Bosniak MA. MR imaging of cystic renal masses. Magn Reson Imaging Clin N Am 2004;12(3):403–12, v.
24. Bosniak MA. The Bosniak renal cyst classification: 25 years later. Radiology 2012;262(3):781–5.
25. Israel GM, Bosniak MA. An update of the Bosniak renal cyst classification system. Urology 2005;66(3):484–8.
26. Birnbaum BA, Hindman N, Lee J, et al. Renal cyst pseudoenhancement: influence of multidetector CT reconstruction algorithm and scanner type in phantom model. Radiology 2007;244(3):767–75.
27. Mileto A, Nelson RC, Marin D, et al. Dual-energy multidetector CT for the characterization of incidental adrenal nodules: diagnostic performance of contrast-enhanced material density analysis. Radiology 2015;274(2):445–54.
28. Holland AE, Goldfarb JW, Edelman RR. Diaphragmatic and cardiac motion during suspended breathing: preliminary experience and implications for breath-hold MR imaging. Radiology 1998;209(2):483–9.

29. Earls JP, Rofsky NM, DeCorato DR, et al. Hepatic arterial-phase dynamic gadolinium-enhanced MR imaging: optimization with a test examination and a power injector. Radiology 1997;202(1):268–73.

30. Hindman NM, Hecht EM, Bosniak MA. Follow-up for Bosniak category 2F cystic renal lesions. Radiology 2014;272(3):757–66.

31. Israel GM, Hindman N, Bosniak MA. Evaluation of cystic renal masses: comparison of CT and MR imaging by using the Bosniak classification system. Radiology 2004;231(2):365–71.

32. Balci NC, Semelka RC, Patt RH, et al. Complex renal cysts: findings on MR imaging. AJR Am J Roentgenol 1999;172(6):1495–500.

33. Hecht EM, Israel GM, Krinsky GA, et al. Renal masses: quantitative analysis of enhancement with signal intensity measurements versus qualitative analysis of enhancement with image subtraction for diagnosing malignancy at MR imaging. Radiology 2004;232(2):373–8.

34. Kim S, Jain M, Harris AB, et al. T1 hyperintense renal lesions: characterization with diffusion-weighted MR imaging versus contrast-enhanced MR imaging. Radiology 2009;251(3):796–807.

35. Heverhagen JT. Noise measurement and estimation in MR imaging experiments. Radiology 2007;245(3): 638–9.

36. Rosenkrantz AB, Wehrli NE, Mussi TC, et al. Complex cystic renal masses: comparison of cyst complexity and Bosniak classification between 1.5 T and 3 T MRI. Eur J Radiol 2014;83(3):503–8.

37. Chandarana H, Block TK, Rosenkrantz AB, et al. Free-breathing radial 3D fat-suppressed T1-weighted gradient echo sequence: a viable alternative for contrast-enhanced liver imaging in patients unable to suspend respiration. Invest Radiol 2011; 46(10):648–53.

38. Chandarana H, Kang SK, Wong S, et al. Diffusion-weighted intravoxel incoherent motion imaging of renal tumors with histopathologic correlation. Invest Radiol 2012;47(12):688–96.

39. Squillaci E, Manenti G, Di Stefano F, et al. Diffusion-weighted MR imaging in the evaluation of renal tumours. J Exp Clin Cancer Res 2004;23(1):39–45.

40. Zhang J, Tehrani YM, Wang L, et al. Renal masses: characterization with diffusion-weighted MR imaging–a preliminary experience. Radiology 2008; 247(2):458–64.

41. Jamis-Dow CA, Choyke PL, Jennings SB, et al. Small (< or = 3-cm) renal masses: detection with CT versus US and pathologic correlation. Radiology 1996;198(3):785–8.

42. Bosniak MA. Difficulties in classifying cystic lesions of the kidney. Urol Radiol 1991;13(2):91–3.

43. Chang YW, Kwon KH, Goo DE, et al. Sonographic differentiation of benign and malignant cystic lesions of the breast. J Ultrasound Med 2007;26(1):47–53.

44. Ascenti G, Mazziotti S, Zimbaro G, et al. Complex cystic renal masses: characterization with contrast-enhanced US. Radiology 2007;243(1):158–65.

45. Clevert DA, Minaifar N, Weckbach S, et al. Multi-slice computed tomography versus contrast-enhanced ultrasound in evaluation of complex cystic renal masses using the Bosniak classification system. Clin Hemorheol Microcirc 2008;39(1–4):171–8.

46. Ignee A, Straub B, Brix D, et al. The value of contrast enhanced ultrasound (CEUS) in the characterisation of patients with renal masses. Clin Hemorheol Microcirc 2010;46(4):275–90.

47. Park BK, Kim B, Kim SH, et al. Assessment of cystic renal masses based on Bosniak classification: comparison of CT and contrast-enhanced US. Eur J Radiol 2007;61(2):310–4.

48. Harisinghani MG, Maher MM, Gervais DA, et al. Incidence of malignancy in complex cystic renal masses (Bosniak category III): should imaging-guided biopsy precede surgery? AJR Am J Roentgenol 2003;180(3):755–8.

49. O'Malley RL, Godoy G, Hecht EM, et al. Bosniak category IIF designation and surgery for complex renal cysts. J Urol 2009;182(3):1091–5.

50. Smith AD, Allen BC, Sanyal R, et al. Outcomes and complications related to the management of Bosniak cystic renal lesions. AJR Am J Roentgenol 2015; 204(5):W550–6.

51. Smith AD, Remer EM, Cox KL, et al. Bosniak category IIF and III cystic renal lesions: outcomes and associations. Radiology 2012;262(1):152–60.

52. Kouba E, Smith A, McRackan D, et al. Watchful waiting for solid renal masses: insight into the natural history and results of delayed intervention. J Urol 2007;177(2):466–70 [discussion: 470].

53. Rendon RA, Stanietzky N, Panzarella T, et al. The natural history of small renal masses. J Urol 2000; 164(4):1143–7.

54. Shuch B, Hanley JM, Lai JC, et al. Adverse health outcomes associated with surgical management of the small renal mass. J Urol 2014;191(2):301–8.

55. Huang WC, Elkin EB, Levey AS, et al. Partial nephrectomy versus radical nephrectomy in patients with small renal tumors–is there a difference in mortality and cardiovascular outcomes? J Urol 2009; 181(1):55–61 [discussion: 61–2].

56. Chawla SN, Crispen PL, Hanlon AL, et al. The natural history of observed enhancing renal masses: meta-analysis and review of the world literature. J Urol 2006;175(2):425–31.

57. Hollenbeck BK, Taub DA, Miller DC, et al. National utilization trends of partial nephrectomy for renal cell carcinoma: a case of underutilization? Urology 2006;67(2):254–9.

58. Webster WS, Thompson RH, Cheville JC, et al. Surgical resection provides excellent outcomes for

patients with cystic clear cell renal cell carcinoma. Urology 2007;70(5):900–4 [discussion: 904].

59. Berland LL, Silverman SG, Gore RM, et al. Managing incidental findings on abdominal CT: white paper of the ACR incidental findings committee. J Am Coll Radiol 2010;7(10):754–73.

60. Thompson RH, Hill JR, Babayev Y, et al. Metastatic renal cell carcinoma risk according to tumor size. J Urol 2009;182(1):41–5.

61. Volpe A, Panzarella T, Rendon RA, et al. The natural history of incidentally detected small renal masses. Cancer 2004;100(4):738–45.

62. Hindman NM. Approach to very small (< 1.5 cm) cystic renal lesions: ignore, observe, or treat? AJR Am J Roentgenol 2015;204(6):1182–9.

63. Silverman SG, Gan YU, Mortele KJ, et al. Renal masses in the adult patient: the role of percutaneous biopsy. Radiology 2006;240(1):6–22.

64. Slywotzky CM, Bosniak MA. Localized cystic disease of the kidney. AJR Am J Roentgenol 2001; 176(4):843–9.

65. Horikawa M, Shinmoto H, Kuroda K, et al. Mixed epithelial and stromal tumor of the kidney with polypoid component extending into renal pelvis and ureter. Acta Radiol Short Rep 2012;1(1):1–5.

66. Wood CG 3rd, Stromberg LJ 3rd, Harmath CB, et al. CT and MR imaging for evaluation of cystic renal lesions and diseases. Radiographics 2015;35(1):125–41.

67. Jevremovic D, Lager DJ, Lewin M. Cystic nephroma (multilocular cyst) and mixed epithelial and stromal tumor of the kidney: a spectrum of the same entity? Ann Diagn Pathol 2006;10(2):77–82.

68. Turbiner J, Amin MB, Humphrey PA, et al. Cystic nephroma and mixed epithelial and stromal tumor of kidney: a detailed clinicopathologic analysis of 34 cases and proposal for renal epithelial and stromal tumor (REST) as a unifying term. Am J Surg Pathol 2007;31(4):489–500.

69. Chowdhury AR, Chakraborty D, Bhattacharya P, et al. Multilocular cystic renal cell carcinoma a diagnostic dilemma: a case report in a 30-year-old woman. Urol Ann 2013;5(2):119–21.

70. Imura J, Ichikawa K, Takeda J, et al. Multilocular cystic renal cell carcinoma: a clinicopathological, immuno- and lectin histochemical study of nine cases. APMIS 2004;112(3):183–91.

71. Brinker DA, Amin MB, de Peralta-Venturina M, et al. Extensively necrotic cystic renal cell carcinoma: a clinicopathologic study with comparison to other cystic and necrotic renal cancers. Am J Surg Pathol 2000;24(7):988–95.

72. Williamson SR, Eble JN, Cheng L, et al. Clear cell papillary renal cell carcinoma: differential diagnosis and extended immunohistochemical profile. Mod Pathol 2013;26(5):697–708.

73. Srigley JR, Delahunt B, Eble JN, et al. The International Society of Urological Pathology (ISUP)

vancouver classification of renal neoplasia. Am J Surg Pathol 2013;37(10):1469–89.

74. MacLennan GT, Farrow GM, Bostwick DG. Low-grade collecting duct carcinoma of the kidney: report of 13 cases of low-grade mucinous tubulocystic renal carcinoma of possible collecting duct origin. Urology 1997;50(5):679–84.

75. Halat S, Eble JN, Grignon DJ, et al. Multilocular cystic renal cell carcinoma is a subtype of clear cell renal cell carcinoma. Mod Pathol 2010;23(7):931–6.

76. Howlader N, Noone AM, Krapcho M, et al, editors. SEER Cancer Statistics Review, 1975-2013, Bethesda, MD, National Cancer Institute, http://seer.cancer.gov/csr/1975_2013/, based on November 2015 SEER data submission, posted to the SEER web site, April 2016.

77. Allory Y, Ouazana D, Boucher E, et al. Papillary renal cell carcinoma. Prognostic value of morphological subtypes in a clinicopathologic study of 43 cases. Virchows Arch 2003;442(4):336–42.

78. Bielsa O, Lloreta J, Gelabert-Mas A. Cystic renal cell carcinoma: pathological features, survival and implications for treatment. Br J Urol 1998;82(1):16–20.

79. Pierorazio PM, Hyams ES, Tsai S, et al. Multiphasic enhancement patterns of small renal masses (</=4 cm) on preoperative computed tomography: utility for distinguishing subtypes of renal cell carcinoma, angiomyolipoma, and oncocytoma. Urology 2013;81(6):1265–71.

80. Young JR, Margolis D, Sauk S, et al. Clear cell renal cell carcinoma: discrimination from other renal cell carcinoma subtypes and oncocytoma at multiphasic multidetector CT. Radiology 2013;267(2):444–53.

81. Pedrosa I, Chou MT, Ngo L, et al. MR classification of renal masses with pathologic correlation. Eur Radiol 2008;18(2):365–75.

82. Ho VB, Allen SF, Hood MN, et al. Renal masses: quantitative assessment of enhancement with dynamic MR imaging. Radiology 2002;224(3):695–700.

83. Goenka AH, Remer EM, Smith AD, et al. Development of a clinical prediction model for assessment of malignancy risk in Bosniak III renal lesions. Urology 2013;82(3):630–5.

84. Mues AC, Haramis G, Badani K, et al. Active surveillance for larger (cT1bN0M0 and cT2N0M0) renal cortical neoplasms. Urology 2010;76(3):620–3.

85. Haramis G, Mues AC, Rosales JC, et al. Natural history of renal cortical neoplasms during active surveillance with follow-up longer than 5 years. Urology 2011;77(4):787–91.

86. Hwang JH, Lee CK, Yu HS, et al. Clinical Outcomes of Bosniak Category IIF Complex Renal Cysts in Korean Patients. Korean J Urol 2012;53(6):386–90.

87. Israel GM, Bosniak MA. Follow-up CT of moderately complex cystic lesions of the kidney (Bosniak category IIF). AJR Am J Roentgenol 2003;181(3): 627–33.

88. Jhaveri K, Gupta P, Elmi A, et al. Cystic renal cell carcinomas: do they grow, metastasize, or recur? AJR Am J Roentgenol 2013;201(2): W292–6.

89. Carrafiello G, Dionigi G, Ierardi AM, et al. Efficacy, safety and effectiveness of image-guided percutaneous microwave ablation in cystic renal lesions Bosniak III or IV after 24 months follow up. Int J Surg 2013;11(Suppl 1):S30–5.

90. Felker ER, Lee-Felker SA, Alpern L, et al. Efficacy of imaging-guided percutaneous radiofrequency ablation for the treatment of biopsy-proven malignant cystic renal masses. AJR Am J Roentgenol 2013; 201(5):1029–35.

Image-Guided Renal Interventions

Sharath K. Bhagavatula, MD*, Paul B. Shyn, MD

KEYWORDS

- Renal mass biopsy • Renal parenchymal biopsy • Renal mass ablation

KEY POINTS

- Renal mass and parenchymal biopsies are safe (<5% minor complication rate and <0.5% major complication rate) with high diagnostic rates.
- Final biopsy pathology results must be compared with preprocedural imaging; rebiopsy or definitive treatment is recommended for discordant or nondiagnostic results.
- The safety and efficacy of renal parenchymal biopsies is optimized by meticulous needle placement confined to the peripheral renal cortex.
- Cryoablation, microwave ablation, and radiofrequency ablation are the most commonly used methods for renal malignancies, each with specific advantages and disadvantages.
- Renal mass ablations are indicated for stage T1a (<4 cm) renal masses in poor surgical candidates; other indications are emerging.

RENAL MASS AND PARENCHYMAL BIOPSIES

Renal mass biopsies (RMB) and renal parenchymal biopsies (RPB) play an increasing role in clinical management. This article discusses the indications, techniques, and clinical considerations for RMB and RPB.

Renal Mass Biopsy Indications

Established indications

Historically, most renal masses were presumed malignant and surgically resected. Accepted indications for RMB were limited to confirmation of metastatic renal disease in patients with known primary malignancies, differentiation of malignancy from infection, evaluation of multiple solid renal masses, and evaluation of unresectable renal masses for prognostication and medical management.[1–4] These indications remain important in current practice (**Table 1**).

Emerging indications

The number of small (<3 cm) incidentally discovered renal lesions has increased dramatically, with a recent study finding 25% of those less than 3 cm and 44% of those less than 1 cm to be benign.[5] Such data have led to a push for biopsies of small masses to decrease the number of unnecessary nephrectomies and preserve renal tissue, particularly when a metastatic, inflammatory, or infectious etiology is suspected.[6]

Reported malignancy rates in indeterminate cystic masses (Bosniak IIF and III) are widely variable, ranging from 31% to 100%.[1,7,8] Therefore, there has been an increasing role of biopsy to characterize these lesions before definitive management.[3,4]

Renal Parenchymal Biopsy Indications

RPB is used to establish a diagnosis for unexplained renal symptoms or to assess chronicity and reversibility of the disease process.

Portions of this article were previously published in March 2017 *Radiologic Clinics*, Volume 55, Issue 2.
Disclosure: The authors have nothing to disclose.
Department of Radiology, Harvard Medical School, Brigham and Women's Hospital, 75 Francis Street, Boston, MA 02115, USA
* Corresponding author.
E-mail address: sbhagavatula@partners.org

Table 1
Common renal mass biopsy indications

Established Indications	Recent and Emerging Indications
Determine metastatic vs primary renal malignancy	Presurgical diagnosis of renal masses (especially <3 cm)
Differentiate infection vs malignancy	Diagnose indeterminate cystic masses (Bosniak IIF and III)
Prognostication/ management in nonsurgical candidates	Confirm malignancy before renal mass ablation

From Bhagavatula SK, Shyn PB. Image-guided renal interventions. Radiol Clin North Am 2017;55(2):360; with permission.

Nephrotic syndrome

In patients with nephrotic syndrome, RPB is commonly performed to evaluate idiopathic and systemic lupus erythematosus-related proteinuria, but is less clinically useful in chronically acquired diabetic proteinuria, in children younger than 6 years of age (>90% have minimal change disease), or in malignancy-related proteinuria.[9,10]

Nephritic syndrome

RPB may be useful in the evaluation of acute nephritic syndrome to diagnose a systemic disease process (eg, microscopic polyangiitis, granulomatosis with polyangiitis, antiglomerular basement membrane antibody disease). RPB is less likely to impact clinical management in patients with post-streptococal glomerulonephritis or endocarditis-related nephritic syndrome.[9,11]

Other indications

RPB is also used to evaluate acute unexplained renal failure, moderate to severe nonnephrotic proteinuria, and suspected renal transplant rejection.[9,11] RPB is often not useful in patients with isolated microscopic hematuria in the absence of proteinuria or renal failure.[9,12]

Differential Diagnosis of Renal Masses

Benign

Commonly biopsied benign entities include oncocytoma (70%), minimal fat angiomyolipoma (18%), and papillary adenoma (4%).[2,5] Other less frequently encountered masses include metanephric adenoma, leiomyoma, and focal pyelonephritis. A mass referred for biopsy may occasionally have imaging characteristics that allow definitive diagnosis of a benign entity (eg, macroscopic fat in

angiomyolipoma) and recognition of such features can avoid unnecessary intervention.

Malignant

Renal cell carcinoma (RCC) can be further categorized by grade and subtype. The Fuhrman classification system offers prognostic and therapeutic implications.[13] Common subtypes include clear cell (80%–90%), papillary (10%–15%), and chromophobe (4%–5%).[14] Chromophobe subtypes share histologic features with oncocytoma with the potential for misdiagnosis.[5,15] Sarcomatoid differentiation may occur with any subtype and portends a worse prognosis.[16,17] Other common malignancies include transitional cell carcinoma and metastases (most commonly lymphoma, lung, and breast).[18]

Preprocedure Workup

Review history and imaging

Before biopsy, the patient's history, underlying disease, and indication for the procedure should be reviewed (**Box 1**). Relevant imaging should also be reviewed to confirm the appropriateness and feasibility of the biopsy.

Box 1
Renal intervention preprocedure checklist

- Confirm appropriate indication.
- Ensure no benign diagnostic features (eg, macroscopic fat in angiomyolipoma).
- Plan approach.
- Review history and physical; allergies.
- Assess pain control (eg, heavy opioid use, recent surgery).
- Assess ability to lie and breathe in desired position.
- Confirm NPO status.
- Anesthesiology consultation, if appropriate.
- Target blood pressure less than 140/90 mm Hg (optional).
- Manage anticoagulation: risk–benefit assessment.
- Review laboratory studies: prefer International Normalized Ratio of less than 1.5; platelets greater than 50,000.
- Check baseline hematocrit.

Abbreviation: NPO, nil per os.
From Bhagavatula SK, Shyn PB. Image-guided renal interventions. Radiol Clin North Am 2017;55(2):360; with permission.

Presedation evaluation

RMB is typically performed under moderate sedation. Patients who are elderly, taking high doses of opioid medications, or have significant cardiovascular, pulmonary, renal, hepatic, metabolic, and neurologic disorders are at increased risk for adverse events from sedation.[19,20]

Patients should be able to lie comfortably in the desired position. Poor pain control, altered mental status, and significant comorbidities (eg, congestive heart failure, chronic obstructive pulmonary disease) can preclude adequate positioning. Finally, the patient should stop eating at least 6 hours before the procedure and stop drinking at least 2 hours before to reduce the risk of aspiration.[21] If a patient is not an appropriate sedation candidate or has conditions precluding appropriate positioning, monitored anesthesia care or general anesthesia should be considered.

Assess coagulation status

The Society for Interventional Radiology guidelines places kidney biopsies in a high bleeding risk category[22]; therefore, a review of the patient's vital signs, medications, and laboratory values is routine. Severe hypertension may increase bleeding risk, but this increased risk is likely minimal.[23]

An International Normalized Ratio of less than 1.5 is generally preferred. Correcting an elevated International Normalized Ratio may require holding warfarin or bridging to heparin beginning at least 5 days before the procedure. Vitamin K or fresh frozen plasma may be considered to expedite the correction in urgent cases. Ideally, platelets should be greater than 50,000/μL, and a platelet transfusion can be considered if this criterion is not met. Withdrawal of therapeutic aspirin and low-molecular-weight heparin 5 days before the procedure and fractionated heparin 24 hours before is preferred.[22] Intravenous unfractionated heparin may be stopped 4 to 6 hours before the procedure.[24] The hematocrit should be assessed beforehand as a baseline in case the patient develops postprocedural bleeding. Withholding or bridging anticoagulant medications used for secondary prophylaxis requires a careful risk–benefit discussion with the physician responsible for managing the anticoagulation. Similarly, the use of blood products to correct laboratory values is a risk–benefit judgment.

Procedure Considerations

Image guidance modality

Ultrasound examination The advantages of ultrasound examination include real-time imaging, the ability to use variable planes and angles of approach, a lack of ionizing radiation, and the relatively low costs and times of the procedure. Disadvantages include a longer learning curve and limited ultrasound windows because of patient size and interposed bowel, lung, or ribs.

Computed tomography and computed tomography fluoroscopy The advantages of computed tomography (CT) with CT fluoroscopy include better spatial and contrast resolution and consistent visualization of the kidney and intervening anatomic structures (**Figs. 1** and **2**). Disadvantages include increased procedural cost, time, and radiation dose.

MRI MRI guidance is uncommon, but is occasionally useful for lesions not visible on other modalities or before MRI–guided renal ablations. The main advantage of MRI is superior soft tissue

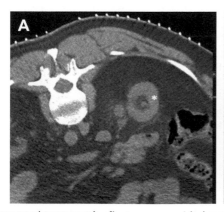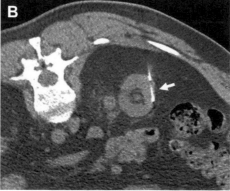

Fig. 1. Computed tomography fluoroscopy-guided renal parenchymal biopsy in a 49-year-old man with a history of multiple myeloma, presenting with worsening renal function, prone oblique position. (*A*) Right lower pole renal cortex (*asterisk*) is targeted. (*B*) Biopsy needle with stylet trough directed peripherally to target cortical glomeruli and avoid renal sinus structures. The stylet trough (*arrow*) should not include the renal capsule. (*From* Bhagavatula SK, Shyn PB. Image-guided renal interventions. Radiol Clin North Am 2017;55(2):361; with permission.)

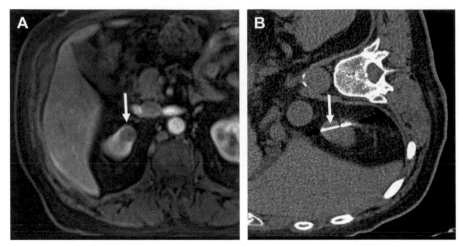

Fig. 2. Computed tomography fluoroscopy-guided biopsy in a 79-year-old man with incidentally discovered renal mass, right lateral decubitus position. (*A*) Contrast-enhanced MRI demonstrates an enhancing 2-cm right upper pole renal mass (*arrow*). (*B*) Biopsy needle tip with stylet extended and trough (*arrow*) centered in the mass before firing. The lateral decubitus position minimizes respiratory motion of the dependent kidney and keeps the dependent lung away from the needle path. (*From* Bhagavatula SK, Shyn PB. Image-guided renal interventions. Radiol Clin North Am 2017;55(2):362; with permission.)

contrast. Disadvantages include a complicated procedural environment, increased procedural cost and time, and a requirement for MRI-compatible devices and equipment.

Patient positioning

Most renal biopsies are performed with the patient in a prone, prone oblique, or lateral decubitus position. This positioning generally allows direct access to the kidneys, although initial imaging should confirm that no intervening structures (eg, bowel, vessels) are in the needle path.

Masses located superiorly in the kidney may be difficult to access without traversing the lung. Ipsilateral side down positioning may decrease ipsilateral lung volume and respiratory diaphragmatic/renal motion that facilitates safe, unimpeded access.[3]

Supine positioning is commonly used for accessing pelvic transplant kidneys. A supine transhepatic approach may occasionally be helpful for right anterior or upper pole renal masses.

Biopsy targeting

In general, the renal hilum should be avoided to prevent inadvertent damage to large vascular structures and the central collecting system. Otherwise, specific targeting strategies differ slightly for solid RMB, cystic RMB, and RPB.

Solid renal mass biopsy In large solid renal masses, it is often preferable to target the peripheral enhancing components, which are less likely to contain necrotic tissue or fluid.[25] In small renal masses, targeting the periphery may not be feasible and could result in the nondiagnostic sampling of adjacent normal parenchyma. Therefore, consensus guidelines for small renal masses prioritize obtaining high-quality samples rather than conforming to a specific targeting pattern (see **Fig. 2**; **Fig. 3**).[4]

Cystic renal mass biopsy Cystic RMB is technically challenging and often yields lower diagnostic rates relative to solid RMB.[18] If a nodular, enhancing component is clearly visualized, this tissue should be targeted. Otherwise, fluid should be aspirated from the cyst and the remaining solid tissue should be sampled. Alternatively, air or contrast may be injected after aspiration to help identify a nodular component for targeting.

Renal parenchymal biopsy The goal of RPB is almost always limited to sampling glomeruli located in the renal cortex. The lower pole cortex is usually targeted, although other regions of the kidney are targeted if the cortex is thicker. The needle should enter the kidney eccentrically such that the deployed stylet remains entirely within the subcapsular cortex and away from the renal medulla, sinuses, and hilum (see **Fig. 1**). Positioning the core biopsy trough in this manner is the key to obtaining diagnostic samples while avoiding bleeding complications.

Needle biopsy techniques

The decision to use a coaxial, tandem, or single needle insertion technique depends on various

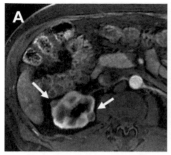 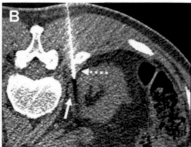 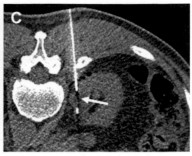

Fig. 3. Computed tomography fluoroscopy-guided renal mass biopsy in a 57-year-old man with multiple incidentally discovered renal masses, prone position. (*A*) Two 1-cm upper pole enhancing masses seen in the medial and lateral right kidney (*arrows*). (*B*) Introducer needle (*dashed arrow*) is advanced to the periphery of the medial mass (*solid arrow*). (*C*) The stylet of the biopsy needle is advanced with the trough (*arrow*) positioned to sample the entire cross-section of the mass. Renal cell carcinoma was confirmed by pathology. (*From* Bhagavatula SK, Shyn PB. Image-guided renal interventions. Radiol Clin North Am 2017;55(2):362; with permission.)

factors, including operator preference, bleeding risk, and lesion size and location. **Table 2** summarizes techniques and advantages of each method.

The decision to use fine needle aspiration, core needle biopsy, or both also depends on multiple factors, and it is important to understand the proper techniques, advantages, and disadvantages of each method (**Table 3**).

Fine needle aspiration Fine needle aspiration samples are obtained using small needles (≤20-G). Once needle position within a lesion is confirmed, negative pressure is applied manually with a syringe. Minimal suction (eg, syringe plunger pulled back approximately 1–2 mL) is sufficient; excessive suction should be avoided because this may lead to bloody, nondiagnostic aspirates. With continuous negative pressure, the needle is advanced and retracted repeatedly with controlled rapid movements, until 1 or 2 drops of blood are visible in the syringe. Sampling may also be performed without suction and with the needle hub open to air ("capillary technique") to minimize aspiration of blood.[11] After biopsy, these samples are placed on slides or in fixative solution for cytologic analysis.

Automated core needle biopsy Automated core needle biopsy samples are obtained using larger needles (≥20-G) with a spring-loaded cutting mechanism. Obtaining a single 18-G core biopsy for small RMB is an attractive strategy that typically samples an entire cross-section of the mass.[4] The core needle biopsy needle is inserted to the proximal edge of the lesion under image guidance with the inner stylet retracted (see

Table 2
Coaxial, tandem, and single needle techniques

	Coaxial Technique	Tandem Needle	Single Needle
Technique	Biopsy needle is passed through a larger introducer needle	Small needle (eg, 22-G) serves as a reference for subsequent biopsy needle passes	Biopsy needle placed directly into the target under image guidance
Advantages	• Multiple biopsies obtained through single introducer needle • May minimize risk of tumor seeding • May reduce risk of bleeding: fewer punctures and introducer needle can tamponade the tract • Potentially shorter procedure time	• Small needle used for initial access • Speeds targeting with subsequent needles • May facilitate sampling multiple regions of mass	• Decreased number of steps • Usually reserved for automated core biopsy of <2 cm mass

From Bhagavatula SK, Shyn PB. Image-guided renal interventions. Radiol Clin North Am 2017;55(2):363; with permission.

Table 3
Fine-needle aspiration versus automated core biopsy

	Fine-Needle Aspiration	Automated Core Biopsy
Needle size	≤20-G	≥20-G
Mechanism	Negative pressure or capillary action collects cellular material during rapid back and forth needle excursion	Spring-loaded outer cutting needle traps tissue in trough of initially deployed inner stylet
Analysis	Cytologic	Histologic
Advantages	• Slightly lower bleeding risk • May allow sampling multiple regions of mass • Potential confirmation of adequacy by on-site cytopathologist	• Higher diagnostic rate and accuracy • Hemodilution of sample is less of a problem • Potentially shorter procedure time

From Bhagavatula SK, Shyn PB. Image-guided renal interventions. Radiol Clin North Am 2017;55(2):364; with permission.

Fig. 3B). The stylet is then advanced further into the lesion. After confirming that the stylet trough is within the mass (see **Fig. 3**C), the biopsy device is fired and a core sample is obtained. If multiple core samples are desired, it may be helpful to slide the introducer needle into the mass over the biopsy needle (before removal) to maintain purchase in the mass. RMB samples are placed in formalin for histologic analysis and RPB samples are typically submitted fresh for light, immunofluorescence, and electron microscopy evaluation.[9,11] On-site pathology assessment of RPB specimens is ideal to confirm adequate numbers of glomeruli for diagnosis.

Efficacy

Renal mass biopsy

RMB effectively differentiates malignant from benign masses with approximately 86% to 100% accuracy.[16,26] Higher diagnostic rates have been associated with larger lesions (>4 cm),[3,27] solid masses,[18] and lesions sampled using core needle biopsy.[28] Core needle biopsy samples obtained with 14-G to 18-G needles have demonstrated higher diagnostic yield relative to 20-G needles.[18,29]

RCC subtyping accuracy ranges from 74% to 98%[2,26,30,31] and Fuhrman grading accuracy ranges from 70% to 83%.[25,31] The cause of the low grading accuracy is likely intratumoral heterogeneity, because up to 82% of tumors contain multiple grades.[15,32,33] Further improvements in RMB will likely be necessary for more accurate grading.[13]

Renal parenchymal biopsy

RPB of native and transplant kidneys has high success rates (>97%)[9,11,34] and affects clinical management in 40% to 60% of cases.[10,31] Needles of 14-G and 16-G are recommended by some

authors[9,35]; however, 18-G needles are also used routinely in our practice and have been shown to have similar efficacy and adequacy.[36]

Complications

Renal biopsies are generally safe, with a less than 5% minor complication rate and less than 0.5% major complication rate.[16]

Bleeding

Postprocedural bleeding is seen in 44% to 91% of RMB[16,37,38] and up to 65% of patients in RPB.[39] Bleeding is typically self-limited, and progression to severe hemorrhage requiring transfusion occurs in fewer than 1% of cases.[16,40] Large needle size (14-G), elevated baseline creatinine (>2.0 mg/dL), patient age (>40 years), and elevated blood pressure (systolic blood pressure of >130 mm Hg) are associated with higher bleeding risk.[40]

Pneumothorax

Pneumothorax may occur during sampling of upper pole lesions. Small pneumothoraces may be followed with serial chest radiographs and commonly resolve without intervention. Clinically significant pneumothoraces requiring chest tube placement are rare (<1%).[16]

Tumor seeding

Tumor seeding is rare, with an estimated incidence of less than 0.01%.[2,16,41] Close attention to the needle track is warranted on postbiopsy imaging. If detected, seeded tumor along the track may potentially be treated with image-guided ablation.[42]

Other complications

Less common complications include arteriovenous fistula, adjacent organ injury, and infection. Although infection is uncommon, nonurgent biopsy should be delayed if a patient has a urinary tract infection or pyelonephritis.

Postbiopsy Management

Immediate postprocedure management

After a biopsy, the patient is observed for approximately 2 to 4 hours (RMB) or 6 to 8 hours (RPB) with regular monitoring of vital signs. After RPB, the hematocrit is checked at 4 to 6 hours, and a urine sample is obtained to assess for gross hematuria and to confirm that the patient is able to void.[24]

Pathology review

The pathology report can demonstrate malignant, benign, or nondiagnostic findings and should be assessed for concordance with imaging findings.[43] A nondiagnostic result in an otherwise suspicious lesion should be reevaluated. Hybrid malignancies containing benign and malignant tissues have been reported, although they are thought to be rare and less aggressive.[15,44] Discordant benign findings should be considered for short interval follow-up imaging, rebiopsy, ablation, or definitive surgical resection, particularly if only fine needle aspiration was performed for the initial sampling.[45]

Nondiagnostic biopsy samples may demonstrate normal renal parenchyma (often seen in small renal masses that are missed), necrotic tissue, or inflammatory tissue.[43] Repeat biopsies have similar diagnostic rates as initial biopsies[4,46] and demonstrate malignancy in more than 50% of patients.[3,43,46] Therefore, rebiopsy is strongly recommended after nondiagnostic results.

Renal mass ablations

Recent literature has demonstrated renal mass ablation (RMA) to be safe and similar in efficacy to surgical resection in carefully selected patients.[47,48] RMA shows significant promise and increasing clinical usefulness as more studies demonstrate its safety and efficacy. This section discusses indications, techniques, and other clinical considerations for RMA.

Indications

RMA is a new treatment modality with emerging longer term outcomes data; therefore, indications are evolving (**Table 4**).

Strong indications

RMA should be strongly considered for stage T1a (<4 cm) renal malignancies in conditions where surgery is considered problematic.[14,48,49] This includes patients with significant surgical risk (eg, major comorbidities, obesity, elderly) or in patients

Table 4 Common thermal ablation indications	
Ablation Strongly Considered	**Ablation May Be Considered**
• Stage T1a (<4 cm) tumors in poor surgical candidates • Stage T1a tumors in patients with risk for multiple RCC (eg, von Hippel-Lindau disease, Birt-Hogg-Dube syndrome) • Stage T1a tumors in patients with solitary kidney	• Stage T1a tumors in healthy patients (eg, patient preference) • Stage T1b (4–7 cm) tumors in poor surgical candidates

Abbreviation: RCC, renal cell carcinoma.

From Bhagavatula SK, Shyn PB. Image-guided renal interventions. Radiol Clin North Am 2017;55(2):365; with permission.

where preservation of nephrons is critical, such as those with known or increased risk of multiple RCC (eg, von Hippel-Lindau disease, Birt-Hogg-Dube syndrome) and those with solitary kidneys.

Relative indications

For stage T1a malignancies in otherwise healthy patients, partial or radical nephrectomy has remained the gold standard treatment; however, RMA is acknowledged as a viable option and will likely have an expanding role in this population as more long-term data become available.[14,49] In stage T1b tumors (4–7 cm), surgery is recommended over ablation; however, guidelines suggest that ablation may be offered as a less invasive alternative, particularly in poor surgical candidates.[49]

Preprocedure Workup

Preprocedure workup, including history and imaging review, presedation evaluation, and coagulation status optimization are similar to the workup for renal biopsies. In addition, careful risk assessment should be performed and preprocedural tumor embolization, ureteral stent placement, hydrodisplacement, or other maneuvers should be considered when indicated to prevent major complications.

Preprocedural risk assessment

The RENAL nephrometry scoring system was initially proposed to quantify surgical risk based on renal mass characteristics (*R*adius, *E*ndophytic/exophytic nature, *N*earness to the renal hilum, *A*nterior/posterior location, and *L*ocation relative to the renal poles).[50] This classification score also correlates with risk of complications and treatment failures following ablation procedures,[51] but was optimized for surgical risk assessment.

The ABLATE classification system was developed specifically for ablation and addresses potential technical challenges before ablation (based on Axial tumor diameter, Bowel proximity, Location, Adjacency to ureter, Touching of the renal sinus fat, and Endophytic/exophytic nature).[52] Tumor embolization is an option to minimize bleeding risk when the axial diameter is larger than 5 cm. Hydrodisplacement or other protective mechanisms may be necessary to prevent bowel injury if the tumor is within 1 cm of the bowel (**Fig. 4**) and a ureteral stent may be necessary if it is within 1 cm of the ureter. Finally, if the tumor is adjacent to the adrenal glands, the patient may require preprocedural α-receptor blockade and careful intraprocedural blood pressure monitoring (arterial line).

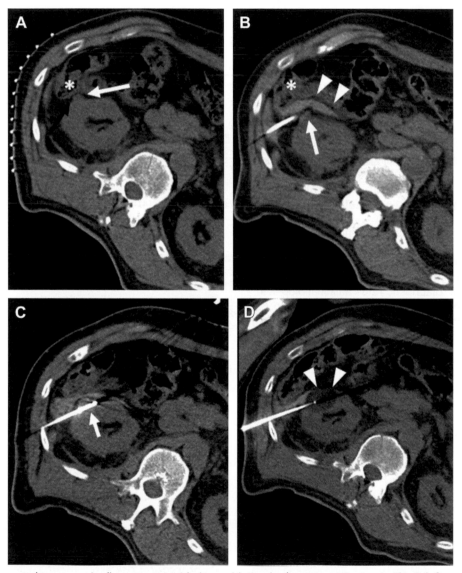

Fig. 4. Computed tomography fluoroscopy-guided cryoablation in the same patient as in **Fig. 3**, left posterior oblique position. (A) A 1-cm exophytic right upper pole mass (*arrow*), in close proximity to adjacent bowel (*asterisk*). (B) Hydrodisplacement with saline and contrast solution (*arrowheads*) injected through a 20-G needle to create separation between the mass (*arrow*) and bowel (*asterisk*). (C) Cryoablation probe (*arrow*) is placed with tip at the distal aspect of the mass. (D) Hypodense ice ball (*arrowheads*) is well seen during 2 freeze–thaw cryoablation cycles. (*From* Bhagavatula SK, Shyn PB. Image-guided renal interventions. Radiol Clin North Am 2017;55(2):366; with permission.)

Preablation biopsy

Pretreatment biopsy is recommended to avoid unnecessary ablation procedures, because up to 37% of tumors referred for ablation may be benign.[1,53] In addition, histology may assist in prognostication and subsequent medical treatment of malignant tumors after ablation.[54]

Methods of Ablation

Cryoablation (CA), microwave ablation (MWA), and radiofrequency ablation (RFA) are the most widely performed renal ablation technologies (**Table 5**). Irreversible electroporation and laser ablation have been used, but remain largely experimental and are not discussed herein.

Cryoablation

Mechanism Rapid expansion of gas (eg, argon) within a CA probe results in cooling of the probe to approximately −190°C.[55] The surrounding tissue is cooled (resulting in an expanding "ice ball"), with cell death resulting from 2 primary mechanisms: direct immediate cellular toxicity during freezing and thawing cycles, and indirect delayed toxicity caused by apoptosis and ischemic injury.[55,56]

Technique Cryoprobe size, number, and placement are determined by the shape and size of the tumor. Sufficient numbers of probes should be used such that they are spaced approximately 1 to 2 cm apart, including peripheral probes located within 1 cm of the outer tumor border.[55]

Probes are most commonly placed under CT or MRI guidance because these modalities allow for optimal visualization of the tumor, adjacent structures, and ice ball. Ultrasound imaging may also be used, but shadowing deep to the ice ball precludes complete visualization of anatomic relationships during ablation.

After probe placement, multiple (at least 2) freeze–thaw cycles are used, each lasting 5 to 20 minutes. Cell death is maximized by rapid freezing to at least −40°C and slow thawing over several minutes.[56] Images should be taken at regular intervals during the procedure to monitor the advancing ice ball and evaluate adjacent structures. The ice ball should extend at least 5 to 10 mm beyond the tumor to ensure complete ablation.[55]

Advantages and disadvantages The main advantage of CA is the ability to monitor the ice ball in real time on all imaging modalities (see **Fig. 4**). CA also causes less pain and is typically preferred in central lesions because it carries a lower risk of collecting structure injury.[57] Compared with RFA and MWA, CA has a longer procedure time (because of multiple probe insertions and multiple freeze–thaw cycles), a slightly increased bleeding risk (because it does not cauterize blood vessels), and higher cost.

Radiofrequency ablation

Mechanism RFA creates an alternating electrical current within the patient, in which the RF probe acts as a point electrode and grounding pads serve as a dispersive electrode. The energy flux at the electrode tip is very high because of the small surface area of the probe, resulting in frictional heating of molecules within the surrounding tissue. Cell death and coagulation necrosis occur rapidly at temperatures of greater than 55°C.[58]

Technique After the RF applicator or applicators are placed in the tumor under image guidance, a single heating cycle is usually used for ablation.

Table 5
Renal mass ablation methods

	Cryoablation	Radiofrequency Ablation	Microwave Ablation
Advantages	• Ablation zone well-monitored with CT or MRI • Less risk when treating central tumors • Less postprocedure pain	• Shorter procedure time (relative to cryoablation) • Cauterizes small blood vessels	• Allows rapid heating of greater amount of tissue • Less prone to heat sink effects
Disadvantages	• Higher cost and longer procedure time • Slight increased bleeding risk	• Ablation zone not well monitored in real time • Unpredictable ablation zone • Prone to heat sink effects	• Ablation zone not well monitored in real time • Higher risk when treating central tumors

From Bhagavatula SK, Shyn PB. Image-guided renal interventions. Radiol Clin North Am 2017;55(2):367; with permission.

Heating duration depends on the tumor and device characteristics with a typical cycle lasting 6 to 15 minutes, generating temperatures of 50°C to 100°C.[58]

Advantages and disadvantages RFA is the most established and least expensive ablation modality, and results in more rapid tissue ablation relative to CA. However, the ablation zone is not well-seen during the procedure. RFA is also susceptible to "heat sink effects" in which blood vessels cool and prevent effective ablation of adjacent tissue, sometimes resulting in a heterogeneous and unpredictable ablation zone. At temperatures exceeding 105°C, tissue charring may interfere with electrical conductivity, resulting in suboptimal ablation.[48,58]

Microwave ablation

Mechanism MWA applies an oscillating electromagnetic field that induces dielectric hysteresis (rapid realignment of polar molecules) to produce heat. Rapid cell death occurs at temperatures greater than 55°C, although maximum temperatures routinely exceed 100°C.[59]

Technique An MWA probe is placed under imaging guidance and tissue is ablated typically during a single heating cycle. Power and duration of heating depend on the size of the tumor and device; a typical treatment uses 45 to 80 W power for 5 to 10 minutes.[47,60] Intraprocedural monitoring of the ablation zone is limited; hypodensity on CT imaging or hyperechogenicity on ultrasound imaging may offer a crude reference.[47]

Advantages and disadvantages As with RFA, MWA cauterizes blood vessels and has lower bleeding rates compared with CA. MWA can rapidly heat a large volume of tissue, ablate through charred/necrotic tissue, and is less prone to heat sink effects.[47,48,59] For these reasons, MWA will likely have a greater clinical role as more data regarding its safety and efficacy become available. The main disadvantages of MWA are the inability to monitor the ablation zone in real time and limited available long-term outcomes data.

Complications

Reported major complication rates range from 3% to 10% in CA, 4.4% to 8.2% in RFA, and 2.5% in MWA, although data for CA and MWA are relatively limited.[47–49,58] CA and RFA seem to have slightly decreased complication rates relative to partial nephrectomy.[49] Many complications associated with renal ablations, including bleeding, adjacent organ injury, and pneumothorax, are uncommon and similar to renal biopsy, as discussed previously. Additional complications include ureteral injury resulting in stricture, urinoma, or fistula; acute kidney injury; and neuromuscular injury, resulting in flank laxity and paresthesias.[61,62] Tumor tract seeding is rare, seen in less than 1% of cases; more commonly, inflammatory nodules can mimic tumor seeding.[63,64]

Follow-Up Imaging

Timing

No evidence-based guidelines exist for imaging follow-up after renal ablation. In general, an initial postablation CT scan or MRI is performed within 1 month to document technical success, exclude complications, and provide a baseline for subsequent studies.[61,65] Early short interval follow-up by 3 to 6 months is recommended because residual unablated tumor is commonly detected within this time interval.[61] Long-term follow-up is also strongly recommended, with gradual reduction in imaging frequency over time. One published surveillance protocol proposes imaging at 1, 3, 6, and 12 months in the first year; every 6 months for the second year; and annually afterward.[61] Our approach is to image at 6 months and annually thereafter for 10 years.

Imaging findings

Nonenhancement, subtle homogeneous enhancement, or peripheral enhancement of the ablation zone is often present after CA and does not indicate malignancy. Eventually, the ablation zone may involute (most commonly seen in CA) or demonstrate a halo appearance. The ablation zone after RFA or MWA usually demonstrates absence of enhancement in the nonviable regions. Nodular or crescentic enhancement contiguous with the ablation margin raises suspicion for disease recurrence, particularly if it persists or enlarges after 3 to 6 months.[48,65] An increase in the size of the ablation zone is also suspicious, even in the absence of enhancement.[66]

Efficacy

RFA and CA have similar efficacy to surgical resection in small T1a RCC.[48,67] Intermediate results prospectively comparing MWA with open nephrectomy in small lesions have also demonstrated similar 5-year RCC-related survival.[47]

Ablation efficacy in larger tumors remains controversial, because no prospective study has compared ablation with nephrectomy. A recent study reported a 5-year postablation survival of 79% for tumors larger than 3 cm, significantly lower than published rates following nephrectomies.[68,69] However, more recent data comparing CA with nephrectomy in masses measuring 3 to 7 cm demonstrate similar survival rates.[67,70]

REFERENCES

1. Sahni VA, Silverman SG. Biopsy of renal masses: when and why. Cancer Imaging 2009;9:44–55.

2. Silverman SG, Gan YU, Mortele KJ, et al. Renal masses in the adult patient: the role of percutaneous biopsy. Radiology 2006;240(1):6–22.

3. Uppot RN, Harisinghani MG, Gervais DA. Imaging-guided percutaneous renal biopsy: rationale and approach. Am J Roentgenol 2010;194(6):1443–9.

4. Tsivian M, Rampersaud EN, del Pilar Laguna Pes M, et al. Small renal mass biopsy - how, what and when: report from an international consensus panel. BJU Int 2014;113(6):854–63.

5. Frank I, Blute ML, Cheville JC, et al. Solid renal tumors: an analysis of pathological features related to tumor size. J Urol 2003;170(6 Pt 1):2217–20.

6. Campbell S, Uzzo RG, Allaf ME, et al. Renal mass and localized renal cancer: AUA guideline. J Urol 2017;198:520–9.

7. Harisinghani MG, Maher MM, Gervais DA, et al. Incidence of malignancy in complex cystic renal masses (Bosniak category III): should imaging-guided biopsy precede surgery? AJR Am J Roentgenol 2003;180(3):755–8.

8. Curry NS, Cochran ST, Bissada NK. Cystic renal masses: accurate Bosniak classification requires adequate renal CT. AJR Am J Roentgenol 2000; 175(2):339–42.

9. Whittier WL, Korbet SM. Indications for and complications of renal biopsy. In: UpToDate, Glassock RJ, Rovin BH, Editors, UpToDate. Accessed December 04, 2017.

10. Richards NT, Darby S, Howie AJ, et al. Knowledge of renal histology alters patient management in over 40% of cases. Nephrol Dial Transplant 1994;9(9): 1255–9. Available at: http://www.ncbi.nlm.nih.gov/pubmed/7816285. Accessed May 3, 2016.

11. Sharma K, Venkatesan A, Swerdlow D, et al. Image-guided adrenal and renal biopsy. Tech Vasc Interv Radiol 2010;13(2):100–9.

12. Fuiano G, Mazza G, Comi N, et al. Current indications for renal biopsy: a questionnaire-based survey. Am J Kidney Dis 2000;35(3):448–57.

13. Rioux-Leclercq N, Karakiewicz PI, Trinh Q-D, et al. Prognostic ability of simplified nuclear grading of renal cell carcinoma. Cancer 2007;109(5):868–74.

14. Ljungberg B, Bensalah K, Canfield S, et al. EAU guidelines on renal cell carcinoma: 2014 update. Eur Urol 2015;67(5):913–24.

15. Tomaszewski JJ, Uzzo RG, Smaldone MC. Heterogeneity and renal mass biopsy: a review of its role and reliability. Cancer Biol Med 2014; 11(3):162–72.

16. Lane BR, Samplaski MK, Herts BR, et al. Renal mass biopsy—A renaissance? J Urol 2008;179(1):20–7.

17. Cheville JC, Lohse CM, Zincke H, et al. Sarcomatoid renal cell carcinoma: an examination of underlying histologic subtype and an analysis of associations with patient outcome. Am J Surg Pathol 2004;28(4): 435–41. Available at: http://www.ncbi.nlm.nih.gov/pubmed/15087662. Accessed May 3, 2016.

18. Rybicki FJ, Shu KM, Cibas ES, et al. Percutaneous biopsy of renal masses: sensitivity and negative predictive value stratified by clinical setting and size of masses. Am J Roentgenol 2003;180(5):1281–7.

19. Waring JP, Baron TH, Hirota WK, et al. Guidelines for conscious sedation and monitoring during gastrointestinal endoscopy. Gastrointest Endosc 2003;58(3): 317–22.

20. Lieberman DA, Wuerker CK, Katon RM. Cardiopulmonary risk of esophagogastroduodenoscopy. Role of endoscope diameter and systemic sedation. Gastroenterology 1985;88(2):468–72. Available at: http://www.ncbi.nlm.nih.gov/pubmed/3965335. Accessed May 3, 2016.

21. Soreide E, Eriksson LI, Hirlekar G, et al. Pre-operative fasting guidelines: an update. Acta Anaesthesiol Scand 2005;49(8):1041–7.

22. Patel IJ, Davidson JC, Nikolic B, et al. Consensus guidelines for periprocedural management of coagulation status and hemostasis risk in percutaneous image-guided interventions. J Vasc Interv Radiol 2012;23(6):727–36.

23. Potretzke TA, Gunderson TM, Aamodt D, et al. Incidence of bleeding complications after percutaneous core needle biopsy in hypertensive patients and comparison to normotensive patients. Abdom Radiol (NY) 2016;41(4):637–42.

24. Hogan JJ, Mocanu M, Berns JS. The native kidney biopsy: update and evidence for best practice. Clin J Am Soc Nephrol 2016;11(4):354–62.

25. Wunderlich H, Hindermann W, Al Mustafa AM, et al. The accuracy of 250 fine needle biopsies of renal tumors. J Urol 2005;174(1):44–6. Available at: http://www.ncbi.nlm.nih.gov/pubmed/15947574. Accessed May 3, 2016.

26. Volpe A, Finelli A, Gill IS, et al. Rationale for percutaneous biopsy and histologic characterisation of renal tumours. Eur Urol 2012;62(3):491–504.

27. Caoili EM, Bude RO, Higgins EJ, et al. Evaluation of sonographically guided percutaneous core biopsy of renal masses. Am J Roentgenol 2002;179(2):373–8.

28. Scanga LR, Maygarden SJ. Utility of fine-needle aspiration and core biopsy with touch preparation in the diagnosis of renal lesions. Cancer Cytopathol 2014;122:182–90.

29. Breda A, Treat EG, Haft-Candell L, et al. Comparison of accuracy of 14-, 18- and 20-G needles in ex-vivo renal mass biopsy: a prospective, blinded study. BJU Int 2010;105(7):940–5.

30. Renshaw AA, Lee KR, Madge R, et al. Accuracy of fine needle aspiration in distinguishing subtypes of renal cell carcinoma. Acta Cytol 1997; 41(4):987–94.

31. Neuzillet Y, Lechevallier E, Andre M, et al. Accuracy and clinical role of fine needle percutaneous biopsy with computerized tomography guidance of small (less than 4. 0 cm) renal masses. J Urol 2004; 171(5):1802–5.

32. Ball MW, Bezerra SM, Gorin MA, et al. Grade heterogeneity in small renal masses: potential implications for renal mass biopsy. J Urol 2015;193(1):36–40.

33. Gerlinger M, Horswell S, Larkin J, et al. Genomic architecture and evolution of clear cell renal cell carcinomas defined by multiregion sequencing. Nat Genet 2014;46(3):225–33.

34. Chunduri S, Whittier WL, Korbet SM. Adequacy and complication rates with 14- vs. 16-gauge automated needles in percutaneous renal biopsy of native kidneys. Semin Dial 2015;28(2):E11–4.

35. Korbet SM, Cameron J, Hicks J, et al. Percutaneous renal biopsy. Semin Nephrol 2002;22(3):254–67.

36. Mahoney MC, Racadio JM, Merhar GL, et al. Safety and efficacy of kidney transplant biopsy: Tru-Cut needle vs sonographically guided biopsy gun. AJR Am J Roentgenol 1993;160(2):325–6.

37. Ralls PW, Barakos JA, Kaptein EM, et al. Renal biopsy-related hemorrhage: frequency and comparison of CT and sonography. J Comput Assist Tomogr 1987;11:1031–4.

38. Lechevallier E, André M, Barriol D, et al. Fine-needle percutaneous biopsy of renal masses with helical CT guidance. Radiology 2000;216(2):506–10.

39. Walker PD. The renal biopsy. Arch Pathol Lab Med 2009;133(2):181–8.

40. Corapi KM, Chen JLT, Balk EM, et al. Bleeding complications of native kidney biopsy: a systematic review and meta-analysis. Am J Kidney Dis 2012; 60(1):62–73.

41. Mullins J, Mullins JK, Rodriguez R. Renal cell carcinoma seeding of a percutaneous biopsy tract. Can Urol Assoc J 2013;7(3–4):E176–9.

42. Sainani NI, Tatli S, Anthony SG, et al. Successful percutaneous radiologic management of renal cell carcinoma tumor seeding caused by percutaneous biopsy performed before ablation. J Vasc Interv Radiol 2013;24:1404–8.

43. Lebret T, Poulain JE, Molinie V, et al. Percutaneous core biopsy for renal masses: indications, accuracy and results. J Urol 2007;178(4):1184–8.

44. Ginzburg S, Uzzo R, Al-Saleem T, et al. Coexisting hybrid malignancy in a solitary sporadic solid benign renal mass: implications for treating patients following renal biopsy. J Urol 2014;191(2): 296–300.

45. Zardawi IM. Renal fine needle aspiration cytology. Acta Cytol 1999;43(2):184–90.

46. Jeon HG, Il Seo S, Jeong BC, et al. Percutaneous kidney biopsy for a small renal mass: a critical appraisal of results. J Urol 2016;195(3):568–73.

47. Yu J, Liang P, Yu X-L, et al. Us-guided percutaneous microwave ablation versus open radical nephrectomy for small renal cell carcinoma: intermediate-term results 1. Radiology 2014;270(3):880–7.

48. Shin BJ, Forris J, Chick B, et al. Contemporary status of percutaneous ablation for the small renal mass. Curr Urol Rep 2016;17:23.

49. Campbell SC, Novick AC, Belldegrun A, et al. Guideline for management of the clinical T1 renal mass. J Urol 2009;182(4):1271–9.

50. Kutikov A, Uzzo RG. The R.E.N.A.L. Nephrometry score: a comprehensive standardized system for quantitating renal tumor size, location and depth. J Urol 2009;182(3):844–53.

51. Schmit GD, Thompson RH, Kurup AN, et al. Usefulness of R.E.N.A.L. nephrometry scoring system for predicting outcomes and complications of percutaneous ablation of 751 renal tumors. J Urol 2013; 189(1):30–5.

52. Schmit GD, Kurup AN, Weisbrod AJ, et al. ABLATE: a renal ablation planning algorithm. AJR Am J Roentgenol 2014;202(4):894–903.

53. Tuncali K, Shankar S, Mortele KJ, et al. Evaluation of patients referred for percutaneous ablation of renal tumors: importance of a preprocedural diagnosis. AJR Am J Roentgenol 2004;183:575–82.

54. Molina AM, Motzer RJ. Clinical practice guidelines for the treatment of metastatic renal cell carcinoma: today and tomorrow. Oncologist 2011;16(Suppl 2): 45–50.

55. Allen BC, Remer EM. Percutaneous cryoablation of renal tumors: patient selection, technique, and postprocedural imaging. Radiographics 2010;30:887–900.

56. Erinjeri JP, Clark TWI. Cryoablation: mechanism of action and devices. J Vasc Interv Radiol 2010;21(8 Suppl):S187–91.

57. Sung GT, Gill IS, Hsu THS, et al. Effect of intentional cryo-injury to the renal collecting system. J Urol 2003;170(2 Pt 1):619–22.

58. Hong K, Georgiades C. Radiofrequency ablation: mechanism of action and devices. J Vasc Interv Radiol 2010;21(8 Suppl):S179–86.

59. Lubner MG, Brace CL, Hinshaw JL, et al. Microwave tumor ablation: mechanism of action, clinical results, and devices. J Vasc Interv Radiol 2010;21(8 Suppl): S192–203.

60. Simon CJ, Dupuy DE, Mayo-Smith WW. Microwave ablation: principles and applications. Radiographics 2005;25(Suppl 1):S69–83.

61. Iannuccilli JD, Grand DJ, Dupuy DE, et al. Percutaneous ablation for small renal masses — imaging follow-up. Semin Intervent Radiol 2014;31:50–63.

62. Bhayani SB, Allaf ME, Su L-M, et al. Neuromuscular complications after percutaneous radiofrequency ablation of renal tumors. Urology 2005;65(3):592.

63. Kurup AN, Morris JM, Schmit GD, et al. Neuroanatomic considerations in percutaneous tumor ablation. Radiographics 2013;33:1195–215.

64. Park BK, Kim CK. Complications of image-guided radiofrequency ablation of renal cell carcinoma: causes, imaging features and prevention methods. Eur Radiol 2009;19(9):2180–90.

65. Atwell TD, Schmit GD, Boorjian SA, et al. Percutaneous ablation of renal masses measuring 3.0 cm and smaller: comparative local control and complications after radiofrequency ablation and cryoablation. Am J Roentgenol 2013;200(2):461–6.

66. Weight CJ, Kaouk JH, Hegarty NJ, et al. Correlation of radiographic imaging and histopathology following cryoablation and radio frequency ablation for renal tumors. J Urol 2008;179(4):1277–81 [discussion: 1281–3].

67. Thompson RH, Atwell T, Schmit G, et al. Comparison of partial nephrectomy and percutaneous ablation for cT1 renal masses. Eur Urol 2015;67(2):252–9.

68. Best SL, Park SK, Youssef RF, et al. Long-term outcomes of renal tumor radio frequency ablation stratified by tumor diameter: size matters. J Urol 2012;187(4):1183–9.

69. Mason RJ, Rendon RA. Partial nephrectomy for T1b renal cell carcinoma: a safe and superior treatment option. Can Urol Assoc J 2012;6(2):128–30.

70. Schmit GD, Atwell TD, Callstrom MR, et al. Percutaneous cryoablation of renal masses ≥3 cm: efficacy and safety in treatment of 108 patients. J Endourol 2010;24(8):1255–62.

Practical Approach to Adrenal Imaging

Khaled M. Elsayes, MD[a],*, Sally Emad-Eldin, MD[b], Ajaykumar C. Morani, MD[a],
Corey T. Jensen, MD[a]

KEYWORDS

- Adrenal • Adenoma • Pheochromocytoma • Adrenocortical carcinoma • Computed tomography
- Magnetic resonance

KEY POINTS

- Noncontrast attenuation less than 10 Hounsfield units is most compatible with a lipid-rich adenoma.
- CT enhancement washout technique is the most sensitive and specific technique for evaluation of adrenal masses exhibiting an attenuation higher than 10 Hounsefield units on noncontrast CT.
- MR imaging is helpful in the setting of a heterogeneous mass or when there is contraindication of iodinated contrast medium (allergy or renal insufficiency).
- Adrenal adenoma is the most common adrenal mass containing intracytoplasmic lipid. Rarely, metastases can contain intracytoplasmic lipid, thus can mimic adenoma on MR imaging.
- Diffuse bilateral gland thickening with preserved adreniform configuration in patients with hypercortisolism is consistent with adrenal hyperplasia.

INTRODUCTION

The adrenal gland can be affected by a variety of pathologies, the majority of which are benign. Adrenal lesions tend to be encountered incidentally when performing imaging for other purposes. Diagnosis of adrenal masses can be challenging, but the imaging characteristics of morphologic and physiologic features can be used to appropriately guide the identification and management of adrenal lesions. This review describes an array of pathologic adrenal conditions discovered through imaging and illustrates their imaging characteristics with the implications for management.

IMAGING TECHNIQUES
Computed Tomography

Computed tomography (CT) is the imaging method most often used to detect and characterize adrenal masses. When an adrenal mass is found incidentally on imaging, a dedicated CT protocol is usually performed to further evaluate the mass. This is particularly true for patients with a history of malignancy. The adrenal mass protocol includes densitometry of the mass on noncontrast CT. Measuring the unenhanced attenuation value of an adrenal mass is crucial for accurate diagnosis of lipid-rich adenoma. An unenhanced attenuation value of less than 10 Hounsfield units (HU) is characteristic. If the mass fits this criterion, no further imaging is required.[1]

Adrenal masses with attenuation values of greater than 10 HU often have a unique contrast enhancement and washout pattern. Adenomas behave differently from other masses, enhancing rapidly after contrast administration and then rapidly washing out. Although most malignant lesions also enhance rapidly, they show a slower

This article was previously published in March 2017 *Radiologic Clinics*, Volume 55, Issue 2.
None of the authors have conflict of interest or financial disclosure.
[a] Department of Diagnostic Radiology, The University of Texas MD Anderson Cancer Center, 1400 Pressler Street Unit 1473, Houston, TX 77030, USA; [b] Department of Diagnostic and Intervention Radiology, Cairo University, Kasr Al-Ainy Street, Cairo 11652, Egypt
* Corresponding author. Department of Diagnostic Radiology, The University of Texas MD Anderson Cancer Center, 1400 Pressler Street, Houston, TX 77030.
E-mail address: KMElsayes@mdanderson.org

urologic.theclinics.com

washout pattern owing to leaky capillaries.[2] The absolute percentage of enhancement washout is calculated by measuring the unenhanced value, the enhanced attenuation at 60 seconds, and enhancement 15 minutes after contrast injection and applying them in the following formula:

$$\frac{\text{Enhanced attenuation value} - \text{delayed attenuation value}}{\text{Enhanced attenuation value} - \text{unenhanced attenuation value}} \times 100$$

Absolute washout measurement requires an unenhanced HU measurement, which is not usually acquired in daily practice. Relative washout can be obtained as an alternative formula when noncontrast phase is not available. Relative enhancement washout is calculated as:

$$\frac{\text{Enhanced attenuation value} - \text{delayed attenuation value}}{\text{Enhanced attenuation value}} \times 100$$

Absolute washout threshold values of greater than or equal to 60% and relative washout threshold values of greater than or equal to 40% have been reported to be highly sensitive (88%–96%) and highly specific (96%–100%) for diagnosing adrenal adenomas (**Fig. 1**).[1,3,4]

Dual-energy computed tomography

Recent technologic advances in dual-energy CT permit nearly simultaneous acquisition of the targeted region at 2 different tube voltages (usually 80 and 140 kVp) during a single breath-hold acquisition. Using a 3-material decomposition algorithm, virtual unenhanced CT images can be reconstructed from contrast-enhanced CT images.[5,6]

Because adrenal lesions display different attenuations at different voltage settings, they are suited for characterization by dual-energy CT.[7] The use of virtual unenhanced images may permit characterization of some adrenal lesions as adenomas, which would be characterized as indeterminate if enhanced images were the only images available.[8]

Lower attenuation of an adrenal lesion at 80 kVp than at 140 kVp has been shown to be a highly specific sign of adrenal adenoma, the diagnostic equivalent of the presence of intracytoplasmic lipid. However, because some adenomas and adrenal metastases show higher attenuation at 80 kVp, the sensitivity of this test is low. Gupta and

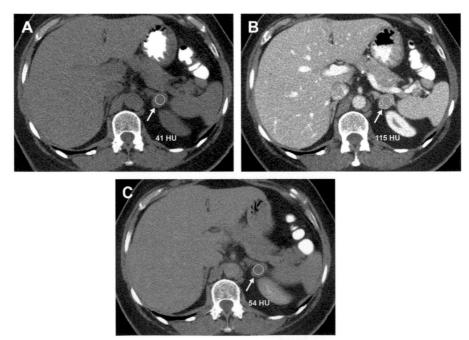

Fig. 1. Lipid-poor adrenal adenoma on computed tomography (CT). Axial nonenhanced CT (*A*), contrast-enhanced CT in venous phase (*B*), and delayed 15 minutes (*C*), demonstrate a well-circumscribed oval mass (*arrows*) involving the left adrenal gland with an attenuation value of 41, 115, and 54 Hounsfield units (HU) on noncontrast, venous, and delayed phase imaging, respectively, yielding an absolute enhancement washout of 82%, characteristic of a lipid-poor adenoma.

colleagues[9] have reported a sensitivity of 50% and a specificity of 100%, whereas Shi and colleagues[10] have reported a sensitivity of 78.6% and a specificity of 100% for dual-energy CT diagnosis of adenoma. The variable presentation of adrenal adenomas on dual-energy CT is likely owing to varying amounts of intracytoplasmic lipid.

Computed tomography perfusion imaging
The application of CT perfusion imaging in adrenal gland tumors is currently undergoing investigation.[11] CT perfusion imaging has been shown to quantitatively differentiate adrenal adenomas from nonadenomas.[11] The CT perfusion parameters (blood flow, blood volume, mean transit time, and permeability surface area product), which reflect adrenal nodule angiogenesis, are quantified.[12] Although adenomas have a higher permeability surface value than nonadenomas, only the blood volume parameter has been shown to have prognostic significance. Blood volume is significantly higher in adenomas than in nonadenomas, with reported sensitivity of 76.9% and specificity of 73.2%.[11,12]

MR Imaging

Chemical shift MR imaging
Chemical shift MR imaging (CS-MR imaging) is the essential MR technique in the evaluation of adrenal lesions. CS-MR imaging uses in-phase (IP) and opposed-phase (OP) T1 gradient-recalled echo pulse sequences.[2] A decrease in signal intensity of the adrenal lesion on OP compared with IP images is characteristic of the presence of intracytoplasmic lipid. Visual analysis of this signal drop is accurate in the diagnosis of most lipid-rich adenomas (**Fig. 2**).[13] The signal intensity drop from IP to OP images is assessed quantitatively through calculation of the signal intensity index (SII). The SII is calculated as:

$$\frac{SI\ on\ IP\ -\ SI\ on\ OP}{SI\ on\ IP} \times 100$$

Where SI is the signal intensity. Using a SII cutoff value of 16.5%, the reported accuracy of CS-MR imaging in distinguishing adenomas from metastatic tumors has been reported as 100% (see **Fig. 2**).[13] Another quantitative chemical-shift method of distinguishing adenomas from malignant tumors is calculation of the adrenal-to-spleen ratio (ASR). The ASR is calculated as:

$$\frac{SI\ adrenal\ OP/spleen\ OP}{SI\ adrenal\ IP/SI\ spleen\ IP} \times 100$$

An ASR of less than or equal to 70 showed 78% sensitivity and 100% specificity for identifying adenomas. However, SII has been found to be a more valid measure than ASR in identifying lipid containing adrenal adenomas.[13–15]

MR imaging has a limited role in characterizing lipid-poor adenomas. Israel and colleagues[16] have reported that CS-MR imaging can identify 60% of adenomas (8/13) that demonstrated greater than 10 HU on unenhanced CT.[16] One study showed that CS-MR imaging is most limited when the unenhanced CT attenuation of the lesion is greater than 30 HU.[17] Sahdev and colleagues[14] reported a sensitivity of 89% for CS-MR imaging in diagnosing lipid-poor adenomas of 10 to 30 HU. Rarely, adrenal metastases, such as those from clear cell renal cell carcinoma or hepatocellular carcinoma, may contain intracytoplasmic lipid and thus show a significant decrease in signal intensity on OP compared with IP images (**Fig. 3**).[18]

Diffusion-weighted MR imaging
The effectiveness of diffusion-weighted imaging (DWI) for the diagnosis of adrenal tumors has been investigated.[15,19] Normal adrenal glands

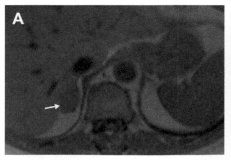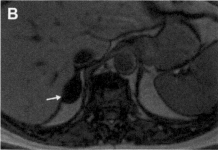

Fig. 2. Adrenal adenoma on MR imaging. Axial in-phase (*A*) and opposed phase (*B*) T1-weighted dual echo gradient echo pulse sequences demonstrate a well-circumscribed oval shaped nodule (*arrow*) involving the right adrenal gland with a significant drop of signal intensity on opposed-phase compared with in-phase (signal intensity index = 791–356/791 = 55%), characteristic of an adenoma.

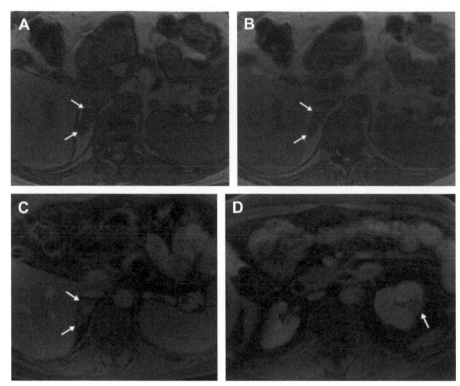

Fig. 3. Lipid-containing metastasis involving the right adrenal gland in a 69-year-old patient with clear cell carcinoma of the left kidney. Axial opposed-phase (OP) (*A*), axial in-phase (IP) (*B*), and axial contrast-enhanced T1-weighted (*C, D*) images demonstrate right adrenal nodules (*arrows in A–C*), which exhibit signal drop in OP compared with IP, and heterogeneous enhancement. Patient also had a heterogeneously enhancing mass in the left kidney (*arrow in D*). Diagnosis was confirmed after left partial nephrectomy and right adrenalectomy.

show high signal intensity with nonpathologic restricted/embedded diffusion on DWI.[20] There is considerable overlap of apparent diffusion coefficient (ADC) values between adenomas and metastatic lesions (**Figs. 4** and **5**). DWI is not useful in the further differentiation of potentially lipid-poor adenomas, indicating that its utility for indeterminate lesions is limited.[15,19,21]

However, pheochromocytomas have relatively higher ADC values than adenomas and metastatic lesions.[22]

MR spectroscopy

Few studies have evaluated the use of MR spectroscopy (MRS) in the characterization of adrenal lesions. The deep location of the adrenal glands

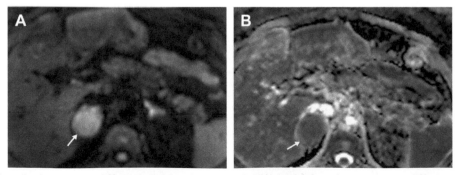

Fig. 4. Adrenal adenoma on diffusion-weighted imaging (DWI). DWI (*A*) and an apparent diffusion coefficient (ADC) map (*B*) demonstrate a right adrenal mass (*arrow*) with restricted diffusion and an ADC value of 1.14 × 10^{-3} mm^2/s.

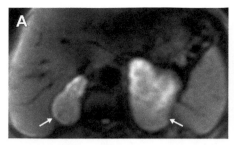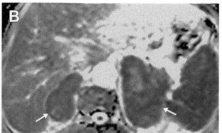

Fig. 5. Adrenal metastases on diffusion-weighted imaging (DWI). DWI (*A*) and an apparent diffusion coefficient (ADC) map (*B*) demonstrate restricted diffusion of the bilateral adrenal masses (*arrows*) with ADC values of 1.062 × 10⁻³ mm²/s and 1.067 × 10⁻³ mm²/s on the left and right sides, respectively. Both adenomas and metastases show restricted (embedded) diffusion; thus, they cannot be differentiated based on diffusion characteristics.

and proximity to regions with significant susceptibility artifact, together with the heterogeneous nature of adrenal masses, limit the feasibility of MRS techniques.[23] On visual analysis of MRS results for the characterization of adrenal lesions, adenomas have only positive lipid peaks in the spectra. There is no difference in metabolic peaks between lipid-rich and lipid-poor adenomas. The presence of a high choline peak supports malignancy.[24]

Quantitative analysis of the metabolic ratios has shown better results. The metabolic ratios are calculated include choline:creatine of 4.0 to 4.3 ppm:creatine, choline:lipid, and lipid:creatine. The first 2 ratios offer the most effective discrimination of adrenal lesions, with the highest sensitivity and specificity.[23,24]

Using a cutoff value of 1.20 for the choline:creatine ratio, adenomas and pheochromocytomas can be distinguished from carcinomas and metastases (92% sensitivity, 96% specificity). In addition, pheochromocytomas and carcinomas can be differentiated from adenomas and metastases by a 4.0 to 4.3 ppm:creatine ratio of greater than 1.50 (87% sensitivity, 98% specificity).[24]

One small series demonstrated that MRS is useful for characterizing pheochromocytomas. These tumors are characterized by a unique spectral peak at 6.8 ppm that may be attributed to the presence of catecholamines.[25]

PET Computed Tomography with ¹⁸FFluorodeoxyglucose

PET with ¹⁸Ffluorodeoxyglucose combined with CT (FDG PET-CT) has shown merit in differentiating adrenal masses, identifying the origin of the mass as adrenal versus nonadrenal, and determining the staging of malignant lesions.[26] It is not, however, used as the primary imaging modality to characterize adrenal lesions.[27] The degree to which qualitative or quantitative PET analysis should be used in the characterization of adrenal lesions remains uncertain. The findings of qualitative PET analyses are interpreted as positive if the FDG uptake of an adrenal lesion is greater than or equal to that of the liver and as negative if lesion uptake is less than that of the liver (**Figs. 6** and **7**).[27] Other reports using quantitative PET analysis to identify adrenal lesions have

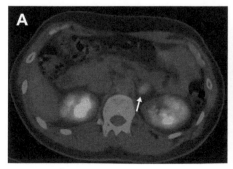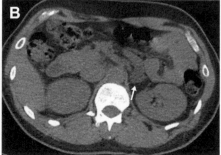

Fig. 6. Adrenal adenoma on PET. Axial fused PET-computed tomography (CT) (*A*), axial noncontrast CT images (*B*) in a 57-year-old man with high-grade lymphoma, show a 2.7-cm mass (*arrow*) involving the left adrenal gland with low grade metabolic activity with maximum standardized uptake value of 3.1, which was similar to the liver background. This was biopsied and pathologically proven to represent an adrenal adenoma.

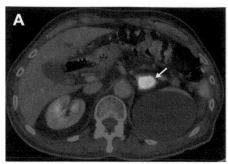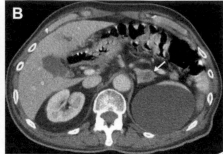

Fig. 7. Adrenal metastasis on PET. Biopsy-proven adrenal metastasis on PET/computed tomography (CT) in a 59-year-old patient with history of lung cancer. Axial fused PET-CT (*A*) and contrast-enhanced CT images (*B*) show a hypermetabolic heterogeneously enhancing 2.3-cm mass (*arrow*) involving the left adrenal with maximum standardized uptake value of 17.1. The increased uptake compared with the liver is more specific for malignancy.

suggested that a maximum standardized uptake value (SUV_{max}) of greater than or equal to 3.1 is useful for differentiating malignant from benign adrenal lesions.[28,29]

The measurement of SUV is subject to variability owing to features such as patient body weight, scanner resolution, image reconstruction method, and time between FDG injection and scan acquisition.[30] Thus, a method that quantifies the ratio of adrenal mass SUV to liver SUV (tumor:liver SUV_{max} ratio) was created to correct some of the variables that affect SUV measurements.[31]

The implementation of a mean CT attenuation threshold greater than 10 HU, with either SUV_{max} greater than 3.1 or tumor:liver SUV ratio greater than 1.0, increases the specificity of FDG PET-CT for identifying metastases without decreasing the sensitivity. Because some adrenal adenomas have moderate FDG uptake above the PET thresholds, both the CT and PET thresholds are applied to improve the overall diagnostic accuracy and decrease the false-positive rate.[28,29] Greater

FDG activity in the tumor than in the liver in some benign adrenal adenomas, adrenal endothelial cysts, and inflammatory lesions (sarcoidosis, tuberculosis) leads to a 5% false-positive rate for PET-CT in the identification of adrenal lesions.[32]

Causes of false-negative results are small (<10 mm) metastatic nodules, adrenal metastatic lesions with hemorrhage or necrosis, and metastases from non–FDG-avid malignancies, including bronchoalveolar carcinoma and carcinoid.[33] PET cannot differentiate between malignant adrenal lesions, such as metastases, adrenocortical carcinoma (**Fig. 8**), or malignant pheochromocytoma, and lymphoma.[2]

ADRENAL MASSES AND SPECTRUM OF IMAGING FEATURES

Adrenal masses can be characterized on the basis of their morphologic features into the following spectrum: intracytoplasmic lipid, fat cells, hemorrhagic, cystic, markedly enhancing,

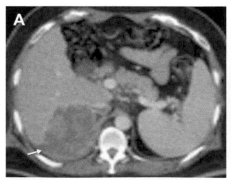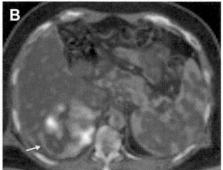

Fig. 8. PET/computed tomography (CT) of a right adrenocortical carcinoma. Axial contrast-enhanced CT (*A*) demonstrates a large (7 × 9 cm) heterogeneously enhancing mass involving the right adrenal gland (*arrow*). On the axial fused PET/CT (*B*), the mass (*arrow*) shows central photopenia suggestive of necrosis, with surrounding hypermetabolic active rim (with maximum standardized uptake value of 10), consistent with peripheral active viable malignancy.

large lobulated heterogeneous mass, calcified, or bilateral adrenal masses.

Adrenal Adenoma

Adrenal adenoma is the most common adrenal lesion, found in 2% to 9% of autopsies.[7] Most adenomas are nonfunctioning; differentiation from functioning adenomas requires clinical and laboratory evaluation in conjunction with imaging. However, other atypical features may provide useful clues. For example, an atrophic contralateral adrenal gland suggests a functioning adenoma, since such atrophy may be owing to suppression of pituitary adrenocorticotropic hormone (ACTH) secretion by elevated cortisol levels.[34]

Adenomas vary in size, with most lesions measuring less than 3 cm in greatest dimension. They are typically well-circumscribed round or oval masses with homogeneous attenuation/signal intensity and enhancement patterns. However, overlap with characteristics of malignant lesions may make these morphologic features insufficient for confirming a diagnosis of adrenal adenoma.[35] Furthermore, some adenomas have an atypical appearance that may include large size, calcification, cystic degeneration, or hemorrhage, thus mimicking the appearance of nonadenomas and making the diagnosis more challenging.[36]

The classic diagnostic feature of adrenal adenoma is the presence of intracytoplasmic lipid. However, 10% to 40% of adenomas are lipid poor, occasionally rendering them almost indistinguishable from other adrenal pathologies.[37] The attenuation of adrenal adenomas on precontrast CT varies according to the amount of intracytoplasmic lipid.[38] The mean attenuation of lipid-rich adenomas ranges from −2 to 16 HU, whereas that of lipid-poor adenomas is higher, measuring 20 to 25 HU.[1,3,16,39] An unenhanced attenuation value of less than 10 HU is characteristic of a lipid-rich adenoma, with reported 71% sensitivity and 98% specificity.[40] When this threshold is not met, washout criteria can be helpful in the identification of these lipid-poor adenomas. Threshold values of greater than 60% for absolute enhancement washout and greater than 40% for relative enhancement washout have been found to be highly sensitive and specific for diagnosing adrenal adenoma, irrespective of lipid content (see Fig. 1).[3,41]

Chemical shift IP and OP pulse sequences is the most reliable MR technique for evaluation of adrenal adenoma. This differentiates adrenal adenomas from metastases with a high sensitivity (81%–100%) and specificity (94%–100%).[42,43]

With CS-MR imaging, most adrenal adenomas demonstrate drop of signal intensity on OP compared with IP images. A decrease in signal intensity of more than 16.5% is diagnostic of an adenoma (see **Fig. 2**).[13] Rarely, foci of fat cells have been reported in adrenal adenomas that were preoperatively diagnosed as myelolipoma on the basis of radiologic findings. The lipomatous tissue may represent fatty degeneration in adrenocortical adenoma or may be an additional neoplastic component of the tumor.[44]

Mimics of Adrenal Adenoma

Various adrenal masses can mimic adrenal adenomas. Although this is not common, misinterpretation may occur mainly because of low attenuation on CT or drop of signal intensity on OP when compared with IP sequence. Simple cyst with attenuation values of less than 10 HU can mimic adrenal lipid-rich adenoma on unenhanced CT. However, they do not enhance on postcontrast series and exhibit markedly increased signal intensity on T2-weighted MR images.

Some metastatic deposits can contain intracytoplasmic lipid, such as those occurring secondary to hepatocellular carcinoma, and clear cell renal cell carcinoma (see **Fig. 3**), and thus can mimic adenoma on MR imaging as they demonstrate drop of signal intensity on OP compared with IP pulse sequences.[18]

Adrenal Metastases

Adrenal metastases are the most common malignant lesions involving the adrenal gland. Although only 2% of adrenal incidentalomas are metastases, the rate is much higher in patients with known malignancy (26%–73%).[2,45] The adrenal gland is a common site of metastasis; common primary tumors that metastasize to the adrenal glands include the lung, breast, kidney, pancreas, and gastrointestinal tract.[46] Isolated adrenal metastasis is less common than bilateral metastases but, if unilateral, they occur more on the left side.[47,48]

On routine CT or MR imaging, the diagnostic features of adrenal metastases can be nonspecific. Metastases tend to be heterogeneous with irregular margins, particularly when large. However, small metastatic lesions may be homogeneous with smooth margins, mimicking benign lesions.[49] Therefore, further evaluation is often needed, especially in cancer patients with no other sites of metastases, given the significant impact on management.[50]

Metastases typically have attenuation values of higher than 10 HU on unenhanced CT. They usually do not demonstrate significant enhancement washout on delayed phase, with absolute enhancement washout less than 60% and relative enhancement washout less than 40% (**Fig. 9**).[1,38,51] One study suggested that any nonhemorrhagic, noncalcified adrenal lesion with an unenhanced CT attenuation 43 HU or greater should be suspicious for metastasis regardless of its contrast washout characteristics.[51]

On MR imaging, metastases usually exhibit low signal intensity on T1-weighted images and high signal intensity on T2-weighted images, with heterogeneous enhancement after administration of contrast material. Metastases typically do not demonstrate signal drop on OP compared to IP pulse sequences, with the exception of metastases containing intracytoplasmic lipid (**Fig. 10**).[52,53]

Collision Tumors

Collision tumors are rare consisting of 2 adjacent but histologically different neoplasms in the same mass without significant histologic admixture.[54] The most frequent adrenal collision tumor comprises an adrenal adenoma and a myelolipoma.[55] Although rare, metastases can occur adjacent to or in an existing adrenal adenoma. In this setting, collision tumor is suspected if there are new findings suggestive of metastatic disease, including an increase in size or development of a new component (**Fig. 11**), together with heterogeneous signal drop on OP images.[36,55]

On CT, an adrenal adenoma complicated by hemorrhage may mimic collision tumor. MR imaging and PET-CT can improve the accuracy of identification of collision tumors' components, thereby avoiding unnecessary biopsy.[54] On MR imaging, the internal component is either a hematoma with characteristic nonenhancing blood products (in case of adrenal adenoma complicated by hemorrhage), or an enhancing metastatic component on top of the adenoma (collision tumor). On PET-CT, the hemorrhagic component of adenomas typically demonstrates no FDG uptake, so it can be distinguished from metastasis.[56,57]

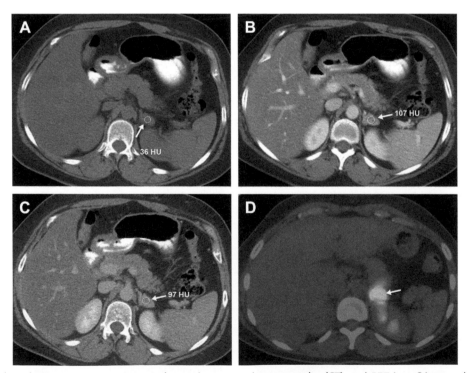

Fig. 9. Adrenal metastasis on contrast-enhanced computed tomography (CT) and PET in a 31-year-old woman with a history of endometrial carcinoma. Axial nonenhanced CT (*A*), contrast-enhanced CT in venous (*B*) and delayed 15 minutes (*C*), demonstrate a well-circumscribed oval mass (*arrows*) involving the left adrenal gland representing metastasis with an attenuation value of 36, 107, and 97 Hounsfield units (HU) on noncontrast, venous, and delayed phase images, respectively, yielding an absolute enhancement washout of 14%. (*D*) Axial fused PET/CT image demonstrates significantly increased uptake (*arrow*).

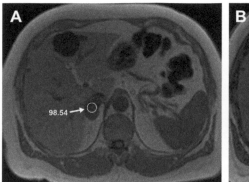
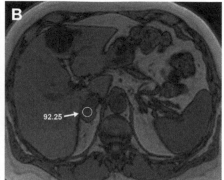

Fig. 10. Adrenal metastasis on MR imaging. Axial in-phase (*A*) and axial opposed-phase images (*B*) demonstrate a lobulated mass (*arrow*) involving the right adrenal gland demonstrating no significant signal drop on out-of-phase compared with in-phase images, proven to represent metastatic deposit in this 59-year-old male patient with a history of lung cancer.

There are case reports of extremely rare types of collision tumors, including adenoma and pheochromocytoma or hemangioma, adrenocortical carcinoma and myelolipoma, or metastases in addition to myelolipoma and lymphoma.[58–60]

Lymphoma

Although rare, lymphoma involving the adrenal gland is more frequently non-Hodgkin lymphoma than Hodgkin lymphoma. Primary adrenal lymphoma is rare, whereas secondary adrenal lymphoma is more common and is frequently associated with other sites of disease, such as the ipsilateral kidney and retroperitoneal lymph nodes. Bilateral adrenal involvement is seen in 50% of patients.[60,61]

Lymphomatous involvement of the adrenal gland may manifest as extensive retroperitoneal disease owing to total engulfment of the adrenal gland, focal discrete masses, or diffuse enlargement of the gland.[42] Occasionally, in the early course of the diffuse infiltrative form, the glands maintain their adreniform configuration and mimic adrenal hyperplasia.[2]

The imaging characteristics of adrenal lymphoma are nonspecific. On CT, lymphoma manifests as homogeneous masses (**Fig. 12**) with washout characteristics similar to those of other malignancies.[62,63] In untreated lymphoma, calcification is uncommon.[64] Lymphoma demonstrates low signal intensity on T1-weighted imaging and heterogeneous high signal intensity on T2-weighted imaging, with mild progressive enhancement after intravenous contrast administration (see **Fig. 11**).[65] Distinguishing adrenal lymphoma from metastases based on imaging alone is not possible.[66] Because of its high cellularity, adrenal lymphoma tends to show diffusion restriction. It also tends to be intensely FDG avid.[67] The degree of FDG uptake in adrenal lymphoma is similar to that of other involved sites.[2]

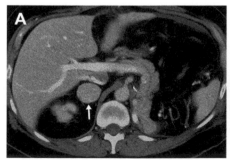
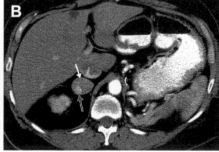

Fig. 11. Coexisting adenoma and metastasis (collision tumor) involving the right adrenal gland in a 67-year-old male patient with renal cell cancer. Axial contrast-enhanced computed tomography (CT) images (*A*) demonstrate a well-circumscribed oval mass involving the right adrenal gland (*arrow*), enhancement washout was consistent with adenoma. (*B*) Follow-up axial contrast-enhanced CT after 2 years demonstrates an enhancing focus (*transparent arrow*), within a right adrenal adenoma (*white arrow*). Surgical pathology confirmed the diagnosis of collision tumor (metastatic focus within an adenoma).

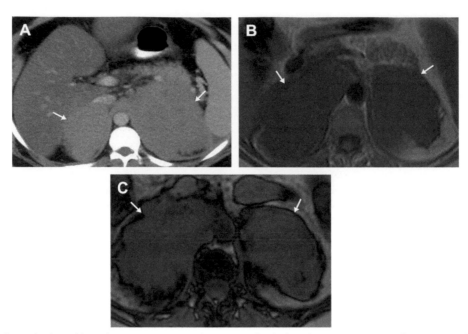

Fig. 12. Bilateral adrenal lymphoma on computed tomography (CT) and MR imaging. Axial contrast-enhanced CT (*A*), T1-weighted in-phase (*B*), and opposed-phase (*C*) images demonstrate bilateral large lobulated adrenal masses (*arrows*), exhibiting homogenous intermediate-low signal intensity of T1-weighted images, no signal drop on out-of-phase compared with in-phase sequence and with mild homogenous postcontrast enhancement.

Myelolipoma

The most common fat cells–containing adrenal mass is myelolipoma, an uncommon benign tumor composed of fatty tissue and hematopoietic tissue that histologically resembles bone marrow.[35] The quantity of fat cells is variable and can be minimal or nearly 100%.[43] Calcification is identified in approximately 20% of adrenal myelolipomas.[68] The overwhelming majority of these masses are asymptomatic. Rarely, large masses cause pain by inducing spontaneous hemorrhage (owing to the myeloid component), necrosis, or mass effect.[43,50] For this reason, surgical excision is recommended for lesions greater than 7 cm in greatest dimension.[69] On CT, the presence of negative-attenuation fat (−20 to −100 HU) in the lesion is virtually diagnostic of myelolipoma (**Fig. 13**).[7] On MR imaging, fat cells are demonstrated as high signal intensity on non–fat-suppressed T1- and T2-weighted images, with signal loss on fat suppression images (**Fig. 14**).

Using CS-MR imaging, voxels containing both fat and water tissue demonstrate lower signal intensity on OP than on IP imaging, leading to India ink artifact at the interface of the fatty components with nonfatty components.[43]

Adrenal lipoma, adrenocortical carcinoma with lipomatous metaplasia, pheochromocytoma, and adrenal teratoma are very rare adrenal lesions that are also reported to demonstrate gross fat cells and may mimic myelolipoma.[36]

In cases of long-standing or improperly treated congenital adrenal hyperplasia, prolonged stimulation of the adrenal cortex by elevated ACTH levels may lead to the characteristic appearance of multiple bilateral adrenal masses with substantial fat cells.[70]

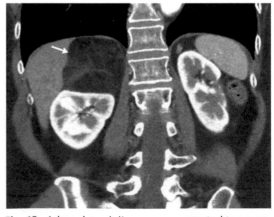

Fig. 13. Adrenal myelolipoma on computed tomography (CT). Coronal reformatted image of contrast-enhanced CT demonstrates a well-circumscribed mass (*arrow*) involving the right adrenal gland exhibiting predominately fat density, which is characteristic of an adrenal myelolipoma.

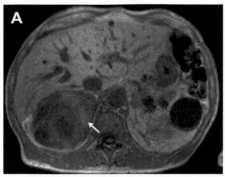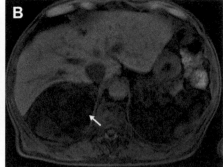

Fig. 14. Adrenal myelolipoma on MR imaging. Axial non–fat-suppressed T1-weighted (*A*) and fat-suppressed T1-weighted (*B*) images demonstrate a well-circumscribed large ovoid mass involving the right adrenal gland with predominately fat signal (*arrows*), which demonstrates drop of signal on fat-suppressed compared with non–fat-suppressed images.

Cystic Adrenal Masses

Adrenal cysts

There are 4 pathologic subtypes of adrenal cysts: vascular or endothelial cysts, pseudocysts, epithelial cysts, and parasitic cysts.[36] Endothelial cysts, also known as simple cysts, are the most common subtype (45%).[71] Endothelial cysts include 2 subtypes: lymphangiomatous (42%) and hemangiomatous cysts (3%).[72]

Simple adrenal cysts are well-defined homogeneous masses with thin walls. They demonstrate fluid attenuation (0–20 HU) on noncontrast CT and thus may be misinterpreted as a lipid-rich adenoma.[73] On MR imaging, their signal is similar to that of fluid, hypointense on T1-weighted images and hyperintense on T2-weighted images. Simple cysts should not demonstrate soft tissue components or internal enhancement on postcontrast CT and MR imaging (**Fig. 15**).

Adrenal pseudocysts typically arise secondary to sequela of a prior episode of hemorrhage; they do not have an epithelial lining and their wall is composed of fibrous tissue.[65] Adrenal pseudocysts have a complex appearance on imaging. They may demonstrate high internal density on CT or blood signal intensity on MR imaging secondary to hemorrhage or hyalinized thrombus, together with thick walls and internal septations. The presence of peripheral curvilinear calcification is characteristic of an adrenal pseudocyst (**Fig. 16**).[74] Given its high sensitivity in detailing the hemorrhagic components and internal septa, MR is superior to other imaging modalities for the identification of adrenal pseudocysts, yet peripheral calcification is best identified on CT.

Parasitic cysts represent 7% of adrenal cysts. For the most part, they occur secondary to echinococcal infection. The imaging appearance depends on the stage of the infection; it varies from simple looking cyst to complex multicystic mass with internal septa. They also can have septal or mural calcification. The presence of daughter cysts in the lumen is characteristic on CT and MR images. Isolated adrenal involvement is extremely rare; the presence of extraadrenal disease is essential to make a proper diagnosis of adrenal hydatid cyst.[75]

Epithelial cysts comprise 9% of adrenal cysts. They lack specific diagnostic features, making them difficult to distinguish from other adrenal cystic lesions.[76]

Occasionally, some adrenal tumors, including pheochromocytoma, adrenocortical carcinoma, metastases, and hemangioma, may go through cystic degeneration and seem to be cystic. Imaging findings that suggest an underlying tumor include an irregular thick wall or nodular septal or mural enhancement.[71]

Of benign cysts, 60% show interval increases in size over time. This should not be interpreted erroneously as a sign of an underlying malignancy or a complication when identified as an isolated finding.[73]

Lymphangioma

Cystic lymphangioma of the adrenal gland is both extremely rare and asymptomatic. A multilocular cyst with thin septa and CT attenuation of simple fluid is most suggestive of a lymphangioma.[36] On MR imaging, adrenal lymphangiomas can be visualized as thin-walled cystic lesions with low signal intensity in T1-weighted imaging and high signal intensity in T2-weighted images without significant postcontrast enhancement.[77]

Pheochromocytoma

Pheochromocytoma is an adrenal medullary paraganglioma arising from chromaffin cells, the predominant cells in the adrenal medulla. Extraadrenal paragangliomas can occur anywhere from

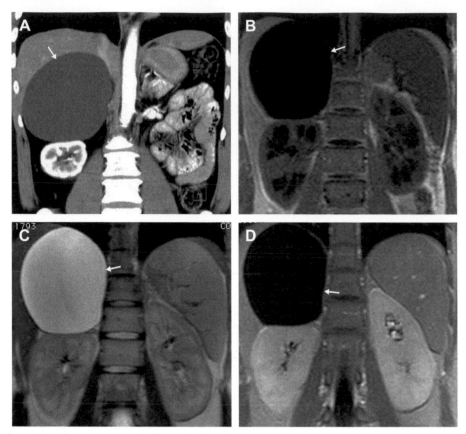

Fig. 15. Adrenal simple cyst. Coronal reformatted contrast enhanced computed tomography image (*A*) demonstrates well-circumscribed fluid attenuation nonenhancing cystic lesion in the right adrenal. Coronal T1-weighted (*B*), T2-weighted (*C*), and postcontrast T1-weighted images (*D*) demonstrate a well-circumscribed cystic lesion involving the right adrenal gland (*arrow*) with hypointense signal on T1-weighted and hyperintense signal on T2-weighted images with no postcontrast enhancement. These features are compatible with a simple adrenal cyst, and no further workup is warranted.

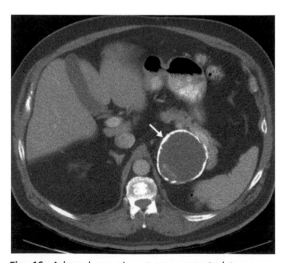

Fig. 16. Adrenal pseudocyst on computed tomography (CT). Axial contrast-enhanced CT demonstrates a well-circumscribed ovoid fluid attenuation lesion involving the left adrenal gland demonstrating dense wall peripheral curvilinear calcification (*arrow*), representing a pseudocyst.

the skull base to the pelvis along the sympathetic chain.[35]

Pheochromocytomas follow the rule of 10s; 10% are bilateral, malignant, extraadrenal, and occur in children.[35] Pheochromocytomas can be associated with various syndromes, including multiple endocrine neoplasia type 2, von Hippel-Lindau disease (**Fig. 17**), neurofibromatosis type 1, Sturge-Weber syndrome, tuberous sclerosis, and familial paraganglioma syndrome.[78] Approximately 10% of pheochromocytomas are asymptomatic. Most patients present with headache, flushing, and palpitations.[79] Patients typically have elevated plasma-free metanephrines, 24-hour levels of urinary metanephrines, or vanillylmandelic acid.[36]

Pheochromocytomas are typically larger than adenomas, yet smaller than adrenocortical carcinomas.[39] Nonfunctioning pheochromocytomas are larger than functioning lesions at presentation.[80] The CT appearance of pheochromocytomas is nonspecific and usually overlaps with

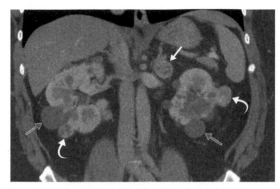

Fig. 17. Left adrenal pheochromocytoma in a 31-year-old patient with von Hippel-Lindau (VHL) syndrome. Coronal reformatted contrast-enhanced computed tomography image demonstrates a heterogeneously enhancing left adrenal mass (*white arrow*), compatible with pheochromocytoma. Note the multiple enhancing solid renal masses owing to multifocal renal cell carcinomas (*curved arrows*) and multiple nonenhancing hypodense renal cysts (*transparent arrows*) in this patient with VHL syndrome.

that of other adrenal masses. Small masses are typically homogeneous, yet larger masses are usually heterogeneous and may show areas of hemorrhage or necrosis.[50] After intravenous contrast administration, most pheochromocytomas demonstrate intense enhancement. The washout characteristics of pheochromocytomas are variable. They typically demonstrate washout values similar to malignant lesions, regardless of whether they are benign or malignant.[39] However, some pheochromocytomas demonstrate significant washout values overlapping with adenoma.[80,81]

On MR imaging, most pheochromocytomas demonstrate high signal intensity on T2-weighted images, which was classically described as a "light bulb" and regarded as characteristic for pheochromocytoma (**Fig. 18**). However, recent studies found that 30% of pheochromocytomas demonstrate intermediate to low signal on T2-weighted images or are inhomogeneous secondary to hemorrhagic, cystic, or myxoid degeneration (**Fig. 19**).[2]

Cystic pheochromocytomas are usually large, typically demonstrating a thick enhancing wall with or without septae (see **Fig. 19**). Some of these tumors are nonfunctioning, with negative biochemical findings.[82] Less than 10% of pheochromocytomas show calcification. Very rarely, pheochromocytomas contain intracytoplasmic fat, with inconsistent signal drop on OP images,

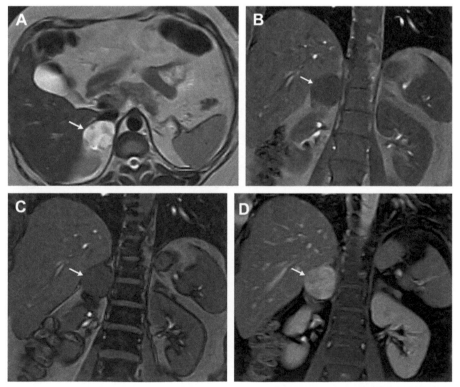

Fig. 18. Pheochromocytoma (*arrows*) on MR imaging. Axial T2-weighted (*A*), axial in-phase (IP) (*B*), and opposed-phase (OP) (*C*) images show right adrenal mass (5 cm) which demonstrates high signal on T2-weighted with lack of signal drop on OP compared with IP imaging. On coronal postcontrast T1-weighted image (*D*), the mass shows intense enhancement. The diagnosis of pheochromocytoma was confirmed on pathology after surgery.

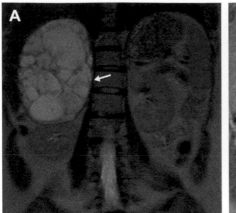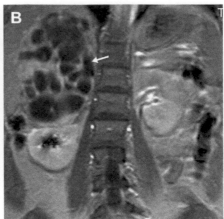

Fig. 19. Cystic pheochromocytoma on MR imaging. Coronal T2-weighted imaging (*A*) and postcontrast coronal T1-weighted imaging (*B*) demonstrate large right adrenal complex cystic lesion (*arrow*), with mural and septal enhancement after contrast administration. The mass is surgically proven to be pheochromocytoma.

potentially mimicking adenoma.[80,83] Conversely, adrenal adenoma typically demonstrates uniform and substantial signal drop. Extensive fatty degeneration in pheochromocytoma can occur rarely and may lead to a large amount of fat cells, which may mimic features of myelolipoma.[37]

Despite the variable imaging appearances of pheochromocytoma, an avidly enhancing mass (3–5 cm in size) with high signal intensity on T2-weighted images and no signal drop on CS-MR imaging is highly suspicious for pheochromocytoma. The presence of local invasion into adjacent structures as well as distant metastases are the only reliable imaging findings for the diagnosis of malignant pheochromocytoma.[35]

Metaiodobenzylguanidine (MIBG) can be useful in the diagnosis of pheochromocytoma. MIBG is particularly helpful in exclusion of bilateral, multifocal, or metastatic disease as well as postoperative recurrence.[84,85]

Adrenocortical carcinoma

Adrenocortical carcinoma is a rare tumor that arises from the adrenal cortex. It shows bimodal age distribution, mainly occurring in children aged 10 years and younger and in adults in their fourth and fifth decades. Approximately 60% of adrenocortical carcinomas are functioning; the functioning form is more common in children than adults.[86,87] Patients often present with Cushing syndrome, virilization, or a combination of both. Feminization and Conn syndrome are much less common.[87,88]

Adrenocortical carcinoma is typically large at presentation, with tumor size greater than 6 cm in greatest dimension. This tumor typically demonstrates heterogeneous appearance on CT and MR

imaging because of the presence of central necrosis and hemorrhage (**Fig. 20**), although smaller lesions may be homogeneous. Calcification is found in 30% of cases.[88] Adrenocortical carcinomas enhance heterogeneously, and CT washout values are similar to those of other malignant adrenal lesions (see **Fig. 20**).[39] The large tumor size and heterogeneity are the most useful features for the diagnosis of these tumors.[7] Very rarely, adrenocortical carcinomas undergo fatty degeneration, producing small foci of intracytoplasmic lipid or fat cells.[89] Vascular invasion of large adrenocortical carcinomas into the inferior vena cava and renal vein is common, particularly in right-sided tumors.[50] Metastases are found frequently at

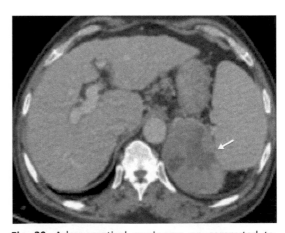

Fig. 20. Adrenocortical carcinoma on computed tomography (CT). Axial contrast-enhanced CT demonstrate a large heterogeneously enhancing mass (*arrow*) involving the left adrenal gland with central necrosis. This was surgically resected and found to represent adrenal cortical carcinoma.

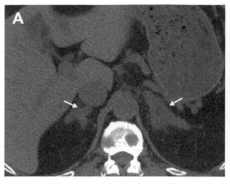
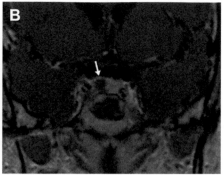

Fig. 21. A 51-year-old man with Cushing disease owing to adrenocorticotropic hormone (ACTH)-dependent/induced adrenal hyperplasia. Axial contrast computed tomography image (*A*) reveal diffuse thickening of the adrenals bilaterally (*arrows*). Coronal-contrast enhanced T1-weighted image through the pituitary reveal a hypoenhancing nodule (*arrow* in *B*) involving the pituitary gland. This was proven to be ACTH-secreting pituitary adenoma after resection.

presentation. The most common sites of metastases are the liver, lungs, bones, and regional lymph nodes.[86,88]

Bilateral Adrenal Lesions

The main differential diagnosis for bilateral adrenal masses includes metastases, lymphoma, granulomatous disease, and hemorrhage, in addition to any other adrenal pathology occurring bilaterally, including adenoma and pheochromocytoma (which is bilateral in 10% of cases). In cortical hyperplasia, adrenal glands can also be diffusely thickened while maintaining their shape, either in a smooth or nodular fashion.

Adrenal cortical hyperplasia
Adrenal cortical hyperplasia is found in patients with Cushing syndrome and, less commonly, in patients with Conn syndrome. It can be ACTH dependent when induced by stimulation of the adrenal cortex by ACTH secreted by a pituitary adenoma (**Fig. 21**) or a rare ectopic tumor such as bronchogenic carcinomas.[90,91] On rare occasions, ACTH-independent adrenal cortical hyperplasia can result from macronodular hyperplasia with marked adrenal nodularity, also known as ACTH-independent macronodular adrenal hyperplasia (**Fig. 22**), which can lead to distortion and marked nodular thickening of the glands.[92] Another cause is primary pigmented nodular adrenocortical disease, in which the adrenal glands are of normal size or slightly enlarged and show small pigmented nodules, with atrophic intervening cortex.[69]

On imaging, adrenal cortical hyperplasia typically appears as smooth to slightly lobular uniform gland enlargement that maintains an adreniform configuration.[90,93] Nodular hyperplasia is identified only if associated with macronodules. These

macronodules appear as small hypodense-to-isodense nodules with atrophic or normal intervening adrenal tissue.[36]

Using a thickness cutoff of 5 mm, CT is shown to have sensitivity and specificity of 47% and 100%, respectively for diagnosis. Using a 3-mm thickness cutoff, better sensitivity (100%) but lower specificity (54%) has been reported.[94]

The attenuation and signal intensity of adrenal cortical hyperplasia are usually similar to that of the normal gland. In a small percentage of cases, however, the precontrast CT attenuation may be lower. Likewise, the signal intensity may also be lower on the OP compared with IP pulse

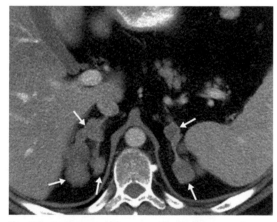

Fig. 22. A 40-year-old man with Cushing syndrome. Axial contrast-enhanced computed tomography images reveal multiple bilateral nodules involving the adrenal glands (*arrows*). Adrenocorticotropic hormone-independent macronodular adrenal hyperplasia was suspected to be the cause of Cushing syndrome based on imaging and biochemical features. It was later confirmed after bilateral adrenalectomy.

sequence, especially in patients with adenomatous cortical nodules.[95]

Adrenal hemorrhage

Adrenal hemorrhage can result from both traumatic and nontraumatic causes, with trauma accounting for 80% of cases. Adrenal hemorrhage is frequently caused by blunt trauma and is usually associated with multiple simultaneous organ injuries.[96] It is usually unilateral (80%) and is more frequently located on the right side. In children, adrenal hemorrhage is sometimes observed in cases of nonaccidental injuries.[97] Nontraumatic adrenal hemorrhage is typically bilateral and associated with causes such as stress (eg, recent surgery, sepsis, organ failure, pregnancy); coagulopathy, including use of an anticoagulant; venous hypertension from adrenal vein or inferior vena cava thrombosis; or hemorrhagic tumor (myelolipoma or, less frequently, adenoma, metastasis, adrenocortical carcinoma, or hemangioma).[98] In rare cases, bilateral adrenal hemorrhage leads to adrenal insufficiency (Addison disease).[99]

In the mildest form of acute adrenal hemorrhage, the gland maintains its adreniform configuration, showing a "tram track" appearance (ie, preserved peripheral enhancement and central hypodensity) together with periadrenal infiltration.[98,100] As bleeding continues, the adrenal gland enlarges, giving the appearance of a mass. CT demonstrates an oval or rounded adrenal mass with an attenuation value greater than simple fluid (ranging from 50–90 HU) (**Fig. 23**).[98] The size and CT density of the adrenal hemorrhage decreases gradually over time, and the majority of cases resolve completely and become undetectable. Chronic hematomas may, however, liquefy and persist as an adrenal pseudocyst or calcification (see **Fig. 16**).[50,101]

MR imaging is the most sensitive and specific modality for diagnosing adrenal hemorrhage. The MR imaging features vary according to the duration of the hematoma.[65] In the acute stage (<7 days), deoxyhemoglobin is isointense to slightly hypointense on T1-weighted images and has low signal intensity on T2-weighted images. In the subacute stage (1–7 weeks), methemoglobin is hyperintense on T1-weighted images. Initially, methemoglobin is intracellular and has low signal intensity on T2-weighted images. With red cell lysis, the methemoglobin becomes extracellular and has high signal intensity on T2-weighted images. In the chronic stage (>7 weeks), the hemorrhage has low signal intensity on both T1-weighted and T2-weighted images because of the presence of hemosiderin, which demonstrates "blooming" on gradient echo sequences.

The presence of an underlying hemorrhagic adrenal tumor should be excluded in patients with no risk factor for hemorrhage. Further imaging with contrast-enhanced CT or MR imaging using a subtraction technique is useful to assess for an enhancing underlying tumor.[35] If a hemorrhage is confirmed, follow-up imaging should be indicated to ensure its decrease in size and resolution.[36]

Hemangioma

Adrenal hemangioma is an extremely rare benign tumor. These tumors are highly vascular, consisting of 2 main types: cavernous and, less frequently, capillary hemangioma. Because of their clinically silent course, they are often very large at presentation.[43]

Characteristic features of hemangiomas include phleboliths and persistent peripheral nodular enhancement either with or without delayed

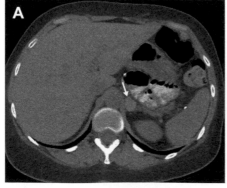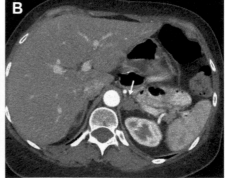

Fig. 23. Left adrenal mass in a 52-year-old patient with acute flank pain. Noncontrast (*A*) and postcontrast (*B*) computed tomography images show a small oval predominantly hyperdense mass (involving the left adrenal gland [*arrow*] exhibiting 79 Hounsfield units) in the left adrenal gland with no significant postcontrast enhancement, compatible with acute hematoma.

central filling.[100] Dystrophic calcification may be present in areas of previous hemorrhage.[36]

On MR imaging, hemangiomas are typically hyperintense on T2-weighted images and hypointense on T1-weighted images. However, they may show central areas of high T1-weighted imaging signal owing to hemorrhage.[93,100] Hemangiomas may be difficult to differentiate from malignant lesions, and a correct diagnosis may be reached only after image-guided biopsy or surgical resection.[36]

Adrenal Masses of Neural Crest Origin

These adrenal tumors are derived from the primordial neural crest cells that form the sympathetic nervous system. They range from malignant (neuroblastoma) to benign (ganglioneuroma); ganglioneuroblastoma is of intermediate malignant potential.

Neuroblastoma
Neuroblastoma is a malignant tumor composed of primitive neuroblasts. The adrenal gland is the most common site of primary neuroblastoma, accounting for 35% to 40% of cases.[102] These tumors are typically found in infants and very young children (mean presentation age, 22 months), and 95% of cases are detected in children younger than 10 years.[103] Neuroblastoma can metastasize to the bones, liver, lymph nodes, and skin. Seventy percent of cases have metastatic disease upon presentation.[104]

On CT, neuroblastoma appears as a large, irregular, heterogenous mass with areas of necrosis or hemorrhage. Coarse amorphous calcification is present in 80% to 90% of cases (**Fig. 24**).[105]

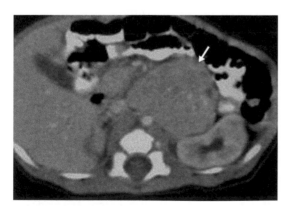

Fig. 24. Adrenal neuroblastoma on computed tomography (CT). Axial unenhanced and contrast-enhanced CT images demonstrate large heterogeneous mass (*arrow*) involving the left adrenal with tiny punctate calcifications. This was surgically resected and proven to represent neuroblastoma.

Encasement and narrowing of adjacent vessels may occur. In aggressive tumors, there can be direct invasion of local soft tissues and organs.[106] Neuroblastoma usually demonstrates heterogeneous low signal intensity on T1-weighted images and high signal intensity on T2-weighted images, with variable and heterogeneous enhancement. Cystic changes demonstrate high signal intensity on T2-weighted images with areas of T1-hyperintense hemorrhage.[106] Gahr and colleagues[107] suggested that DWI is effective for the differentiation of neuroblastoma, ganglioneuroblastoma and ganglioneuroma. They found that the ADC values of ganglioneuroma and ganglioneuroblastoma are significantly higher than those of neuroblastomas. No ganglioneuroma or ganglioneuroblastoma had an ADC value of less than $1.1 \times 10^{-3} mm^2/s$.

Ganglioneuroma
Ganglioneuroma is a rare benign neoplasm composed of Schwann cells and ganglion cells. These tumors grow slowly and are often discovered incidentally. They have a good prognosis after surgical resection.[104] They are most often seen in young adults; 60% of patients are younger than 20 years at the time of diagnosis. These tumors are more common in the posterior mediastinum and retroperitoneum than in the adrenal gland (20%–30% of cases).[76]

Adrenal ganglioneuroma is typically seen as a well-circumscribed, mildly enhancing, lobulated, hypodense mass on CT. Areas of necrosis and hemorrhage have been described. Twenty percent to 30% of cases show discrete punctate calcifications.[106] On MR imaging, ganglioneuroma typically demonstrates homogenous low signal intensity on T1-weighted images and mildly to moderately high signal intensity on T2-weighted images, depending on its content of myxoid stroma (**Fig. 25**).[104] A whorled appearance of T2 hyperintensity has been described owing to interlacing bundles of longitudinal and transverse Schwann cells or collagen fibers.[108] Contrast-enhanced CT and MR imaging typically demonstrate slight enhancement with progressive enhancement on delayed phase.[109]

Ganglioneuroblastoma
Ganglioneuroblastoma is an intermediate-grade tumor composed of mature ganglion cells and primitive neuroblasts. Ganglioneuroblastoma typically occurs in the pediatric population, with a mean presentation age of 2 to 4 years, and a rare incidence in individuals older than 10 years.[110] Ganglioneuroblastomas are generally smaller and more well-defined than neuroblastoma at

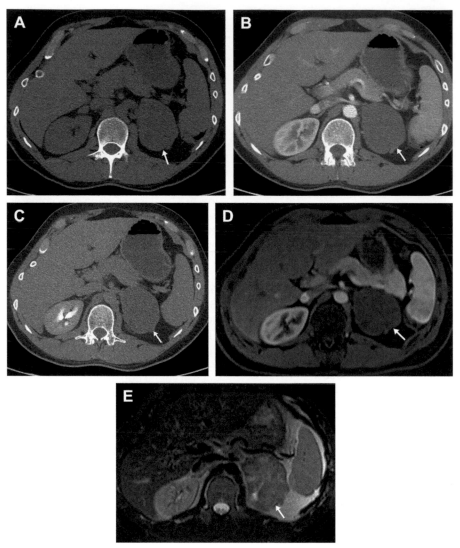

Fig. 25. Adrenal ganglioneuroma on computed tomography (CT) and MR imaging. Axial nonenhanced CT (*A*), contrast-enhanced CT in venous (*B*), and delayed 15 minutes (*C*), demonstrate a well-circumscribed oval mass (*arrows*) involving the left adrenal gland with an attenuation value of 19, 35, and 38 Hounsfield units on noncontrast, venous, and delayed phase imaging, respectively, indicating slight progressive enhancement owing to the myxoid stroma. Axial contrast enhanced T1-weighted imaging (*D*) and T2-weighted imaging (*E*) demonstrates a low signal intensity on T1-weighted imaging with slight postcontrast enhancement (*arrow*) and mildly increased signal intensity on T2-weighted images (*arrow*).

diagnosis.[111] Imaging appearance vary and can be predominantly solid or cystic.[108] These tumors usually demonstrate intermediate signal intensity on T1-weighted images and heterogeneously high signal intensity on T2-weighted images, with heterogeneous moderate contrast enhancement.[112]

Adrenal Calcification

Adrenal calcification can be observed in a variety of lesions, including adrenal cyst, adenoma, adrenocortical carcinoma, myelolipoma, pheochromocytoma, adrenal hemorrhage, and chronic granulomatous diseases. Calcification in an adrenal mass is overall nonspecific. Ancillary CT findings may help to indicate an underlying etiology of calcification. For example, diffuse bilateral calcification in normal-sized or atrophic glands is suggestive of an old hemorrhage or granulomatous infection. The pattern of calcification can be helpful, as in the case of adrenal pseudocyst, which demonstrates peripheral curvilinear calcification. To narrow the differential diagnosis, the pattern of calcification in an adrenal mass must be correlated with other imaging features such as size, homogeneity, enhancement pattern, and margins.[113]

Tuberculosis and histoplasmosis are granulomatous diseases that can affect adrenal glands. In the early acute stages of granulomatous diseases, bilateral enlargement, with or without contour preservation, can be seen. After intravenous administration of contrast, peripheral marginal enhancement with a nonenhancing necrotic center can be noted.[114] Chronic infection is characterized typically by calcification, which may be associated with significant gland destruction and subsequent adrenal insufficiency (Addison disease).[42]

Another cause of adrenal gland calcification is Wolman disease, a rare recessive autosomal inborn error of metabolism. It leads to fat accumulation in multiple organs such as the liver, spleen, lymph nodes, small bowel, and adrenal cortex. A characteristic of Wolman disease is the presence of dense punctuate calcifications in bilaterally enlarged adrenal glands that maintain adeniform shape.[111]

Key Teaching Points and a Practical Approach to Diagnosis

- In imaging evaluation of adrenal mass, the most important utility is to differentiate between adenomas and nonadenomatous adrenal masses.
- CT washout technique is the most sensitive and specific for characterization of adrenal adenoma.
- Noncontrast attenuation less than 10 Hounsfield units is most compatible with a lipid-rich adenoma.
- Absolute percentage washout of greater than or equal to 60%, and relative percentage washout of greater than or equal to 40% are highly sensitive and specific for lipid-poor adenoma.
- MR imaging is helpful in the setting of a heterogeneous mass, or when there is contraindication of iodinated contrast medium (allergy or renal insufficiency).
- Chemical shift IP and OP pulse sequences are useful for diagnosing lipid-rich and most lipid-poor adenomas. It is limited at characterizing cases of lipid-poor adenomas with noncontrast CT attenuation of greater than 30 HU.
- Various morphologic patterns can help to make a specific diagnosis, for example:
  o Adrenal adenoma is the most common adrenal mass containing intracytoplasmic lipid.
    ■ Rarely, metastases secondary to clear cell renal cell carcinoma and hepatocellular carcinoma can contain intracytoplasmic lipid, thus can mimic adenoma on chemical shift MR imaging.
    ■ Simple cyst can also mimic adenoma on unenhanced CT.
  o The presence of fat cells in an adrenal mass is consistent with myelolipoma.
    ■ Rarely, bilateral fatty masses can be seen in congenital adrenal hyperplasia
    ■ Very rarely, adrenocortical carcinoma contains fat cells.
- Adrenal mass with a simple fluid attenuation is consistent with a simple cyst.
  o Complex features including calcification can be seen in pseudocysts. Pseudocyst can have heterogeneous complex features, thus may mimic malignancy.
- Avidly enhancing adrenal lesion with a high signal intensity of T2-weighted images raises the suspicion of pheochromocytoma. Biochemical evidence can be helpful in the majority of cases.
- Lesion with hemorrhagic CT density or MR imaging signal intensity is suggestive of adrenal hemorrhage. However, in patients with no risk factor for nontraumatic hemorrhage, hemorrhagic adrenal tumor has to be excluded (contrast-enhanced MR imaging with subtraction technique and/or follow-up).
- Diffuse bilateral gland thickening with preserved adreniform configuration, in patients with hypercortisolism (Cushing) is suggestive of adrenal hyperplasia. Other causes of diffuse gland enlargement include lymphoma, metastases or adrenal hemorrhage.
- Adrenal calcification can be seen in both benign and malignant lesions. Curvilinear calcification suggests an adrenal pseudocyst. Bilateral calcification in atrophic or normal sized adrenal glands is usually the sequela of previous hemorrhage or granulomatous infection.

SUMMARY

Proper imaging, combined with detailed clinical evaluation, provides robust assessment of adrenal pathologies. The small incidental adrenal nodules are overwhelmingly benign, making further evaluation and treatment often unnecessary. Some tumors such as lipid-rich adenoma and myelolipoma have characteristic features that can be diagnosed accurately, thus preventing further unnecessary workup. Many indeterminate lesions can be considered benign if stability for greater than 1 year can be shown; if no prior images are available and characteristics are indeterminate, a 12-month follow-up evaluation is suggested. When imaging or clinical factors are more suspicious, additional noninvasive imaging such as FDG PET-CT can be a useful adjunct. Finally, when a lesion remains indeterminate, adrenal biopsy may be considered; resection may be prudent when masses are greater than 4 cm because of the higher chance of malignancy.

REFERENCES

1. Caoili EM, Korobkin M, Francis IR, et al. Adrenal masses: characterization with combined unenhanced and delayed enhanced CT. Radiology 2002;222(3):629–33.
2. Blake MA, Cronin CG, Boland GW. Adrenal imaging. AJR Am J Roentgenol 2010;194(6):1450–60.
3. Caoili EM, Korobkin M, Francis IR, et al. Delayed enhanced CT of lipid-poor adrenal adenomas. AJR Am J Roentgenol 2000;175(5):1411–5.
4. Park BK, Kim CK, Kim B, et al. Comparison of delayed enhanced CT and chemical shift MR for evaluating hyperattenuating incidental adrenal masses. Radiology 2007;243(3):760–5.
5. Petersilka M, Bruder H, Krauss B, et al. Technical principles of dual source CT. Eur J Radiol 2008; 68(3):362–8.
6. Graser A, Johnson TR, Chandarana H, et al. Dual energy CT: preliminary observations and potential clinical applications in the abdomen. Eur Radiol 2009;19(1):13–23.
7. Korivi BR, Elsayes KM, de Castro SF, et al. An update of practical CT adrenal imaging: what physicians need to know. Curr Radiol Rep 2015; 3(4):1–11.
8. Coursey CA, Nelson RC, Boll DT, et al. Dual-energy multidetector CT: how does it work, what can it tell us, and when can we use it in abdominopelvic imaging? Radiographics 2010;30(4):1037–55.
9. Gupta RT, Ho LM, Marin D, et al. Dual-energy CT for characterization of adrenal nodules: initial experience. AJR Am J Roentgenol 2010;194(6): 1479–83.
10. Shi JW, Dai HZ, Shen L, et al. Dual-energy CT: clinical application in differentiating an adrenal adenoma from a metastasis. Acta Radiol 2014;55(4): 505–12.
11. Qin HY, Sun HR, Li YJ, et al. Application of CT perfusion imaging to the histological differentiation of adrenal gland tumors. Eur J Radiol 2012;81(3): 502–7.
12. Qin HY, Sun H, Wang X, et al. Correlation between CT perfusion parameters and microvessel density and vascular endothelial growth factor in adrenal tumors. PLoS One 2013;8(11):e79911.
13. Fujiyoshi F, Nakajo M, Fukukura Y, et al. Characterization of adrenal tumors by chemical shift fast low-angle shot MR imaging: comparison of four methods of quantitative evaluation. AJR Am J Roentgenol 2003;180(6):1649–57.
14. Sahdev A, Willatt J, Francis IR, et al. The indeterminate adrenal lesion. Cancer 2010;10:102–13.
15. Miller FH, Wang Y, McCarthy RJ, et al. Utility of diffusion-weighted MRI in characterization of adrenal lesions. AJR Am J Roentgenol 2010;194(2): W179–85.
16. Israel GM, Korobkin M, Wang C, et al. Comparison of unenhanced CT and chemical shift MRI in evaluating lipid-rich adrenal adenomas. AJR Am J Roentgenol 2004;183(1):215–9.
17. Haider MA, Ghai S, Jhaveri K, et al. Chemical shift MR imaging of hyperattenuating (>10 HU) adrenal masses: does it still have a role? Radiology 2004; 231(3):711–6.
18. Gabriel H, Pizzitola V, McComb EN, et al. Adrenal lesions with heterogeneous suppression on chemical shift imaging: clinical implications. J Magn Reson Imaging 2004;19(3):308–16.
19. Sandrasegaran K, Patel AA, Ramaswamy R, et al. Characterization of adrenal masses with diffusion-weighted imaging. AJR Am J Roentgenol 2011; 197(1):132–8.
20. Morani AC, Elsayes KM, Liu PS, et al. Abdominal applications of diffusion-weighted magnetic resonance imaging: where do we stand. World J Radiol 2013;5(3):68–80.
21. El-Kalioubie M, Emad-Eldin S, Abdelaziz O. Diffusion-weighted MRI in adrenal lesions: a warranted adjunct? Egypt J Radiol Nucl Med 2016;47(2): 599–606.
22. Tsushima Y, Takahashi-Taketomi A, Endo K. Diagnostic utility of diffusion-weighted MR imaging and apparent diffusion coefficient value for the diagnosis of adrenal tumors. J Magn Reson Imaging 2009;29(1):112–7.
23. Melo HJ, Goldman SM, Szejnfeld J, et al. Application of a protocol for magnetic resonance spectroscopy of adrenal glands: an experiment with over 100 cases. Radiol Bras 2014;47(6):333–41.
24. Faria JF, Goldman SM, Szejnfeld J, et al. Adrenal masses: characterization with in vivo proton MR spectroscopy–initial experience. Radiology 2007; 245(3):788–97.
25. Kim S, Salibi N, Hardie AD, et al. Characterization of adrenal pheochromocytoma using respiratory-triggered proton MR spectroscopy: initial experience. AJR Am J Roentgenol 2009;192(2):450–4.
26. Wong KK, Arabi M, Bou-Assaly W, et al. Evaluation of incidentally discovered adrenal masses with PET and PET/CT. Eur J Radiol 2012;81(3):441–50.
27. Boland GW, Dwamena BA, Jagtiani Sangwaiya M, et al. Characterization of adrenal masses by using

FDG PET: a systematic review and meta-analysis of diagnostic test performance. Radiology 2011; 259(1):117–26.

28. Metser U, Miller E, Lerman H, et al. 18F-FDG PET/CT in the evaluation of adrenal masses. J Nucl Med 2006;47(1):32–7.

29. Brady MJ, Thomas J, Wong TZ, et al. Adrenal nodules at FDG PET/CT in patients known to have or suspected of having lung cancer: a proposal for an efficient diagnostic algorithm. Radiology 2009; 250(2):523–30.

30. Vikram R, Yeung HD, Macapinlac HA, et al. Utility of PET/CT in differentiating benign from malignant adrenal nodules in patients with cancer. AJR Am J Roentgenol 2008;191(5):1545–51.

31. Kunikowska J, Matyskiel R, Toutounchi S, et al. What parameters from 18F-FDG PET/CT are useful in evaluation of adrenal lesions? Eur J Nucl Med Mol Imaging 2014;41(12):2273–80.

32. Chong S, Lee KS, Kim HY, et al. Integrated PET-CT for the characterization of adrenal gland lesions in cancer patients: diagnostic efficacy and interpretation pitfalls. Radiographics 2006;26(6):1811–24 [discussion: 1824–16].

33. Jana S, Zhang T, Milstein DM, et al. FDG-PET and CT characterization of adrenal lesions in cancer patients. Eur J Nucl Med Mol Imaging 2006; 33(1):29–35.

34. Reznek RH, Armstrong P. The adrenal gland. Clin Endocrinol (Oxf) 1994;40(5):561–76.

35. Taffel M, Haji-Momenian S, Nikolaidis P, et al. Adrenal imaging: a comprehensive review. Radiol Clin North Am 2012;50(2):219–43.

36. Lattin GE Jr, Sturgill ED, Tujo CA, et al. From the radiologic pathology archives: adrenal tumors and tumor-like conditions in the adult: radiologic-pathologic correlation. Radiographics 2014;34(3): 805–29.

37. Adam SZ, Nikolaidis P, Horowitz JM, et al. Chemical shift MR imaging of the adrenal gland: principles, pitfalls, and applications. Radiographics 2016;36(2):414–32.

38. Korobkin M, Giordano TJ, Brodeur FJ, et al. Adrenal adenomas: relationship between histologic lipid and CT and MR findings. Radiology 1996;200(3): 743–7.

39. Szolar DH, Korobkin M, Reittner P, et al. Adrenocortical carcinomas and adrenal pheochromocytomas: mass and enhancement loss evaluation at delayed contrast-enhanced CT. Radiology 2005; 234(2):479–85.

40. Boland GW, Lee MJ, Gazelle GS, et al. Characterization of adrenal masses using unenhanced CT: an analysis of the CT literature. AJR Am J Roentgenol 1998;171(1):201–4.

41. Johnson PT, Horton KM, Fishman EK. Adrenal imaging with multidetector CT: evidence-based protocol optimization and interpretative practice. Radiographics 2009;29(5):1319–31.

42. Mayo-Smith WW, Boland GW, Noto RB, et al. State-of-the-art adrenal imaging. Radiographics 2001; 21(4):995–1012.

43. Boland GW, Blake MA, Hahn PF, et al. Incidental adrenal lesions: principles, techniques, and algorithms for imaging characterization. Radiology 2008;249(3):756–75.

44. Papotti M, Sapino A, Mazza E, et al. Lipomatous changes in adrenocortical adenomas: report of two cases. Endocr Pathol 1996;7(3):223–8.

45. Barzon L, Sonino N, Fallo F, et al. Prevalence and natural history of adrenal incidentalomas. Eur J Endocrinol 2003;149(4):273–85.

46. DeAtkine AB, Dunnick NR. The adrenal glands. Semin Oncol 1991;18(2):131–9.

47. Lee JE, Evans DB, Hickey RC, et al. Unknown primary cancer presenting as an adrenal mass: frequency and implications for diagnostic evaluation of adrenal incidentalomas. Surgery 1998;124(6): 1115–22.

48. Lam KY, Lo CY. Metastatic tumours of the adrenal glands: a 30-year experience in a teaching hospital. Clin Endocrinol (Oxf) 2002;56(1):95–101.

49. Song JH, Grand DJ, Beland MD, et al. Morphologic features of 211 adrenal masses at initial contrast-enhanced CT: can we differentiate benign from malignant lesions using imaging features alone? AJR Am J Roentgenol 2013;201(6):1248–53.

50. Song JH, Mayo-Smith WW. Current status of imaging for adrenal gland tumors. Surg Oncol Clin N Am 2014;23(4):847–61.

51. Blake MA, Kalra MK, Sweeney AT, et al. Distinguishing benign from malignant adrenal masses: multi-detector row CT protocol with 10-minute delay. Radiology 2006;238(2):578–85.

52. Namimoto T, Yamashita Y, Mitsuzaki K, et al. Adrenal masses: quantification of fat content with double-echo chemical shift in-phase and opposed-phase FLASH MR images for differentiation of adrenal adenomas. Radiology 2001;218(3):642–6.

53. Korobkin M, Lombardi TJ, Aisen AM, et al. Characterization of adrenal masses with chemical shift and gadolinium-enhanced MR imaging. Radiology 1995;197(2):411–8.

54. Otal P, Escourrou G, Mazerolles C, et al. Imaging features of uncommon adrenal masses with histopathologic correlation. Radiographics 1999;19(3): 569–81.

55. Schwartz LH, Macari M, Huvos AG, et al. Collision tumors of the adrenal gland: demonstration and characterization at MR imaging. Radiology 1996; 201(3):757–60.

56. Katabathina VS, Flaherty E, Kaza R, et al. Adrenal collision tumors and their mimics: multimodality imaging findings. Cancer 2013;13(4):602–10.

57. Tappouni R, DeJohn L. AJR teaching file: enlarging adrenal mass previously characterized as an adenoma. AJR Am J Roentgenol 2009;192(6 Suppl):S125–7.

58. Anderson SB, Webb MD, Banks KP. Adrenal collision tumor diagnosed by F-18 fluorodeoxyglucose PET/CT. Clin Nucl Med 2010;35(6):414–7.

59. Bertolini F, Rossi G, Fiocchi F, et al. Primary adrenal gland carcinosarcoma associated with metastatic rectal cancer: a hitherto unreported collision tumor. Tumori 2011;97(5):27e–30e.

60. Hagspiel KD. Manifestation of Hodgkin's lymphoma in an adrenal myelolipoma. Eur Radiol 2005;15(8):1757–9.

61. Glazer HS, Lee JK, Balfe DM, et al. Non-Hodgkin lymphoma: computed tomographic demonstration of unusual extranodal involvement. Radiology 1983;149(1):211–7.

62. Young WF Jr. Clinical practice. The incidentally discovered adrenal mass. N Engl J Med 2007;356(6):601–10.

63. Sohaib SA, Reznek RH. Adrenal imaging. BJU Int 2000;86(Suppl 1):95–110.

64. Zhou L, Peng W, Wang C, et al. Primary adrenal lymphoma: radiological; pathological, clinical correlation. Eur J Radiol 2012;81(3):401–5.

65. Elsayes KM, Mukundan G, Narra VR, et al. Adrenal masses: MR imaging features with pathologic correlation. Radiographics 2004;24(Suppl 1):S73–86.

66. Rashidi A, Fisher SI. Primary adrenal lymphoma: a systematic review. Ann Hematol 2013;92(12):1583–93.

67. Kumar R, Xiu Y, Mavi A, et al. FDG-PET imaging in primary bilateral adrenal lymphoma: a case report and review of the literature. Clin Nucl Med 2005;30(4):222–30.

68. Rao P, Kenney PJ, Wagner BJ, et al. Imaging and pathologic features of myelolipoma. Radiographics 1997;17(6):1373–85.

69. Lack EE. Tumors of the adrenal glands and extraadrenal paraganglia. Atlas of tumor pathology. Washington, DC: American Registry of Pathology; 2007.

70. Ioannidis O, Papaemmanouil S, Chatzopoulos S, et al. Giant bilateral symptomatic adrenal myelolipomas associated with congenital adrenal hyperplasia. Pathol Oncol Res 2011;17(3):775–8.

71. Sanal HT, Kocaoglu M, Yildirim D, et al. Imaging features of benign adrenal cysts. Eur J Radiol 2006;60(3):465–9.

72. Foster DG. Adrenal cysts. Review of literature and report of case. Arch Surg 1966;92(1):131–43.

73. Ricci Z, Chernyak V, Hsu K, et al. Adrenal cysts: natural history by long-term imaging follow-up. AJR Am J Roentgenol 2013;201(5):1009–16.

74. Rozenblit A, Morehouse HT, Amis ES Jr. Cystic adrenal lesions: CT features. Radiology 1996;201(2):541–8.

75. Polat P, Kantarci M, Alper F, et al. Hydatid disease from head to toe. Radiographics 2003;23(2):475–94 [quiz: 536–7].

76. Guo YK, Yang ZG, Li Y, et al. Uncommon adrenal masses: CT and MRI features with histopathologic correlation. Eur J Radiol 2007;62(3):359–70.

77. Touiti D, Deligne E, Cherras A, et al. Cystic lymphangioma in the adrenal gland: a case report. Ann Urol (Paris) 2003;37(4):170–2 [in French].

78. Mittendorf EA, Evans DB, Lee JE, et al. Pheochromocytoma: advances in genetics, diagnosis, localization, and treatment. Hematol Oncol Clin North Am 2007;21(3):509–25, ix.

79. Johnson PT, Horton KM, Fishman EK. Adrenal mass imaging with multidetector CT: pathologic conditions, pearls, and pitfalls. Radiographics 2009;29(5):1333–51.

80. Blake MA, Krishnamoorthy SK, Boland GW, et al. Low-density pheochromocytoma on CT: a mimicker of adrenal adenoma. AJR Am J Roentgenol 2003;181(6):1663–8.

81. Park BK, Kim B, Ko K, et al. Adrenal masses falsely diagnosed as adenomas on unenhanced and delayed contrast-enhanced computed tomography: pathological correlation. Eur Radiol 2006;16(3):642–7.

82. Andreoni C, Krebs RK, Bruna PC, et al. Cystic phaeochromocytoma is a distinctive subgroup with special clinical, imaging and histological features that might mislead the diagnosis. BJU Int 2008;101(3):345–50.

83. Schieda N, Alrashed A, Flood TA, et al. Comparison of quantitative MRI and CT washout analysis for differentiation of adrenal pheochromocytoma from adrenal adenoma. AJR Am J Roentgenol 2016;206(6):1141–8.

84. Maurea S, Klain M, Mainolfi C, et al. The diagnostic role of radionuclide imaging in evaluation of patients with nonhypersecreting adrenal masses. J Nucl Med 2001;42(6):884–92.

85. Tenenbaum F, Lumbroso J, Schlumberger M, et al. Comparison of radiolabeled octreotide and meta-iodobenzylguanidine (MIBG) scintigraphy in malignant pheochromocytoma. J Nucl Med 1995;36(1):1–6.

86. Ng L, Libertino JM. Adrenocortical carcinoma: diagnosis, evaluation and treatment. J Urol 2003;169(1):5–11.

87. Icard P, Goudet P, Charpenay C, et al. Adrenocortical carcinomas: surgical trends and results of a 253-patient series from the French Association of Endocrine Surgeons study group. World J Surg 2001;25(7):891–7.

88. Reznek RH, Narayanan P. Primary adrenal malignancy. In: Husband JE, Reznek RH, editors. Husband & Reznek's imaging in oncology. 3rd edition. London (UK): Informa Healthcare; 2010. p. 280–98.

89. Schlund JF, Kenney PJ, Brown ED, et al. Adreno-cortical carcinoma: MR imaging appearance with current techniques. J Magn Reson Imaging 1995; 5(2):171–4.

90. Sohaib SA, Hanson JA, Newell-Price JD, et al. CT appearance of the adrenal glands in adrenocorti-cotrophic hormone-dependent Cushing's syndrome. AJR Am J Roentgenol 1999;172(4):997–1002.

91. Doppman JL, Chrousos GP, Papanicolaou DA, et al. Adrenocorticotropin-independent macronod-ular adrenal hyperplasia: an uncommon cause of primary adrenal hypercortisolism. Radiology 2000;216(3):797–802.

92. Dobbie JW. Adrenocortical nodular hyperplasia: the ageing adrenal. J Pathol 1969;99(1):1–18.

93. Lockhart ME, Smith JK, Kenney PJ. Imaging of ad-renal masses. Eur J Radiol 2002;41(2):95–112.

94. Lingam RK, Sohaib SA, Vlahos I, et al. CT of pri-mary hyperaldosteronism (Conn's syndrome): the value of measuring the adrenal gland. AJR Am J Roentgenol 2003;181(3):843–9.

95. Lumachi F, Zucchetta P, Marzola MC, et al. Usefulness of CT scan, MRI and radiocholesterol scintigraphy for adrenal imaging in Cushing's syndrome. Nucl Med Commun 2002;23(5): 469–73.

96. Rana AI, Kenney PJ, Lockhart ME, et al. Adrenal gland hematomas in trauma patients. Radiology 2004;230(3):669–75.

97. Nimkin K, Teeger S, Wallach MT, et al. Adrenal hemorrhage in abused children: imaging and post-mortem findings. AJR Am J Roentgenol 1994; 162(3):661–3.

98. Jordan E, Poder L, Courtier J, et al. Imaging of non-traumatic adrenal hemorrhage. AJR Am J Roent-genol 2012;199(1):W91–8.

99. Ten S, New M, Maclaren N. Clinical review 130: Ad-dison's disease 2001. J Clin Endocrinol Metab 2001;86(7):2909–22.

100. Kawashima A, Sandler CM, Ernst RD, et al. Imag-ing of nontraumatic hemorrhage of the adrenal gland. Radiographics 1999;19(4):949–63.

101. Huelsen-Katz AM, Schouten BJ, Jardine DL, et al. Pictorial evolution of bilateral adrenal haemor-rhage. Intern Med J 2010;40(1):87–8.

102. Papaioannou G, McHugh K. Neuroblastoma in childhood: review and radiological findings. Can-cer 2005;5:116–27.

103. Brossard J, Bernstein ML, Lemieux B. Neuroblas-toma: an enigmatic disease. Br Med Bull 1996; 52(4):787–801.

104. Rha SE, Byun JY, Jung SE, et al. Neurogenic tu-mors in the abdomen: tumor types and imaging characteristics. Radiographics 2003;23(1):29–43.

105. Abramson SJ. Adrenal neoplasms in children. Ra-diol Clin North Am 1997;35(6):1415–53.

106. Lonergan GJ, Schwab CM, Suarez ES, et al. Neu-roblastoma, ganglioneuroblastoma, and ganglio-neuroma: radiologic-pathologic correlation. Radiographics 2002;22(4):911–34.

107. Gahr N, Darge K, Hahn G, et al. Diffusion-weighted MRI for differentiation of neuroblastoma and gan-glioneuroblastoma/ganglioneuroma. Eur J Radiol 2011;79(3):443–6.

108. Rajiah P, Sinha R, Cuevas C, et al. Imaging of un-common retroperitoneal masses. Radiographics 2011;31(4):949–76.

109. Scherer A, Niehues T, Engelbrecht V, et al. Imaging diagnosis of retroperitoneal ganglioneuroma in childhood. Pediatr Radiol 2001;31(2):106–10.

110. Yamanaka M, Saitoh F, Saitoh H, et al. Primary retroperitoneal ganglioneuroblastoma in an adult. Int J Urol 2001;8(3):130–2.

111. Westra SJ, Zaninovic AC, Hall TR, et al. Imaging of the adrenal gland in children. Radiographics 1994; 14(6):1323–40.

112. McLoughlin RF, Bilbey JH. Tumors of the adrenal gland: findings on CT and MR imaging. AJR Am J Roentgenol 1994;163(6):1413–8.

113. Paterson A. Adrenal pathology in childhood: a spectrum of disease. Eur Radiol 2002;12(10): 2491–508.

114. Guo YK, Yang ZG, Li Y, et al. Addison's disease due to adrenal tuberculosis: contrast-enhanced CT features and clinical duration correlation. Eur J Radiol 2007;62(1):126–31.

Upper and Lower Tract Urothelial Imaging Using Computed Tomography Urography

Siva P. Raman, MD*, Elliot K. Fishman, MD

KEYWORDS

- Transitional cell carcinoma • Computed tomography (CT) • Kidney • Ureter • Bladder
- Single-bolus • Split-bolus

KEY POINTS

- Appropriate technique is critical in the diagnosis of urothelial tumors anywhere in the urinary tract, because subtle or small tumors may be virtually impossible to identify without appropriate distension and the correct phase of contrast.
- There are several options when designing a computed tomography (CT) urography protocol, the most important of which are the single-bolus and split-bolus techniques, which offer a trade-off between maximal sensitivity and increased radiation dose.
- The most important CT imaging features of urothelial malignancy (whether in the urinary bladder, ureters, or intrarenal collecting systems) include focal urothelial thickening, urothelial hyperenhancement, a focal nodule/mass, asymmetric collecting system dilatation, and urothelial calcification.

INTRODUCTION

Computed tomography (CT) urography is the best noninvasive method of evaluating the upper urinary tract for urothelial malignancies, most importantly transitional cell carcinoma. In particular, CT urography has proved to be effective in the assessment of the upper urinary tracts in patients who present with painless hematuria, with sensitivities of more than 90%.[1] Accordingly, CT urography is now a widely accepted part of the routine evaluation of patients who present with hematuria, serving as the primary means of screening the upper urinary tract for malignancy. Just as importantly, although CT has historically been considered purely as a means of evaluating the upper urinary tracts (ie, intrarenal collecting systems and ureters), with the evaluation of the bladder having largely been left to the domain of direct visualization under cystoscopy, it has increasingly become evident that many bladder tumors are readily visible on CT, provided that the proper CT protocols are used and that the bladder is appropriately evaluated during image review. Although cystoscopy is (rightly) recommended on a routine basis for patients who present with gross hematuria, many patients, particularly when presenting in the emergency room setting, do not go on to undergo cystoscopy and are subsequently lost to follow-up, making careful examination of the bladder increasingly important when evaluating patients with CT on their initial presentations.

This article was previously published in March 2017 *Radiologic Clinics*, Volume 55, Issue 2.
Department of Radiology, Johns Hopkins University, JHOC 3251, 601 North Caroline Street, Baltimore, MD 21287, USA
* Corresponding author.
E-mail address: srsraman3@gmail.com

Urol Clin N Am 45 (2018) 389–405
https://doi.org/10.1016/j.ucl.2018.03.004

However, the utility of CT urography, whether in the upper or lower urinary tract, is heavily contingent on the use of optimized CT protocols and proper image acquisition techniques, because poor technique can create significant barriers to making a correct radiologic interpretation, particularly given that identification of subtle tumors can be nearly impossible in the absence of good collecting system distension and opacification. Moreover, although standard axial image review may be sufficient in most other parts of the abdomen and pelvis, evaluation of the collecting systems and ureters presents a prime example of an application for which standard axial images may not be sufficient to identify many subtle urothelial tumors, and for which the use of multiplanar reformations and three-dimensional (3D) imaging techniques may be helpful (or even necessary) for the identification of small or difficult-to-see lesions.

This article focuses primarily on the appropriate protocols for optimizing CT urography acquisitions, including a discussion of the many different protocol options available, both in terms of contrast administration and the timing of imaging acquisitions, as well as the use of several ancillary techniques designed to increase collecting system distension and opacification. In addition, this this article discusses the imaging findings that should raise concern for urothelial carcinoma at each of the 3 segments of the urinary tract, namely the intrarenal collecting systems, ureters, and the bladder, and the best means of using 3D reconstructions at each of these 3 sites for augmenting standard axial image review.

BACKGROUND

Urothelial carcinoma of the upper urinary tract (including the intrarenal collecting systems, renal pelvis, and ureters) is uncommon, although the renal pelvis is probably the second most common location for urothelial carcinoma following the bladder. Although exact numbers are difficult to obtain for the incidence of upper urinary tract tumors given their rarity, it is thought that roughly 2300 patients in the United States were diagnosed with transitional cell carcinoma of the ureter (with 700 deaths) in 2008. Upper tract tumors account for only 5% of all urothelial carcinomas and ~15% of all renal tumors.[2] The major risk factors for urothelial carcinoma of the upper urinary tract include male gender, increasing age, cigarette smoking and tobacco use, phenacetin abuse, exposure to certain chemicals and drugs (such as cyclophosphamide), chronic hydronephrosis, and a history of prior recurrent or severe urinary tract infections. Patients with upper tract tumors most commonly present with hematuria (microscopic or gross) or flank pain, although many tumors (~20%) may be discovered incidentally.[3]

In contrast, bladder cancer is very common, representing the most common primary malignancy of the urinary tract, with more than 70,000 new cases and more than 14,000 deaths in 2010.[4] Almost all bladder cancers represent transitional cell carcinomas, although other possible subtypes include squamous cell carcinoma, adenocarcinoma, and rare mucinous neoplasms. Risk factors for bladder cancer are similar to those of upper tract malignancy, including age, male gender, smoking, repeated urinary tract infections, chronic urinary obstruction, and chemical carcinogens. As with upper tract malignancies, these tumors commonly present with hematuria, although macroscopic or gross hematuria is a much bigger risk factor than microscopic hematuria. Other less common presenting symptoms include urinary urgency, urinary frequency, or symptoms caused by metastatic disease.[3–5]

One of the unique features of transitional cell carcinoma, regardless of whether it arises in the upper or lower urinary tract, is its strong tendency for both recurrence and multifocality, with almost 4% of patients with bladder cancer going on to develop a transitional cell carcinoma in the upper urinary tract.[3–5]

TECHNIQUE

In general, when designing a CT urography protocol, the primary goals of the study are to maximize opacification and distension of the collecting systems and ureters in the delayed excretory phase, so as to increase sensitivity for transitional cell carcinoma, while still having sufficient sensitivity to identify a variety of other abnormalities that may potentially cause hematuria, including renal stones and renal cell carcinoma. Accordingly, there must be a balance between acquiring images of sufficient quality in several different phases so as to maximize sensitivity for significant disorder, while at the same time minimizing radiation dose. The 2 most important CT urography protocols in wide clinical use are[1] the single-bolus technique and[2] split-bolus technique.[6–8]

The single-bolus technique is the most widely used protocol across a spectrum of different clinical practices, and entails giving a single full-strength dose of intravenous contrast (typically roughly 120 mL of Omnipaque-350), followed by the acquisition of separate arterial, venous, and delayed excretory phase images (**Fig. 1**). Given that the entirety of the contrast dose contributes toward the excretory phase and is excreted into

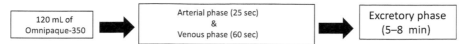

Fig. 1. Typical single-bolus technique protocol.

the intrarenal collecting systems and ureters, this protocol, in theory, maximizes distention and opacification of the collecting systems, including the distal ureters, which are notoriously the most difficult segment of the collecting systems to distend. At the same time, given that multiple different phases of contrast are acquired (ie, arterial, venous, and delayed), this protocol is almost certainly the most sensitive for renal cell carcinoma (regardless of subtype), and the inclusion of noncontrast images can maximize sensitivity for renal and ureteral stones. In addition, this technique is the simplest to perform for technologists, requiring only a single injection of intravenous contrast, at least partially accounting for the widespread popularity of this protocol option. However, given that at least 3 separate contrast phases are acquired (and usually 4 phases when noncontrast images are obtained), this protocol option does have a higher radiation dose compared with the split-bolus technique. It could be argued that this increased radiation dose is a major disadvantage of this protocol option when imaging young patients, in whom the likelihood of either renal cell carcinoma or transitional cell carcinoma is significantly lower.[6–9] Despite the higher radiation doses associated with the single-bolus technique, newer scanner technologies offer some potential in terms of reducing radiation dose, such as the creation of virtual noncontrast images (rather than acquiring a separate noncontrast phase) when studies are acquired using a dual-energy scanner.[2,10–12]

The other major alternative to the single-bolus technique is the split-bolus technique, which involves dividing the contrast dose into 2 separate administrations, such as initially administering 50 mL of intravenous contrast, followed by a second administration of roughly 80 mL of intravenous contrast 5 minutes later, and subsequently acquiring a single set of images at 7 minutes if the kidneys show enhancement of the renal parenchyma in the nephrographic phase and opacification of the collecting

systems and ureters in the excretory phase (**Fig. 2**). This protocol has become increasingly popular as concerns regarding radiation dose have become more prevalent, and it has the advantage of combining 2 separate contrast phases (nephrographic and excretory phases) into a single acquisition, thereby reducing the total number of phases acquired, and, accordingly, reducing the total radiation dose. In theory, instead of acquiring a total of 4 phases (as with the single-bolus technique), this technique might allow clinicians to acquire a total of only 2 or 3 phases (such as noncontrast, arterial, and combined nephrographic/excretory). However, there are significant concerns about this protocol with regard to the robustness of collecting system distention and opacification, particularly given that only a fraction of the total administered contrast dose is excreted into the collecting system, likely reducing the degree of collecting system distention and, in theory, reducing sensitivity for subtle transitional cell carcinomas. A study by Dillman and colleagues[9] found inferior urinary tract distension with the split-bolus technique. In our own experience, this protocol is particularly problematic when evaluating the ureters, with poor distention of the distal ureters.[6–8,13] Another potential disadvantage of this protocol is decreased sensitivity for small or subtle renal cell carcinomas, because only 2 postcontrast phases are available for evaluation of the renal parenchyma, as opposed to 3 phases in the single-bolus technique.

There is a third protocol option, which to our knowledge is used at almost no institution across the country, known as the triple bolus technique. This technique involves splitting the total contrast dose into 3 separate administrations, and subsequently acquiring a combined corticomedullary-nephrographic-excretory phase. As with the split-bolus technique, this protocol option considerably diminishes the total radiation dose as a result of reducing the total number of

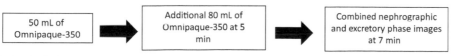

Fig. 2. Typical split-bolus technique protocol.

acquired contrast phases, at the significant expense of poor collecting system distention and opacification. Just as importantly, this protocol is poor in terms of evaluating for renal cell carcinoma, given the absence of dedicated arterial phase images, which are the most sensitive for clear cell renal cell carcinoma. To our knowledge, this is purely a protocol of academic interest, and is not practically used at any major institution.[2]

Regardless of which of the major contrast administration protocols are used, there are several additional ancillary techniques that have been described in the literature (each of which has been shown to have variable efficacy), designed to potentially improve the degree of collecting system distention. Of these, the 2 techniques with the most supporting data are the use of a diuretic (ie, intravenous Lasix) before the study, and the administration of either oral or intravenous hydration. There is little doubt that intravenous Lasix (usually a nominal dose of only 10–20 mg) improves excretion into the collecting systems (providing better distention), and, in addition, dilutes the contrast entering the collecting system, allowing radiologists to see through the dense contrast and identify subtle sites of urothelial thickening or nodularity. In a study by Sanyal and colleagues[14] in 2007, Lasix administration resulted in significant improvements in ureteral distension and opacification, particularly in the distal ureters, classically the most difficult portion of the ureter to fill with contrast. Another study, by Silverman and colleagues,[15] suggested significant improvements in distension with Lasix that were substantially greater than those seen from hydration alone. There is a great deal of data supporting the use of Lasix, but there is also little doubt that the routine administration of Lasix can potentially slow down work flow (particularly at a busy practice), and requires nursing support in order to administer the medication and take into account medication allergies and other contraindications. An alternative technique that is much less problematic in terms of daily work flow is hydration. Hydration has been shown in the literature to have good efficacy in terms of improving distention and also diluting contrast, and can be done either with the administration of intravenous fluids (typically only 100–250 mL of saline administered as a bolus before the study) or having the patient drink water (usually roughly 500–1000 mL) before the study, both of which have been shown to produce good results.[6,8,16–19] A study by Szolar and colleagues[18] suggested that simple hydration of patients before the study resulted in significant improvements in distension of the entire upper urinary tract and also reduced contrast attenuation values of the excreted urine.[2]

Data in the literature supporting several other additional techniques are less robust, including such practices as placing a compression belt over the abdomen or imaging the patient in the prone position. In particular, both of these techniques have not been proved to significantly improve distention of either the intrarenal collecting systems or the ureters, and additionally both techniques create several issues in terms of patient work flow. For example, placing a compression belt over the abdomen requires 2 separate acquisitions during the excretory phase, including a single acquisition with a compression belt inflated (in order to trap contrast in the intrarenal collecting systems) and a second acquisition once the compression belt is deflated, allowing contrast to flow into the ureters and bladder. The acquisition of 2 separate sets of images potentially can slow workflow, increase complexity for technologists, and increase radiation dose. There is evidence that the use of a compression belt may have some benefit in terms of distending the intrarenal collecting systems and proximal ureters, but its benefits in terms of distending the distal ureters (the most difficult to distend using standard techniques) are less convincing.[17] The literature with regard to the use of compression belts is mixed at best, because a study by Caoili and colleagues[19] suggested no significant benefit anywhere in the urinary tract from using a compression belt. Prone positioning theoretically allows contrast to flow dependently into the proximal portions of the collecting system (particularly the intrarenal collecting systems). However, prone positioning can be uncomfortable for patients, particularly when obese or when there is other abdominal disorder (such as patients who have undergone recent surgeries). In particular, this technique requires patients to lie prone for at least 4 to 5 minutes, which is an uncomfortable position that many patients are unable to tolerate. Perhaps most importantly, there is little strong evidence in the literature to suggest that prone positioning is effective in improving distension.[14,16] A study by Wang and colleagues[20] in 2009 suggested the opposite, with their review of 114 patients imaged either in the prone or supine position suggesting superior distension with supine positioning.

In addition, there are a few selected institutions that have chosen to make a radical change to their CT urography technique, using a larger volume of more dilute contrast (eg, 200 mL of diluted Omnipaque-200), rather than the standard dose (120 mL) of Omnipaque-350. The theory behind this technique is that the larger volume of contrast increases excretion into the collecting systems and ureters, whereas the more dilute contrast agent makes it easier to see through the contrast in the collecting systems to identify subtle filling defects or urothelial thickening. However, the problem with this technique is that it assumes that the only cause for a patient's hematuria is transitional cell carcinoma, thereby ignoring any other potential causes of hematuria that might be identified on a CT scan. In particular, images acquired using this technique have a dull, washed-out appearance with poor contrast enhancement of the parenchymal organs, and it is almost certainly true that this technique is much less sensitive for renal cell carcinoma.

At our own institution, in patients who present with hematuria, we have made the decision that our primary goal is to maximize sensitivity for all renal malignancies (ie, both renal cell carcinoma and transitional cell carcinoma), and to make the diagnosis on the first attempt (rather than having patients be imaged repeatedly without a clear diagnosis being made). Accordingly, at our own institution we have decided to use the single-bolus technique, and in patients more than 35 years of age (at maximal risk for the development renal malignancies), we acquire 4-phase studies with separate noncontrast, arterial, venous, and delayed phase acquisitions. We know that the single-bolus technique carries a slightly higher radiation dose, although we think that its greater diagnostic efficacy, as well as recent technological improvements in scanner design that have reduced radiation dose, have made this an acceptable compromise. In our protocol, arterial phase images are typically acquired using bolus tracking (with the region of interest placed in the abdominal aorta), whereas venous and delayed phase images are acquired at a fixed delay (usually roughly 50–60 seconds for the venous phase and roughly 4 minutes for the delayed excretory phase). The delayed excretory phase is traditionally acquired roughly 4 minutes following the injection of intravenous contrast, because a more lengthy delay can potentially introduce a large amount of highly dense contrast agent within the collecting systems, making it difficult to see through the contrast to identify subtle filling defects or urothelial thickening, as well as producing beam hardening artifact, which can make it difficult to diagnose lesions within the adjacent renal parenchyma. The exact length of the delay for the excretory phase is a fine balancing act: a

longer delay improves distension, particularly of the distal ureter, but runs the risk of making the study uninterpretable as a result of dense contrast pooling in the proximal collecting systems and producing massive streak and beam hardening artifact.[19] The arterial and delayed phase images are acquired through the entire abdomen and pelvis (encompassing the kidneys, ureters, and bladder), whereas the noncontrast and venous phase images are only acquired through the kidneys, thereby allowing us to obtain opacified and unopacified images through the ureters and bladder.

In patients less than 35 years old, ostensibly at much lesser risk of developing renal malignancies, we acquire only noncontrast, arterial, and delayed phase images, because the odds of the patient having either a renal parenchymal lesion or a significant abnormality in the other parenchymal organs of the upper abdomen are much less, making venous phase acquisitions of less value. In addition, given the shortage of evidence for many of the ancillary techniques discussed previously, we do not use compression belts, prone positioning, or alternative doses or volumes of intravenous contrast. Despite knowing that intravenous Lasix can be advantageous in distending the collecting system and improving excretion, our own experience has been that the administration of diuretics can be problematic in terms of daily work flow, and introduces another layer of complexity in terms of dealing with medication administration and medication allergies, as well as requiring a nurse to administer the medication on a daily basis. In our experience, concordant with data in the literature, oral hydration is roughly equivalent to any of the other techniques described in the literature, and accordingly we have patients ingest roughly 500 mL of water immediately before the study, and we have found this to work well in terms of improving collecting system distention.[6,8,19]

In addition, at our institution we have made a conscious effort to improve our ability to diagnose bladder malignancies in patients who present with unexplained hematuria, particularly in the emergency room setting, and our goal is to maximize distention of the bladder before the CT scan (even with the understanding that CT is less sensitive for bladder malignancies compared with cystoscopy). This goal is part of the rationale for our administration of oral hydration before the study, because there is improved excretion of both contrast and urine into the collecting systems, ureters, and bladder, improving bladder distention and the ability to evaluate the entirety of the bladder wall. In addition, our standard protocols include the acquisition of both arterial and delayed phase images through the entirety of the abdomen and pelvis, including the bladder. Accordingly, we acquire images through the bladder in the arterial phase when the bladder is unopacified with urine, maximizing our ability to evaluate the bladder wall for subtle urothelial thickening or hyperenhancement, a finding that can easily be obscured on the delayed excretory phase images as a result of beam hardening artifact from dense excreted contrast. In our experience, many subtle bladder malignancies are easy to overlook on the delayed excretory phase, especially when located in the dependent posterior portion of the bladder adjacent to layering contrast, and such malignancies (particularly presenting with only mild focal bladder wall thickening rather than a polyploid mass) are much easier to identify on the arterial phase if the bladder is filled with unopacified, low density urine. In addition, many bladder malignancies (and most transitional cell carcinomas in general) show arterial hyperenhancement, and tend to be more conspicuous in the arterial phase.[6,8]

IMAGE RECONSTRUCTION

At our own institution, all source axial images are acquired using thin collimation (0.5–0.75 mm), with coronal and sagittal reformations automatically created at the scanner for standard radiologist review. Subsequently, the source axial images (0.5 mm) are sent to an independent workstation for generation of 2 separate sets of 3D reconstructions, including maximum intensity projection (MIP) images and volume-rendered reconstructions. The MIP technique involves taking the highest attenuation voxels in a data set and projecting these voxels into a 3D display, which can be interactively rotated or manipulated by the interpreting radiologist. MIP images are particularly useful in evaluating the collecting systems and ureters, providing a good global overview of the high-density contrast within the collecting systems, and highlighting subtle sites of urothelial thickening, luminal narrowing, calyceal destruction, or asymmetric hydronephrosis/hydroureter. In particular, our own experience has suggested that these reconstructions are particularly helpful in evaluating the ureters, where subtle urothelial thickening or even ureteral strictures are easy to overlook on the source axial images (and are commonly missed), whereas these abnormalities tend to be more conspicuous using a coronal MIP reconstruction. In particular, MIP images allow the entirety of the collecting systems and ureters to be viewed at a single glance (providing a global overview of the collecting systems), which is a great advantage compared with standard axial image review, in which the intrarenal collecting systems and ureters are constantly moving in and out of plane, making careful evaluation difficult. In contrast, volume-rendered reconstruction is a more computationally intense reconstruction algorithm that entails assigning a specific color and transparency to each voxel in a data set based on its attenuation and relationship to other adjacent voxels, thereby creating a 3D display that can be manipulated by the radiologist in real time. Volume-rendered images allow the data set to be viewed from multiple discrete perspectives, making it useful to identify subtle sites of urothelial thickening, and, in particular, to evaluate obstructed collecting systems in which there is minimal excretion of contrast into the collecting system and for which MIP reconstructions may be of minimal utility.[6,8,21]

IMAGING OF BLADDER MALIGNANCIES

There is little doubt that cystoscopy is a better diagnostic test for evaluation of bladder malignancies than CT. Nevertheless, there is some evidence in the literature suggesting that CT is a better modality than is commonly thought for the identification of bladder cancers, particularly when proper technique is used to ensure that the bladder is well distended.[22,23] In a study by Sadow and colleagues,[24] a large number of patients underwent both CT urography and cystoscopy within 6 months of each other, and CT urography had a sensitivity of 79% and a specificity of 94%. Another study, by Turney and colleagues,[25] of patients who underwent both cystoscopy and CT urography found sensitivities and specificities that were even better, ranging up to 0.93 and 0.99 respectively.[26,27]

The success of these studies is heavily contingent on using proper technique, and if the bladder is largely decompressed, there is almost no way of identifying even large bladder tumors. Alternatively, if the bladder is well distended and the proper technique is used, these studies suggest that even subtle tumors can be diagnosed (**Figs. 3–9**). First and foremost, with regard to technique, although the delayed excretory phase has traditionally been considered the most important contrast phase for identifying bladder malignancies, it is important to remember that most bladder malignancies are fundamentally hypervascular tumors. A study by Kim and colleagues[28] of bladder tumors on multiphase imaging found that bladder malignancies

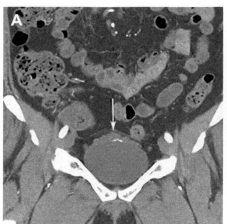
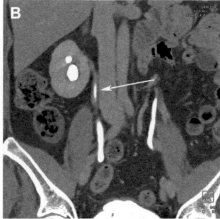

Fig. 3. (*A*) Contrast-enhanced coronal CT image shows focal wall thickening (*arrow*) along the superior wall of the bladder with associated mucosal hyperemia, consistent with the patient's known primary bladder malignancy in this location. (*B*) Contrast-enhanced coronal CT in the delayed excretory phase in the same patient shows focal urothelial thickening (*arrow*) of the proximal ureter, consistent with upper tract malignancy. Transitional cell carcinomas are commonly multifocal, and the presence of a malignancy in one part of the urinary tract should prompt a careful search for other sites of disease.

showed Hounsfield attenuation values well over 100 (usually in the arterial or venous phase), and then slowly washed out contrast over time. Accordingly, these tumors are most likely to be conspicuous in terms of their enhancement on the arterial phase of imaging. As a result, one of the most important imaging features in identifying a bladder malignancy is the presence of focal hyperenhancement or hypervascularity of the bladder urothelium, a finding that can often be difficult to appreciate on the delayed excretory phase images as a result of immediately adjacent high-density contrast material, which may obscure the urothelium and abnormal enhancement as a result of beam hardening artifact (see **Figs. 6** and **8**). This possibility is a primary

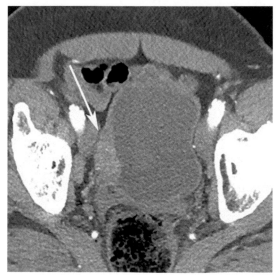

Fig. 4. Contrast-enhanced axial CT image shows focal severe wall thickening (*arrow*) along the right lateral margin of the bladder, a finding that rightly prompted cystoscopy, which confirmed the diagnosis of bladder cancer.

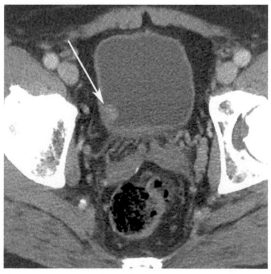

Fig. 5. Contrast-enhanced axial CT image shows a focal polypoid nodule (*arrow*) in the right posterolateral aspect of the bladder, confirmed to represent a bladder cancer at cystoscopy.

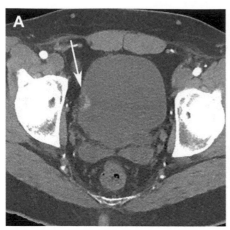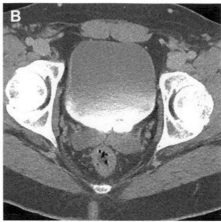

Fig. 6. (*A*) Axial contrast-enhanced CT image in the arterial phase shows focal nodular wall thickening (*arrow*) along the right lateral wall of the bladder, which is prominently hypervascular. (*B*) However, this same site of abnormality is not clearly visualized on the delayed excretory phase images. This example shows how bladder malignancies can be obscured by adjacent excreted contrast within the bladder on the delayed excretory phase, and are typically more conspicuous on the arterial phase images in which the hypervascularity of these tumors can aid in detection.

rationale for the inclusion of the bladder on the arterial phase images (before the excretion of high-density contrast material into the bladder lumen), because this phase maximizes distention of the bladder with low-density urine, and maximizes the chances of identifying subtle urothelial hyperenhancement or thickening. A study by Helenius and colleagues[29] found the corticomedullary phase to be the most sensitive (rather than the excretory phase) for the identification of bladder malignancies.

Other important signs of bladder malignancy include focal (rather than diffuse) bladder wall thickening or a discrete bladder nodule/mass.

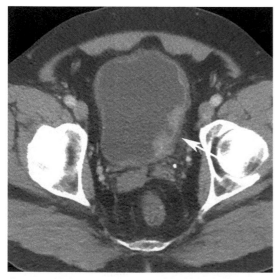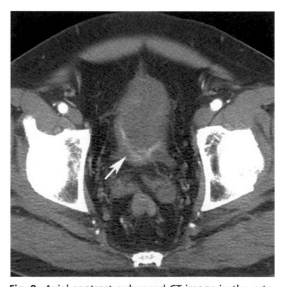

Fig. 7. Axial contrast-enhanced CT image shows multiple nodular sites of wall thickening (*arrow*) and enhancement along the left lateral margin and posterior wall of the bladder. Any focal nodular wall thickening of this kind should elicit strong concern for malignancy, and should prompt cystoscopy.

Fig. 8. Axial contrast-enhanced CT image in the arterial phase shows prominent wall thickening with significant hypervascularity (*arrow*). Many transitional cell carcinomas of the bladder are hypervascular in the arterial phase, making it important to include early phase images through the bladder in any CT urography protocol.

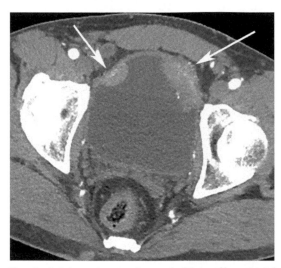

Fig. 9. Axial contrast-enhanced CT in the arterial phase shows 2 discrete sites (*arrows*) of polyploid nodularity in the anterior aspect of the bladder, each of which represents a transitional cell carcinoma. These tumors are often multifocal, and it is common to see multiple discrete nodules within the bladder in patients with a primary bladder malignancy.

Diffuse bladder wall thickening is very unlikely to represent malignancy, and most often represents infectious cystitis or an artificially thickened bladder wall caused by bladder decompression. However, the presence of focal or asymmetric bladder wall thickening should always raise concern for malignancy, and should prompt further evaluation with cystoscopy (see **Fig. 4**). Just as importantly, a discrete bladder nodule or mass should definitively be considered suspicious for malignancy (see **Figs. 5** and **9**). In theory, a blood clot or hematoma within the bladder lumen could mimic the presence of a bladder malignancy, although, unlike hematoma, a true bladder malignancy should show some degree of enhancement over the multiple phases of the study, whereas hematoma should remain unchanged in attenuation from one contrast phase to another. In addition, the presence of any abnormal calcification within the bladder wall, particularly when associated with focal thickening, is another sign of malignancy, because transitional cell carcinoma anywhere within the urinary tract can show internal punctate or dystrophic calcification (see **Fig. 3**).[6]

IMAGING OF URETERAL MALIGNANCIES

Tumors of the ureter are notoriously difficult to identify, particularly in their earliest stages before the development of frank urinary tract obstruction. This difficulty in identification is compounded by problems of technique, because the distal portions of the ureters are almost always the most difficult to adequately distend or fill with contrast on the excretory phase of CT urography, and this is the most common location for the development of ureteral malignancies (ie, distal ureter). Nevertheless, paying attention to several primary and secondary signs of malignancy can allow improvements in diagnostic efficacy, even for subtle tumors (**Figs. 10–19**). The most common imaging manifestation of transitional cell carcinoma in the ureters is urothelial thickening, particularly focal thickening or a short-segment ureteral stricture. Similar to other sites in the urinary tract, diffuse or bilateral urothelial thickening in the ureters is unlikely to represent malignancy, and is much more likely to represent an ascending urinary tract infection (particularly when associated with diffuse bladder wall thickening secondary to cystitis) (see **Figs. 17** and **19**).

As in the bladder, using all available contrast phases is important for adequate evaluation, because subtle sites of urothelial thickening can be obscured on the delayed excretory phase images as a result of high-density contrast within the ureteral lumen and resultant beam hardening artifact. Accordingly, some sites of subtle urothelial thickening may be more apparent on the arterial phase images as a result of associated hypervascularity and enhancement (see **Fig. 15**). In general, any type of urothelial thickening, when focal, should raise concern for malignancy, with many ureteral tumors showing irregular, nodular soft tissue thickening, rather than circumferential or smooth wall thickening.

As with other portions of the urinary tract, transitional cell carcinomas in the ureter are often hypervascular, making it critical that the field of view includes the entirety of the ureters during the arterial phase acquisition (see **Fig. 15**). Any focal or irregular urothelial hyperenhancement should raise concern for malignancy, and, in some instances, there may be associated tumor neovascularity. Other signs of malignancy are similar to those at other sites in the urinary tract, including the presence of ureteral calcifications or a discrete filling defect/mass, both of which are uncommon manifestations of ureteral transitional cell carcinoma, particularly in the earliest stages of the disease. The most important means of identifying a ureteral tumor is the presence of asymmetric hydronephrosis and hydroureter, with even subtle differences in the distention of the collecting systems and ureters between the right and left sides potentially

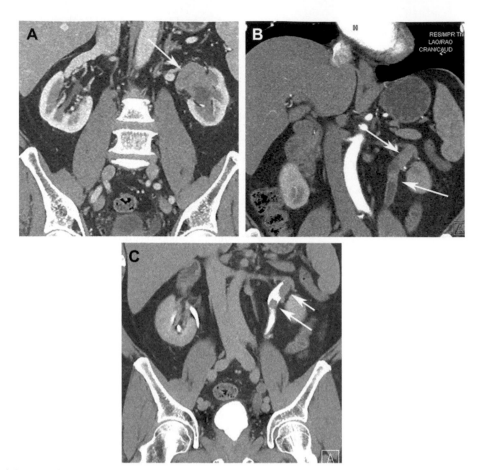

Fig. 10. (*A*) Coronal contrast-enhanced CT image shows avidly enhancing tumor (*arrow*) filling the left renal pelvis and the left intrarenal collecting system, representing the patient's primary urothelial malignancy. (*B, C*) Coronal arterial phase and delayed excretory phase images show multiple discrete enhancing nodules (*arrows*) within the proximal ureter, compatible with additional sites of tumor. This example shows the typical multifocality of these tumors.

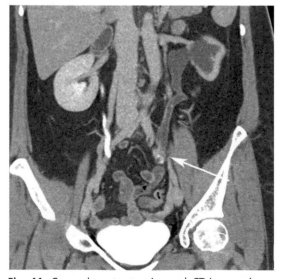

Fig. 11. Coronal contrast-enhanced CT image shows severe left-sided hydronephrosis and hydroureter. The site of transition in the left ureter is identified at the level of the pelvic inlet, where a discrete enhancing nodule (*arrow*) with some calcification is noted, representing the patient's primary ureteral malignancy.

serving as a clue as to the presence of an early tumor. This is one area in which the use of MIP images can be helpful in terms of providing a global overview of the ureters and collecting systems, and highlighting subtle differences in ureteral distention. Whenever asymmetric hydronephrosis or hydroureter is identified, the ureter should then be followed along its course to identify a potential transition point or change in caliber that might suggest an obstructing tumor (see **Figs. 11–14**).[8]

IMAGING OF INTRARENAL COLLECTING SYSTEM MALIGNANCIES

The findings of malignancy in the intrarenal collecting system are similar to those in the ureter and bladder, with the presence of urothelial thickening, nodularity, a discrete soft tissue mass, or focal calcification; all imaging features that suggest the presence of a transitional cell carcinoma (**Figs. 20–27**). Unlike the ureters or bladder, where the arterial phase images are probably the most important for the identification of

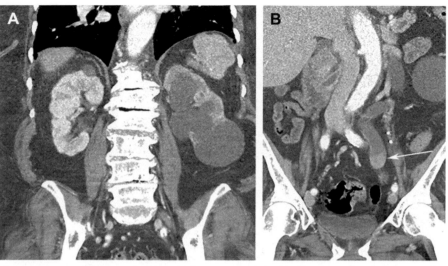

Fig. 12. (*A*) Coronal contrast-enhanced CT image shows severe left-sided hydronephrosis, whereas the right-sided collecting system is normal in caliber. Any unexplained hydronephrosis or hydroureter of this kind should prompt a careful search for an obstructing tumor. (*B*) Coronal contrast-enhanced CT image in the same patient shows an obstructing mass (*arrow*) in the left midureter, representing a transitional cell carcinoma.

tumors, the delayed excretory phase is critical for the diagnosis of transitional cell carcinomas within the intrarenal collecting system, because subtle urothelial tumors can be difficult to distinguish in the corticomedullary phase of imaging as a result of the adjacent hypodense medullary pyramids. In addition, 3D imaging (particularly MIP images) can be particularly helpful in evaluating the intrarenal collecting systems, because the amputation of a calyx or focal calyceal destruction can be much easier to appreciate when using a global coronal MIP overview, rather than relying on the source axial images alone.[7,30–33]

Overall, studies evaluating the utility of CT urography in the detection of upper tract urothelial

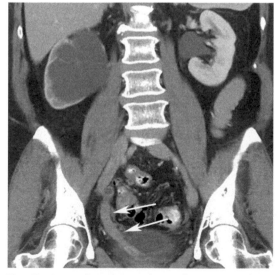

Fig. 13. Coronal contrast-enhanced CT image shows severe right-sided hydronephrosis, whereas the left collecting system is essentially normal. There is a long, enhancing filling defect (*arrows*) within the right distal ureter, which expands the ureter and extends into the right ureterovesical junction, compatible with a distal ureteral transitional cell carcinoma.

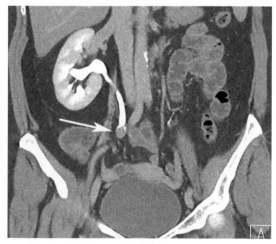

Fig. 14. Coronal contrast-enhanced CT image in the delayed excretory phase shows a focal nodular filling defect (*arrow*) in the right midureter, resulting in mild proximal hydronephrosis and hydroureter, representing a transitional cell carcinoma.

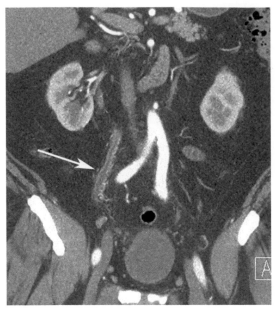

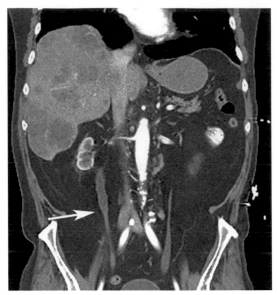

Fig. 15. Coronal contrast-enhanced CT image shows a long segment of wall thickening (*arrow*) and urothelial hyperenhancement of the right midureter, with multiple tiny tumor vessels extending to this hyperemic segment of the ureteral wall. This finding was ultimately discovered to represent a transitional cell carcinoma.

Fig. 16. Coronal contrast-enhanced CT shows significant dilatation of the right proximal and midureter, with abrupt narrowing (*arrow*) of the right midureter at a site of thickening. This finding represents the classic goblet sign associated with transitional cell carcinoma as a result of an obstructing ureteral tumor. Note the presence of extensive metastatic disease to the liver.

malignancies (ie, intrarenal collecting systems, renal pelvis, and ureters) have found that CT is quite sensitive and specific in its ability to identify urothelial carcinoma, with a study by Chlapoutakis and colleagues[34] showing sensitivities ranging from 80% to 100% and a specificities ranging from 93% to 100%. In particular, CT urography is definitively superior to other more traditional imaging modalities (such as excretory urography or retrograde pyelography) for the diagnosis of upper

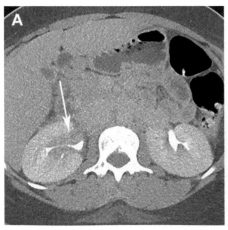

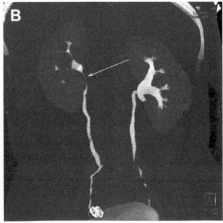

Fig. 17. (*A*) Axial contrast-enhanced CT in the delayed excretory phase shows focal severe urothelial thickening (*arrow*) in the right renal pelvis and proximal ureter, resulting in narrowing of the collecting system at this site. (*B*) Coronal contrast-enhanced CT with MIP reconstruction in the delayed excretory phase shows that this tumor results in severe narrowing (*arrow*) of the proximal ureter and renal pelvis.

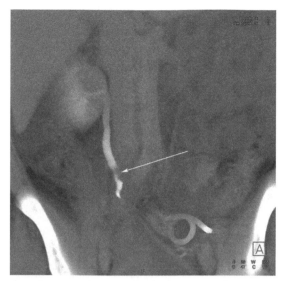

Fig. 18. Coronal contrast-enhanced CT with volume-rendered reconstruction shows a focal filling defect (*arrow*) in the right distal ureter, resulting in mild proximal hydroureter, ultimately discovered to represent a transitional cell carcinoma.

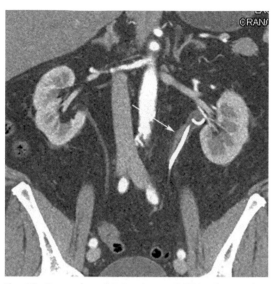

Fig. 19. Coronal contrast-enhanced CT in the cortico-medullary phase shows severe urothelial thickening (*arrow*) surrounding the margins of a nephroureteral stent, representing the patient's known transitional cell carcinoma. Although the presence of a stent or other instrumentation can make diagnosis more difficult, it does not necessarily preclude identification of the tumor.

tract malignancy, and should be the first noninvasive test of choice for diagnosis.[35–37]

MIMICS OF MALIGNANCY

The presence of focal wall thickening or a discrete nodule/mass should raise concern for the presence of malignancy anywhere in the upper or lower urinary tract and should prompt

further evaluation with direct visualization. Nevertheless, there are multiple benign entities that could potentially mimic findings of malignancy. In particular, urothelial thickening is a common finding, and, when bilateral and diffuse throughout the collecting systems, is much more likely to be the sequela of infection, rather than

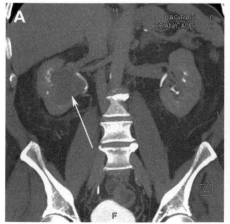
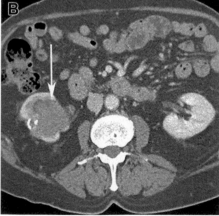

Fig. 20. (*A*) Coronal contrast-enhanced CT in the delayed excretory phase with volume-rendered reconstruction shows a large filling defect (*arrow*) distending the right renal pelvis and extending into the intrarenal collecting system. (*B*) Axial contrast-enhanced CT in the nephrographic phase shows that this filling defect (*arrow*) represents a large enhancing mass, compatible with a transitional cell carcinoma.

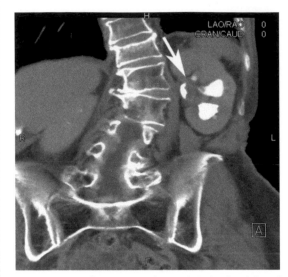

Fig. 21. Coronal contrast-enhanced CT in the delayed excretory phase shows a filling defect (*arrow*) in the left renal pelvis extending into the intrarenal collecting system, representing this patient's primary transitional cell carcinoma.

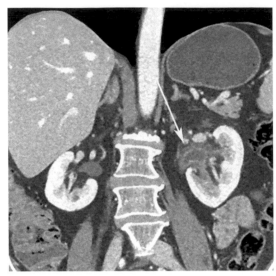

Fig. 23. Coronal contrast-enhanced CT shows focal urothelial thickening (*arrow*) and hyperemia in the left renal pelvis extending into the calyceal system, associated with subtle surrounding stranding and induration. Although such a finding could theoretically represent infection, the relative focality of this thickening, with sparing of the other portions of the collecting system, raises concern for malignancy, and this was ultimately found to represent a transitional cell carcinoma.

tumor, particularly when the wall thickening is smooth and regular. In addition, wall thickening along the margins of instrumentation (such as ureteral stent) is another common finding, and usually reflects reactive inflammatory wall thickening secondary to the stent. Diffuse wall thickening of the bladder is another common finding as a result of underdistention or cystitis, and the possibility of bladder cancer should not

necessarily be evoked unless focal or asymmetric wall thickening can be convincingly identified.

In contrast, benign entities are much less likely to present as a focal nodule or mass, although in

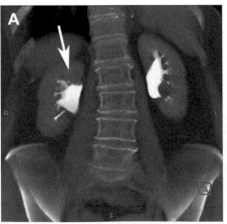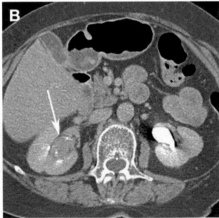

Fig. 22. (*A*) Coronal contrast-enhanced CT in the delayed excretory phase with volume-rendered reconstruction shows a focal filling defect (*arrow*) in the right upper pole collecting system extending into the calyces, a finding that should prompt careful search for a primary transitional cell carcinoma on the source axial images. (*B*) Axial contrast-enhanced CT in the delayed excretory phase in the same patient shows that the previously seen filling defect represents a focal enhancing polyploid mass (*arrow*), compatible with a transitional cell carcinoma.

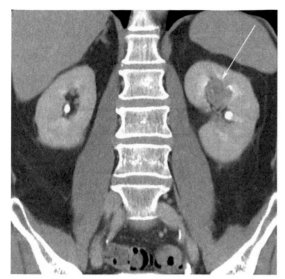

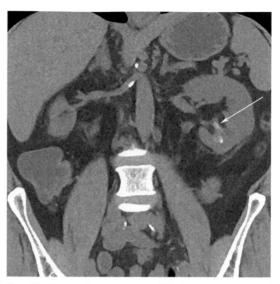

Fig. 24. Coronal contrast-enhanced CT in the delayed excretory phase shows a focal filling defect (*arrow*) distending the left upper pole calyces, representing a transitional cell carcinoma.

Fig. 26. Coronal noncontrast CT shows an area of abnormal calcification (*arrow*) within the left lower pole calyx in a patient with a known bladder cancer. The patient could not receive intravenous contrast, but this was ultimately discovered on direct visualization to represent a site of recurrent upper tract transitional cell carcinoma. The presence of calcification in the urothelium should always raise concern for tumor.

rare instances blood clots within the upper or lower urinary tract can appear nodular and masslike, and could potentially mimic a malignancy. However, in most cases, blood clots are completely intraluminal (and completely surrounded by contrast material on the delayed excretory phase images), unlike tumors, which show an attachment to the adjacent wall, and should show no apparent enhancement on multiphase imaging. Other benign causes of

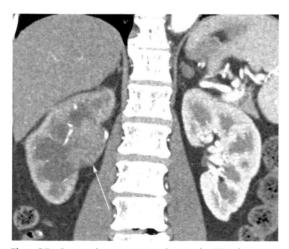

Fig. 25. Coronal contrast-enhanced CT shows a large enhancing filling defect (*arrow*) in the right renal pelvis extending into the calyces, with associated diffuse hypoenhancement of the right kidney, representing a large transitional cell carcinoma.

intraluminal filling defects or nodules include sloughed papilla (ie, papillary necrosis), fungus balls, or even rare entities such as pyeloureteritis cystica. Given this overlap between benign and malignant entities, it is not surprising that the positive predictive value of CT urography for upper tract urinary malignancy may be as low as 53% (with a positive predictive value of only 46% for urothelial thickening), although this increases in patients with a discrete mass, for which the positive productive value may be as high as 83%.[1,2,38] In particular, the literature suggests that urothelial thickening in the intrarenal collecting systems is more commonly caused by inflammatory or infectious conditions than in the ureters, and is more likely to represent malignancy.[38] In addition, perhaps the most common mimic of malignancy in the ureter is the presence of either a ureteral kink or a vessel immediately crossing over the ureter, resulting in compression of the ureter and resulting in a pseudo–filling defect. This interpretive error is most common when viewing 3D images (either MIP images or volume-rendered images), but tends to be more obvious when viewing the source axial images (particularly when cross-referenced to the arterial phase images before excretion of contrast).

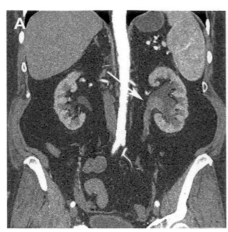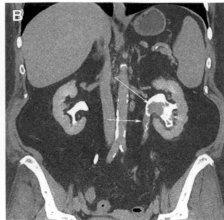

Fig. 27. (*A*) Coronal contrast-enhanced CT image shows an enhancing tumor (*arrow*) extending from the left renal pelvis into the proximal ureter. (*B*) This same tumor is visualized as a filling defect (*arrows*) highlighted against the surrounding high-density excreted contrast on the delayed phase image, representing a primary transitional cell carcinoma.

SUMMARY

The identification of transitional cell carcinomas throughout the upper and lower urinary tract (including the intrarenal collecting systems, ureters, and bladder) can be very difficult, and relies on several subtle imaging features. However, it is important to be cognizant that the identification of these imaging features is heavily contingent on proper imaging technique and protocol design. Failure to acquire the correct contrast enhancement phases, or, alternatively, failure to adequately distend the collecting system, can make identification of even large tumors difficult.

REFERENCES

1. Sadow CA, Wheeler SC, Kim J, et al. Positive predictive value of CT urography in the evaluation of upper tract urothelial cancer. AJR Am J Roentgenol 2010; 195(5):W337–43.
2. Caoili EM, Cohan RH. CT urography in evaluation of urothelial tumors of the kidney. Abdom Radiol (NY) 2016;41(6):1100–7.
3. Vikram R, Sandler CM, Ng CS. Imaging and staging of transitional cell carcinoma: part 1, lower urinary tract. AJR Am J Roentgenol 2009;192(6):1481–7.
4. Lee EK, Dickstein RJ, Kamta AM. Imaging of urothelial cancers: what the urologist needs to know. AJR Am J Roentgenol 2011;196(6):1249–54.
5. Vikram R, Sandler CM, Ng CS. Imaging and staging of transitional cell carcinoma: part 2, upper urinary tract. AJR Am J Roentgenol 2009;192(6):1488–93.
6. Raman SP, Fishman EK. Bladder malignancies on CT: the underrated role of CT in diagnosis. AJR Am J Roentgenol 2014;203(2):347–54.
7. Raman SP, Horton KM, Fishman EK. Transitional cell carcinoma of the upper urinary tract: optimizing image interpretation with 3D reconstructions. Abdom Imaging 2012;37(6):1129–40.
8. Raman SP, Horton KM, Fishman EK. MDCT evaluation of ureteral tumors: advantages of 3D reconstruction and volume visualization. AJR Am J Roentgenol 2013;201(6):1239–47.
9. Dillman JR, Caoili EM, Cohan RH, et al. Comparison of urinary tract distension and opacification using single-bolus 3-phase vs split-bolus 2-phase multidetector row CT urography. J Comput Assist Tomogr 2007;31(5):750–7.
10. Takeuchi M, Kawai T, Ito M, et al. Split-bolus CT-urography using dual-energy CT: feasibility, image quality and dose reduction. Eur J Radiol 2012; 81(11):3160–5.
11. Chen CY, Tsai TH, Jaw TS, et al. Diagnostic performance of split-bolus portal venous phase dual-energy CT urography in patients with hematuria. AJR Am J Roentgenol 2016;206(5):1013–22.
12. Kaza RK, Platt JF. Renal applications of dual-energy CT. Abdom Radiol (NY) 2016;41(6):1122–32.
13. Chow LC, Kwan SW, Olcott EW, et al. Split-bolus MDCT urography with synchronous nephrographic and excretory phase enhancement. AJR Am J Roentgenol 2007;189(2):314–22.
14. Sanyal R, Deshmukh A, Singh Sheorain V, et al. CT urography: a comparison of strategies for upper urinary tract opacification. Eur Radiol 2007;17(5). 1262–6.
15. Silverman SG, Akbar SA, Mortele KJ, et al. Multidetector row CT urography of normal urinary collecting system: furosemide versus saline as adjunct to contrast medium. Radiology 2006; 240(3):749–55.

16. McTavish JD, Jinzaki M, Zou KH, et al. Multi-detector row CT urography: comparison of strategies for depicting the normal urinary collecting system. Radiology 2002;225(3):783–90.

17. Sun H, Xue HD, Liu W, et al. Effects of saline administration, abdominal compression, and prolongation of acquisition delay on image quality improvement of CT urography. Chin Med Sci J 2013;27(4):201–6.

18. Szolar DH, Tillich M, Preidler KW. Multi-detector CT urography: effect of oral hydration and contrast medium volume on renal parenchymal enhancement and urinary tract opacification–a quantitative and qualitative analysis. Eur Radiol 2010;20(9):2146–52.

19. Caoili EM, Inampudi P, Cohan RH, et al. Optimization of multi-detector row CT urography: effect of compression, saline administration, and prolongation of acquisition delay. Radiology 2005;235(1):116–23.

20. Wang ZJ, Coakley FV, Joe BN, et al. Multidetector row CT urography: does supine or prone positioning produce better pelvecalyceal and ureteral opacification? Clin Imaging 2009;33(5):369–73.

21. Calhoun PS, Kuszyk BS, Heath DG, et al. Three-dimensional volume rendering of spiral CT data: theory and method. Radiographics 1999;19(3):745–64.

22. Capalbo E, Kluzer A, Peli M, et al. Bladder cancer diagnosis: the role of CT urography. Tumori 2015;101(4):412–7.

23. Park SB, Kim JK, Lee HJ, et al. Hematuria: portal venous phase multi detector row CT of the bladder–a prospective study. Radiology 2007;245(3):798–805.

24. Sadow CA, Silverman SG, O'Leary MP, et al. Bladder cancer detection with CT urography in an academic medical center. Radiology 2008;249(1):195–202.

25. Turney BW, Willatt JM, Nixon D, et al. Computed tomography urography for diagnosing bladder cancer. BJU Int 2006;98(2):345–8.

26. Blick CG, Nazir SA, Mallett S, et al. Evaluation of diagnostic strategies for bladder cancer using computed tomography (CT) urography, flexible cystoscopy and voided urine cytology: results for 778 patients from a hospital haematuria clinic. BJU Int 2012;110(1):84–94.

27. Knox MK, Cowan NC, Rivers-Bowerman MD, et al. Evaluation of multidetector computed tomography urography and ultrasonography for diagnosing bladder cancer. Clin Radiol 2008;63(12):1317–25.

28. Kim JK, Park SY, Ahn HJ, et al. Bladder cancer: analysis of multi-detector row helical CT enhancement pattern and accuracy in tumor detection and perivesical staging. Radiology 2004;231(3):725–31.

29. Helenius M, Dahlman P, Lonnemark M, et al. Comparison of post contrast CT urography phases in bladder cancer detection. Eur Radiol 2016;26(2):585–91.

30. Kawamoto S, Horton KM, Fishman EK. Transitional cell neoplasm of the upper urinary tract: evaluation with MDCT. AJR Am J Roentgenol 2008;191(2):416–22.

31. Caoili EM, Cohan RH, Inampudi P, et al. MDCT urography of upper tract urothelial neoplasms. AJR Am J Roentgenol 2005;184(6):1873–81.

32. Urban BA, Buckley J, Soyer P, et al. CT appearance of transitional cell carcinoma of the renal pelvis: Part 2. Advanced-stage disease. AJR Am J Roentgenol 1997;169(1):163–8.

33. Urban BA, Buckley J, Soyer P, et al. CT appearance of transitional cell carcinoma of the renal pelvis: Part 1. Early-stage disease. AJR Am J Roentgenol 1997;169(1):157–61.

34. Chlapoutakis K, Theocharopoulos N, Yarmenitis S, et al. Performance of computed tomographic urography in diagnosis of upper urinary tract urothelial carcinoma, in patients presenting with hematuria: systematic review and meta-analysis. Eur J Radiol 2010;73(2):334–8.

35. Jinzaki M, Matsumoto K, Kikuchi E, et al. Comparison of CT urography and excretory urography in the detection and localization of urothelial carcinoma of the upper urinary tract. AJR Am J Roentgenol 2011;196(5):1102–9.

36. Mueller-Lisse UG, Mueller-Lisse UL, Hinterberger J, et al. Multidetector-row computed tomography (MDCT) in patients with a history of previous urothelial cancer or painless macroscopic haematuria. Eur Radiol 2007;17(11):2794–803.

37. Sudakoff GS, Dunn DP, Guralnick ML, et al. Multidetector computerized tomography urography as the primary imaging modality for detecting urinary tract neoplasms in patients with asymptomatic hematuria. J Urol 2008;179(3):862–7 [discussion: 7].

38. Xu AD, Ng CS, Kamat A, et al. Significance of upper urinary tract urothelial thickening and filling defect seen on MDCT urography in patients with a history of urothelial neoplasms. AJR Am J Roentgenol 2010;195(4):959–65.

Diffusion-Weighted Genitourinary Imaging

Martin H. Maurer, MD, Kirsi Hannele Härmä, MD, Harriet Thoeny, MD*

KEYWORDS

- Diffusion-weighted imaging • Genitourinary imaging • Magnetic resonance imaging
- Prostate cancer • Bladder cancer • Renal cell carcinoma

KEY POINTS

- Diffusion-weighted MR imaging (DW-MR imaging) allows the detection of early microstructural and functional changes in the genitourinary tract with a high sensitivity and specificity.
- In the kidneys, DW-MR imaging permits further differentiation between benign and malignant lesions compared with conventional cross-sectional imaging.
- DW-MR imaging improves the preoperative workup of bladder cancer in distinguishing between superficial and muscle-invasive urothelial cancers.
- In the pelvis, DW-MR imaging allows detection of lymph nodes metastases even in normal-sized lymph nodes.
- In addition to conventional T2-weighted imaging, DW-MR imaging improves tumor detection in the prostate (mainly the peripheral zone [PZ]) and recurrent tumor in patients after radiation therapy.

INTRODUCTION

In the urogenital tract, cross-sectional imaging methods like computed tomography (CT) and MR imaging are established techniques that allow a comprehensive morphologic overview of all parts of the genitourinary tract to detect and stage different malignant lesions (eg, renal cell carcinoma (RCC), prostate and bladder cancers, pelvic lymph node staging). However, conventional cross-sectional imaging methods have limitations concerning a proper differentiation between benign and malignant lesions and may have a reduced value in patients with an impaired renal function when contrast media cannot be applied.

Diffusion-weighted MR imaging (DW-MR imaging) measures the microscopic mobility of water molecules in biologic tissues, which highly depends on the cellularity within the different tissues and thus allows the detection of biologic abnormalities without the use of contrast media.[1] At first, the clinical use of DW-MR imaging was within the brain to detect microstructural changes in brain tissue after a stroke before morphologic changes can be detected with conventional cross-sectional imaging techniques.[2,3] Although DW-MR imaging has become the gold standard in the early diagnosis of stroke, extracranial applications have been limited initially owing to artifacts caused by physiologic movement of the lung, heart, and bowels.[4] Nevertheless, extensive developments in the technique of DW-MR imaging now allow application in various parts of the abdomen and pelvis, with the potential for the detection, characterization, and treatment monitoring of different malignant lesions.[5–8] This review provides an overview of the possible applications of DW-MR imaging in the urogenital tract with focus on the kidneys, bladder, and prostate, as well in the characterization of pelvic lymph nodes.

This article was previously published in March 2017 *Radiologic Clinics*, Volume 55, Issue 2.
Department of Radiology, Inselspital, Bern University Hospital, University of Bern, Freiburgstrasse 10, Bern 3010, Switzerland
* Corresponding author.
E-mail address: harriet.thoeny@insel.ch

Urol Clin N Am 45 (2018) 407–425
https://doi.org/10.1016/j.ucl.2018.03.003
0094-0143/18/© 2017 Elsevier Inc. All rights reserved.

IMAGING TECHNIQUE OF DIFFUSION-WEIGHTED MR IMAGING

Because DW-MR imaging visualizes the Brownian motion of water molecules in different human tissues, the degree of such a motion of molecules is known as diffusion.[9] DW-MR imaging measures the path length traveled by water molecules within a certain time period. The imaging procedure is based on an application of 2 diffusion-sensitizing gradients, which have an opposed polarity.[10] The usual effect on water molecules that do not move is a complete rephrasing. However, in substances with moving water molecules, the random displacement of molecules between the gradient pulses with opposed polarity leads to a signal loss that correlates with the degree of water mobility. The image in DW-MR imaging is based both on the amplitude of random movement of water molecules and on the duration and strength of the paired gradients, which determine the b-value. In practice, the b-value usually is varied by a variation of the gradient strength. An acquisition of at least 2 b-values (usually between 0 and 1000 s/mm^2) allows the calculation of apparent diffusion coefficient (ADC) maps. ADC maps are generated from ADC values voxel by voxel based on the equation $ADC = \log [(S_0/S_1)/(b_1/b_0)]$. Here, S_0 is the signal intensity on the unweighted b_0 image (without a diffusion sensitizing gradient) and S_1 is the signal intensity on the DW-MR image with a higher b-value. The b-value is the gradient factor of the diffusion-sensitizing gradient measured in seconds per square millimeter (s/mm^2). In tissues with tightly packed cells like malignancies, Brownian motion is less than in an environment with a lesser degree of compartmentalization and, therefore, diffusion is impeded, appearing bright on DW-MR images and darker in the ADC map.[11] The extend of diffusion impediment can be measured objectively on the ADC map.

DW-MR imaging can be performed on nearly all currently available clinical MR scanners and is usually integrated in a conventional cross-sectional imaging protocol. Under free breathing, the extra time that is needed for the acquisition of axial DW-MR imaging sequences is approximately 4 minutes.

In this discussion, the use of DW-MR imaging in genitourinary imaging is described with a focus on its application in the kidneys, prostate, bladder, and pelvic lymph nodes. Imaging protocols for DW-MR imaging used in our institution are listed in **Table 1**.

IMAGE INTERPRETATION

DW-MR imaging sequences can be analyzed both qualitatively and quantitatively. Usually, the first step in image analysis is a visual qualitative assessment. In relation to their cellularity, different tissues show a different appearance using various b-values. Tumors with tightly packed cells show a lesser signal attenuation of the signal (ie, they seem to be hyperintense) when using higher b-values (eg, $\geq$800 s/mm^2) than normal parenchymal tissue or free fluid. However, a typical pitfall in the qualitative interpretation is the so-called T2 shine-through effect of some normal tissues like the PZ of the prostate, which shows a high signal intensity also in higher b-values, because the signal intensity does not only depend on the diffusion on water molecules within a tissue, but also on the intrinsic T2 relaxation time of the specific tissue (**Fig. 1**).[12,13]

A possible misinterpretation of the imaging material owing to the T2 shine-through effect can be avoided by comparing areas with a high intensity in images with high b-values with the corresponding ADC map. In the ADC map, a high signal in corresponding areas of high signal intensity in the b-value DW-MR imaging image indicate a T2 shine-through effect. In contrast, a signal attenuation in corresponding areas in the ADC maps indicates a high cellularity of a tissue like in solid tumors (eg, renal cell carcinoma (RCC), **Fig. 2**) or pus-filled structures like the renal pelvis (**Fig. 3**).

A quantitative analysis of DW-MR images can be performed by a calculation of the ADC value within specific regions of a tissue. Therefore, a region of interest (ROI) is drawn manually within a tissue region that is to be evaluated in a b-value image and is then copied to the corresponding region in the ADC map, because tumor margins may be difficult to identify within the ADC map. For a quantification, summary statistics like the mean value with in the ROI can be used. Furthermore, ROIs can be analyzed on a voxel-by-voxel basis and their distribution within the ROI can be displayed by histograms that visualize the heterogeneity within different tissues like tumor tissue.

APPLICATIONS OF DIFFUSION-WEIGHTED MR IMAGING IN THE GENITOURINARY TRACT
Kidney

Cross-sectional imaging (CT and MR imaging) combined with intravenous contrast medium administration allows a reliable detection and characterization of most focal renal masses. However, the differentiation between cystic lesions like complicated cysts and cystic RCC, solid lesions like oncocytomas and RCCs, as well as between different subtypes of RCCs remains challenging. In various cases, DW-MR imaging can be helpful for further differentiation, because ADC values in

Table 1
Imaging protocols for diffusion-weighted imaging in the kidneys, pelvis (bladder and lymph nodes), and the prostate at different field strengths (1.5 and 3 T) of the MR scanner

Body Region	Scan Parameters
Kidneys	1.5 T field strength: Coil: body array b-Values: 50, 400 (2 averages), 800 (4 averages) Slice thickness: 5 mm Gap between slices: 1 mm Repetition time: 7300 ms Echo time: 54 ms Matrix: 134 × 108 Parallel imaging technique: GRAPPA (acceleration factor = 2) Fat suppression technique: SPAIR Direction of diffusion gradients: 3-scan trace 3 T field strength: Coil: body array b-Values: 50, 300 (2 averages), 800 (4 averages) Slice thickness: 5 mm Gap between slices: 1 mm Repetition time: 8000 ms Echo time: 48 ms Matrix: 134 × 108 Parallel imaging technique: GRAPPA (acceleration factor = 3) Fat suppression technique: SPAIR Direction of diffusion gradients: 4-scan trace
Bladder/pelvis	1.5 T field strength: Coil: body array b-Values: 50 (2 averages), 300 (3 averages), 800 (5 averages) Slice thickness: 5 mm Gap between slices: 1 mm Repetition time: 7900 ms Echo time: 56 ms Matrix: 134 × 108 Parallel imaging technique: GRAPPA (acceleration factor = 2) Fat suppression technique: SPAIR Direction of diffusion gradients: 3-scan trace

(continued on next page)

Table 1
(continued)

Body Region	Scan Parameters
	3 T field strength: Coil: body array *b*-Values: 50, 300 (2 averages), 800 (4 averages) Slice thickness: 5 mm Gap between slices: 1 mm Repetition time: 7800 ms Echo time: 48 ms Matrix: 134 × 108 Parallel imaging technique: GRAPPA (acceleration factor = 3) Fat suppression technique: SPAIR Direction of diffusion gradients: 4-scan trace
Prostate	3 T only Whole pelvis: Coil: body array *b*-Values: 0, 500 (2 averages), 1000 (4 averages) Slice thickness: 5 mm Gap between slices: 0 mm Repetition time: 8200 ms Echo time: 50 ms Matrix: 134 × 108 Parallel imaging technique: GRAPPA (acceleration factor = 3) Fat suppression technique: SPAIR Direction of diffusion gradients: 4-scan trace Zoom in prostate: Coil: body array *b*-Values: 0 (2 averages), 500 (4 averages), 1000 (8 averages), 2000 (10 averages) Slice thickness: 3.5 mm Gap between slices: 0 mm Repetition time: 4400 ms Echo time: 94 ms Matrix: 134 × 108 Parallel imaging technique: none Fat suppression technique: SPAIR Direction of diffusion gradients: 4-scan trace

Abbreviations: GRAPPA, generalized autocalibrating partially parallel acquisition; SPAIR, spectral attenuated inversion recovery.

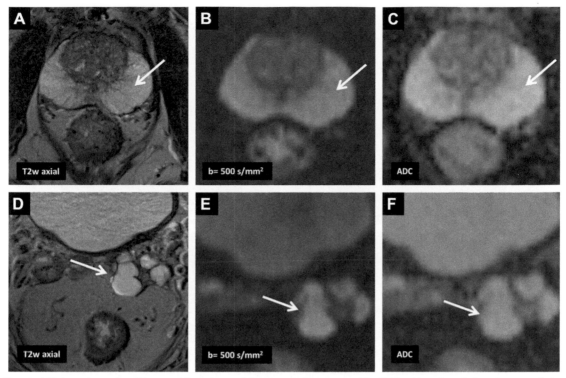

Fig. 1. MR imaging of a 55-year-old patient with a normal prostate. (*A, B*) The broad peripheral zone of the prostate shows a high signal intensity both in T2-weighted (T2w) imaging and in diffusion-weighted (DW) MR imaging with a *b*-value of 500 s/mm² (*arrows*) as a result of the "T2w shine through effect." (*C*) On the apparent diffusion coefficient (ADC) image, the peripheral zone keeps a high signal confirming that the high signal in the *b*-value MR image was due to the T2w shine through effect. (*D–F*) In the same patient, the left seminal vesicle seems to be prominent (*arrows*) in the T2w image and shows a high signal in DWI image at a *b*-value of 500 s/mm². The high signal also in the ADC image again confirms a T2w shine through effect.

benign and malignant lesions as well as in malignant subtypes differ.

In general, solid lesions are expected to have low ADC values owing to their high cellular density, which impedes the free diffusion of water molecules, whereas benign lesions lose signal with higher *b*-values and show high ADC values.[14] This general rule has been confirmed by several studies that have shown high ADC values in cystic renal masses, whereas solid masses had lower ADC values[15–20] (see **Fig. 2**).

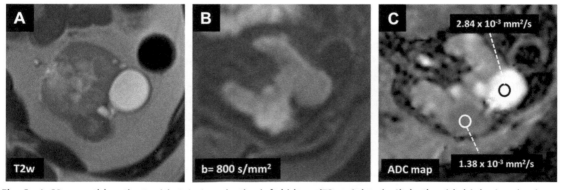

Fig. 2. A 69-year-old patient with 2 lesions in the left kidney (T2-weighted, *A*), both with high signal using a *b*-value of 800 mm²/s, (*B*). In the apparent diffusion coefficient (ADC) map, the more medial located lesion that turned out to be a renal cell carcinoma shows a much lower value of 1.38×10^{-3} mm²/s (*white ring*) than the more lateral lesion (2.84×10^{-3} mm²/s, *black ring*), which was proven to be a simple cyst (*C*).

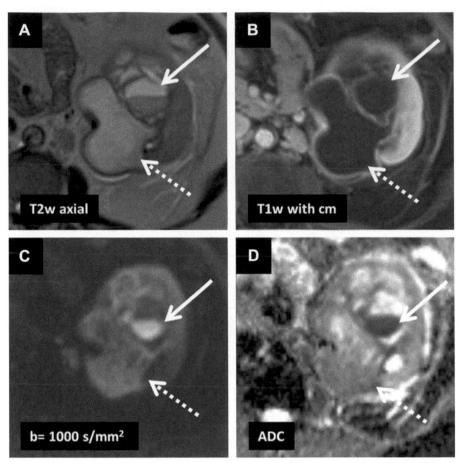

Fig. 3. A 60-year-old woman with left flank pain, fever, and general weakness underwent MR imaging with the suspicion of a xanthogranulomatous pyelonephritis. (*A*) The T2-weighted (T2w) axial image shows the renal pelvis (*dotted arrow*) and an adjacent cystic structure (*arrow*) with a level of sedimentation. (*B*) After the administration of contrast medium (cm), the renal pelvis (*dotted arrow*) and the adjacent cystic structure (*arrow*) show a mild contrast enhancement of their wall, but no central enhancement. (*C*) In diffusion-weighted MR imaging with a *b*-value of 1000 s/mm², there is a moderate signal within the renal pelvis (*dotted arrow*), but a high signal in the lower part of sedimentation in the cystic structure (*arrow*). (*D*) The apparent diffusion coefficient (ADC) image shows an intermediate signal in the renal pelvic (*dotted arrow*) indicating an empyema of the renal pelvic with high cellularity. The adjacent cystic lesion (*arrow*) was also pus filled with a high cellular segmentation. The patient was treated with a percutaneous drainage of the left renal pelvis (the microbiological examination revealed an infection with *Escherichia coli*) and antibiotics for 2 weeks and recovered fully.

A recent metaanalysis by Lassel and colleagues[21] compared ADC values for different renal lesions on a large scale. Altogether, they included 17 studies (with different *b*-values ranging between 0 and 1000 s/mm²) with 764 patients and found overall significantly lower ADC values in RCCs than in benign lesions ($1.61 \pm 0.08 \times 10^{-3}$ mm²/s vs $2.10 \pm 0.09 \times 10^{-3}$ mm²/s). Cysts had the highest ADC values (average of $3.27 \pm 0.11 \times 10^{-3}$ mm²/s), followed by normal renal tissue ($2.26 \pm 0.10 \times 10^{-3}$ mm²/s) and oncocytomas ($2.01 \pm 0.08 \times 10^{-3}$ mm²/s). The lowest ADC values were found for RCC, angiomyolipomas (AML) and urothelial tumors. Interestingly, the authors also found that ADC measurements do allow to distinguish between oncocytomas and malignant lesions like RCCs. Because oncocytomas represent up to 14% of all renal lesions and their appearance can resemble that of RCCs on conventional MR imaging, there is a strong need to distinguish them from RCCs, because the management of both lesion types involves either partial or total nephrectomy and the resection of oncocytomas may be unnecessary. In contrast, the authors did not find a difference between AMLs and various malignancies within their pooled data. However, because AMLs usually show macroscopic fat, conventional MR imaging techniques like opposed-phase

MR imaging and attenuation values equal to fat in CT usually allow the proper identification of AML. An exception is the small proportions of lipid-poor AMLs. In these cases, it was suggested that AMLs with a low fat content show a more heterogeneous DW-MR imaging pattern that may help to distinguish them from RCCs.[22]

RCCs have 3 common histopathologic subtypes, namely, clear cell (about 75%), papillary (10%–15%), and chromophobic (about 5%) RCC.[23] All 3 subtypes differ in their histopathologic features and their clinical outcome; patients with a chromophobic and papillary RCC were shown to have a better prognosis than those with a clear cell RCC.[24] For this reason, the value of DW-MR imaging with the aim to allow a differentiation between different RCC subtypes has been investigated in different studies with overall contrasting results. Using b-values of 0 and 800 s/mm^2, Wang and colleagues[25] found clear cell RCC to have significantly higher ADC values compared with both papillary and chromophobic RCC ($P<.001$) and were able to differentiate between each pair of subtype. Similarly, in a study by Choi and colleagues[26] on 27 patients, clear cell RCCs (1.81×10^{-3} mm^2/s) showed significantly higher ADC values than did papillary (1.29×10^{-3} mm^2/s) and chromophobe RCCs (1.55×10^{-3} mm^2/s; $P<.01$), however, there was no difference when comparing papillary with chromophobic RCCs. In contrast, in a study from Sandrasegaran and colleagues,[19] there were no significant differences in ADC values in clear cell RCCs and non–clear cell RCCs. Using DW-MR imaging with b-values of 0, 300, and 1000 s/mm^2 in a group of patients with clear cell RCCs (n = 25), papillary RCCs (n = 6), and chromophobe RCCs (n = 1), clear cell RCCs even had significantly lower ADC values ($P = .0004$) than non–clear cell RCCs. Rosenkrantz and colleagues[27] investigated a further use of DW-MR imaging for the differentiation of clear cell RCCs as the most common RCC subtype and were able to distinguish between high-grade and low-grade RCC because high-grade clear cell RCCs showed significantly lower ADC values than low-grade clear cell RCCs both for combinations of b-values of 0 and 400 s/mm^2 and of 0 and 800 s/mm^2.

In patients undergoing contrast-enhanced cross-sectional imaging, renal impairment is a common problem and contrast medium administration should be avoided in those patients with a risk for nephropathy owing to iodinated CT contrast media or a nephrogenic systemic fibrosis with certain MR contrast media.[28] More recently, there is an ongoing discussion on gadolinium depositions within the dentate nucleus and globus pallidus after repeated administrations of gadolinium-based contrast agents.[29,30] When contrast media cannot be administered to patients, DW-MR imaging may replace contrast-enhanced cross-sectional imaging. In a study of 64 patients with 109 renal lesions (81 benign lesions and 28 RCCs), the sensitivity (86%) and specificity (80%) of DW-MR imaging for diagnosing a malignant lesion was only slightly lower than for contrast-enhanced MR imaging (sensitivity, 100%; specificity, 89%).[15] In complex cystic renal masses, DW-MR imaging showed a similar diagnostic performance to predict a malignant lesion (sensitivity, 71%; specificity, 91%) than contrast-enhanced imaging (sensitivity, 65%; specificity, 96%). Therefore, DW-MR imaging can be a meaningful alternative imaging technique in patients with impaired renal function.

Attempts have been made to use changes in ADC values in RCCs to predict a tumor response to newly developed antiangiogenic drugs like sorafenib. Jeon and colleagues[31] showed that in xenograft models (n = 9 mice) ADC values in RCC increased progressively and significantly within 1 week after beginning an oral therapy with 40 mg Sorafenib/kg body weight from $0.243 \pm 0.191 \times 10^{-3}$ mm^2/s (pretherapy baseline) to $0.550 \pm 0.164 \times 10^{-3}$ mm^2/s (7 days after therapy; $P = .004$). They concluded that DW-MR imaging may offer the potential for an early assessment of therapeutic response to sorafenib in clinical trials as early as 1 week after the beginning of the treatment. Further studies showed antitumor activity and prolonged median progression-free survival in patients with advanced clear cell RCCs.[32,33] Bharwani and colleagues[34] analyzed the impact of DWI as a surrogate marker of response to sunitinib in metastatic RCC in 20 patients. They found significant changes in the whole tumor ADC in 47% of all patients after therapy, but no correlation with the outcome.

Bladder

Malignant tumors of the bladder are most commonly urothelial carcinomas; far less common are squamous cell carcinomas, adenocarcinomas, or sarcomas.[35] The different T stages include carcinomas in situ (Tis), T1 tumors that invade the subepithelial connective tissue, T2 tumors with an invasion of the superficial muscle (T2a) and the deep muscle (T2b), T3 tumors with a microscopic (T3a) or microscopic (T3b) invasion of the perivesical tissue, and T4 tumors that invade the adjacent prostate, uterus or vagina (T4a) or the pelvic or abdominal wall (T4b).

Ideally, imaging techniques should be able to provide a proper detection of malignant lesions and a differentiation between different tumor stages (**Fig. 4**). To distinguish between stage T1 and stages T2 or higher is of particular importance, as superficial T1 tumors can be treated with transurethral resection, whereas invasive tumors of stage T2 or higher usually require a radical cystectomy, a radiation therapy or chemotherapy, or their combination.[36-38]

However, with conventional MR imaging, staging accuracy was found to be an only moderately accurate tool in assessing the T stage.[39,40] In conventional MR imaging, malignant tumors of the bladder wall appear like the regular muscle layers of the bladder wall in T1-weighted sequences, but are usually slightly hyperintense on T2-weighted (T2w) images.[41] Although in some cases discrimination of different muscle layers is possible that might allow to separate T2a (invasion to superficial muscle) from T2b stages (invasion of deep muscle), a proper and reliable differentiation between T1 stages and invasive tumor stages of T2 and higher is usually not possible with conventional T2w MR imaging.

Therefore, several studies investigated the additional value of DW-MR imaging and its combination with T2w imaging in identifying the correct tumor stage.[42] In 106 patients, El-Assmy and colleagues[43] found an overall staging accuracy of only 39.6% using T2w imaging for differentiating superficial from invasive tumors, whereas the accuracy was 63.6% to separate superficial from invasive tumors. On a stage by stage basis, the accuracy of DW-MR imaging in correlation with the histopathologic finding was 63.6% for tumor stage T1, 75.7% for stage T2, 93.7% stage T3, and 87.5% for tumor stage T4.

Another study revealed an overall accuracy of correctly diagnosing the T stage of 67% for T2w imaging alone, of 79% for T2w and contrast-enhanced imaging, of 88% for T2w plus DW-MR imaging, and of 92% when combining all 3 imaging techniques.[44] A recent study by Ohgiya and colleagues[45] showed that the specificity and accuracy in differentiating T1 tumors from T2 and higher stage tumors were significantly higher when using T2w combined with DW-MR imaging than with T2w imaging alone (specificity, 83.3% vs 50%, P = .02; accuracy, 84.6% vs 66.7%, P = .02). A similar result was revealed by Wu and colleagues,[46] who found a higher specificity of T2w combined with DWI than with DW-MR imaging alone ($P<.05$) when differentiating Tis to T1 tumor stages from T2 to T4 tumor stages.

Beside the tumor stages, attempts have been made to analyze the histologic grading of malignant bladder tumors noninvasively, because grading correlates with invasiveness and clinical outcome.[44] One study of 121 patients aimed to investigate whether ADC values provide useful information on the clinical aggressiveness of a tumor, because ADC values have been shown to be significantly lower in high-grade disease (median 0.79×10^{-3} mm^2/s) compared with low-grade tumors (median 0.99×10^{-3} mm^2/s; $P<.0001$).[47] Moreover, patients in this study with higher T stages exhibited significantly lower ADC values ($P<.0001$). Similar results have been shown by Takeuchi and colleagues[44] using a tumor classification with 3 grades.[48] Differences in the ADC values were significant between both G1 and G3 and between G2 and G3 tumors, but not between G1 and G2 tumors. In another study, in 39 patients with 60 bladder tumors, ADC values for muscle-invasive and G3 grade bladder cancers were

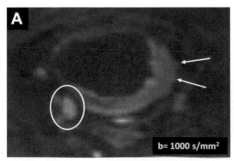
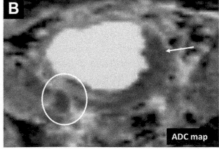

Fig. 4. MR images of a 57-year-old female patient with muscle invasive urothelial cancer of the bladder and lymph node metastasis. (*A*) Axial diffusion-weighted MR image acquired at a *b*-value of 1000 s/mm^2 showing a thickened hyperintense bladder wall with irregular borders on the lateral side (*arrows*), suggesting infiltration of the perivesical fat. There is also an enlarged, hyperintense lymph node in the right internal iliac region suspicious of a lymph node metastasis (*circle*). (*B*) On the corresponding apparent diffusion coefficient (ADC) map (*arrow*) the bladder tumor as well as the lymph node metastasis (*circle*) are hypointense and have the same ADC value of 785×10^{-6} mm^2/s. Urothelial bladder cancer stage pT3b and lymph node metastasis have been confirmed by histology.

significantly lower than those of non–muscle-invasive and G1 grade cancers ($P<.01$), both when conventional full field-of-view and reduced field-of-view DW-MR imaging techniques were used.[49] Avcu and colleagues[50] reported similar results with ADC values that were significantly lower in high-grade malignant urinary bladder tumors compared with low-grade lesions ($0.918 \pm 0.2 \times 10^{-3}$ mm^2/s vs $1.281 \pm 0.18 \times 10^{-3}$ mm^2/s; $P<.01$).

Attempts have been made to provide an early prediction of response to induction chemotherapy in patients with muscle-invasive bladder cancer. Patients with a complete response to induction chemoradiotherapy (CRT) may avoid to be treated with radical cystectomy without compromising their oncologic outcome.[51,52] In a first study on this topic in 20 patients with muscle-invasive bladder cancer who previously underwent a low-dose CRT, Yoshida and colleagues[53] compared different imaging techniques to predict a complete response based on histopathology and found that DW-MR imaging had a significantly higher specificity (92%) and accuracy (80%) than conventional T2w imaging (45% and 44%) or dynamic contrast-enhanced (DCE)-MR imaging (18% and 33%). The same authors later modified the study setting with the aim to predict sensitivity to CRT in patients with muscle-invasive bladder cancers.[54] The tumors of 13 patients with a pathologic complete response to CRT initially showed significantly lower ADC values than patients with tumors that were CRT resistant (median, 0.63×10^{-3} mm^2/s vs 0.84×10^{-3} mm^2/s; $P<.0001$).

Finally, DW-MR imaging has been shown to be superior to DCE-MR imaging in differentiating recurrent tumor from chronic inflammation and fibrosis in patients after cystectomy or transurethral resection of bladder cancer. In a group of 11 patients with suspected tumor recurrence, Wang and colleagues[25] found significantly higher accuracies, sensitivities, specificities, and positive predictive values of DW-MR imaging compared with DCE-MR imaging for detecting recurrent tumors and proposed to include diffusion-weighted imaging (DWI) in the MR imaging protocol after bladder cancer surgery.

Prostate

The use of DWI as part of a multiparametric imaging concept for the prostate has been studied extensively on the aspects of detection and localization of prostate cancers; for the characterization of malignant lesions, local staging, treatment response; and for the detection of local tumor recurrence.[55,56] Multiparametric MR imaging of the prostate consists of high-resolution T2w sequences, DWI with at least 2 b-values and DCE sequences according to the Prostate Imaging and Reporting and Data System (PI-RADS) version 2 guideline.[57]

For the detection of prostate cancer, transrectal ultrasound imaging is the current standard also allowing image guidance for biopsies. Although transrectal ultrasound imaging provides a very good depiction of the PZ, where most malignant lesions are located; however, the tumor detection in the transitional zone (TZ) and anterior parts of the prostate remain challenging. Several studies evaluated the usefulness of DW-MR imaging compared with conventional T2w sequences to detect prostate cancers primarily in the PZ and also in the TZ.[58–64] In these studies, the sensitivity (range, 71%–89%) and specificity (range, 61%–91%) of tumor detection increased significantly when DW-MR imaging and T2w imaging are combined, compared with the sole use of T2w imaging (sensitivity, 49%–88%; specificity, 57%–84%).

A metaanalysis of the role of DW-MR imaging in combination with T2w imaging revealed in 7 out of 10 studies where T2w imaging in combination with DW-MR imaging versus T2w imaging alone was analyzed a higher sensitivity and specificity in tumor detection when both techniques were combined compared with T2w imaging alone (sensitivity, 0.72 vs 0.62; specificity, 0.81 vs 0.77).[65] However, a recent metaanalysis on the overall value of DWI as a single noninvasive method in the detection of prostate cancer including 21 studies showed a pooled sensitivity of 0.62 and a specificity of 0.90, respectively.[66] The overall lower sensitivity in tumor detection may be caused by the fact that most studies that were included did not differentiate between tumor detection in the PZ and TZ. However, tumor detection in the TZ is even more difficult because both tumor tissue and common benign hyperplastic nodules show a high cellularity. A recent study outlined the limitations of DW-MR imaging in the detection of malignant lesions in the central parts of the prostate in 38 foci of carcinoma, 38 foci of stromal hyperplasia, and 38 foci of glandular hyperplasia. Although significant differences in the mean ADCs (1.05 vs 1.27 vs 1.73×10^{-3} mm^2/s) were found in the 3 different types of lesions, there was substantial overlap.[67] Another study with 28 patients with malignant lesions in the TZ focused on the value of T2w imaging compared with multiprametric MR imaging (T2w, DW-MR imaging with b-values of 50, 500, and 800 s/mm^2, and DCE) exclusively in lesions in the TZ and did not find an improvement in cancer detection and localization accuracy when multiparametric MR imaging was used compared with T2w imaging.[68] The differences in the value of ADC maps is reflected by the recently updated guideline of the PI-RADS.[57] In the current version 2 of these guidelines, DW-MR imaging is the key component in multiparametric MR imaging in detecting and in the category assessment of significant cancer lesions in the PZ, whereas T2w imaging remains the most important sequence for detecting significant cancer lesions in the transition zone (**Fig. 5**).

Because the ADC map and the high b-value image serve as the primary image set for evaluating suspect areas in the prostate when using DW-MR imaging for tumor detection, at least 2 b-values are necessary. A recent study on the gain of higher b-values than the usual b-values up to 1000 s/mm^2 revealed that computed b-values in the range of 1500 to 2500 s/mm^2 are optimal for prostate cancer detection, but that higher values of 3000 to 5000 s/mm^2 were associated with a lower diagnostic performance.[69]

Besides tumor detection, attempts have been made for further characterization of tumor grading and aggressiveness.[70–72] Jung and colleagues[73] analyzed the value of DW-MR imaging in addition to T2w imaging in assessing tumor aggressiveness of malignant lesions in the TZ. In 156 consecutive patients, they found that mean ADC values were correlated inversely with Gleason scores (1.10 for tumors Gleason 3 + 3, 0.98 for 3 + 4, 0.87 for 4 + 3, and 0.75 for 4 + 4, respectively) of tumors in the TZ. Similar results with inverse relationships of ADC value and Gleason score were seen in several other studies with 110, 57, 51, and 48 patients, respectively with biopsy-proven prostate cancer.[74–77] A study on the assessment of tumor aggressiveness using DW-MR imaging in 22 patients (median Gleason score of 7; range, 6–9) revealed that the intrapatient-normalized ADC ratios between malignant lesions and normal tissue both in the PZ and in the TZ were significantly lower in high-risk tumors compared with low-risk tumors ($P<.001$). Furthermore, the 2 ratios had a better diagnostic performance (central zone: area under the curve [AUC], 0.77; sensitivity, 82.2%; specificity, 66.7%; and PZ: AUC, 0.90; sensitivity, 93.7%; specificity 80%) than stand-alone tumor ADCs (AUC, 0.75;

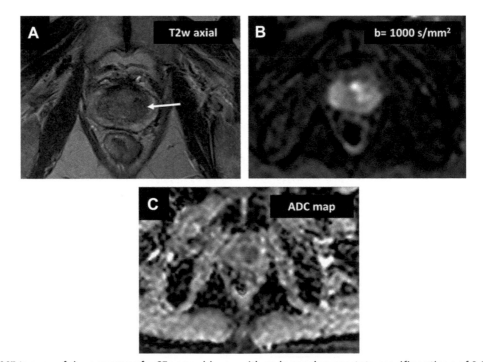

Fig. 5. MR images of the prostate of a 65-year-old man with an increasing prostate-specific antigen of 9.9 ng/mL. (*A*) Axial T2-weighted image at the midlevel of the prostate showing an ill-defined hyopintense lesion in the transition zone on the left (*arrow*) with an erased charcol sign, suggestive of the presence of a significant prostate cancer. (*B*) Axial diffusion-weighted MR image acquired at a b-value of 1000 s/mm^2 showing the suspicious lesion on (*A*) as an ill-defined hyperintense lesion with a hypointense signal on the corresponding apparent diffusion coefficient (ADC) map in (*C*) and an ADC-value of 698 × 10^{-6} mm^2/s. These findings correspond with a Prostate Imaging Reporting and Data System assessment category of 4 (lesion is <1.5 cm). MR/transrectal ultrasound fusion–guided biopsy confirmed a significant prostate cancer with a Gleason score of 3 + 4 = 7 on histology.

sensitivity, 72.7%; specificity, 70.6%) for identifying high-risk lesions. These intrapatient-normalized ADC ratios may be better to detect high-grade tumors than tumor ADCs alone.[78] Donati and colleagues[79] evaluated different ADC parameters from a whole-lesion assessment of DW-MR imaging to differentiate low-grade from intermediate-grade and high-grade cancer lesions. They found that the 10th percentile correlated best with the Gleason score and may be the best option to differentiate low-grade from intermediate-grade and high-grade cancers. Although malignant lesions altogether show significantly lower ADC values than normal tissue at least in the PZ of the prostate gland, there remain no universal cutoff values for a reliable detection of prostate cancer owing to different sequence protocols, vendor specifications, and different b-values being used.

For local tumor staging, the detection of capsule infiltration or extracapsular extension, seminal vesicle infiltration, or invasion of pelvic lymph nodes is essential because these are major negative prognostic factors[80] (**Fig. 6**). Usually, high-resolution T2w sequences and postcontrast sequences allow to evaluate an infiltration of the prostate capsule or an extracapsular infiltration owing to their high spatial resolution. However, in a group of 47 patients, DW-MR imaging was shown to have a sensitivity of 72%, a specificity of 77%, and a positive predictive value of 86% to detect extracapsular extension of prostate cancers.[81] In another group of 40 patients, thereof 23 had extracapsular extension of the tumor, DWI, and ADC mapping added to T2w imaging significantly improved the accuracy for preoperative detection of extracapsular extension for both readers ($P<.05$).[82] Furthermore, a recent study by Giganti and colleagues[83] on 101 patients with the aim to predict extracapsular extension based on DWI found the ADC to be a potential biomarker to predict extracapsular extension in prostate cancer.

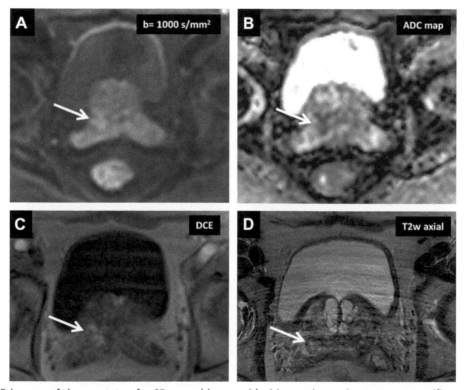

Fig. 6. MR images of the prostate of a 65-year-old man with rising an increasing prostate-specific antigen. (A) Axial diffusion-weighted MR image acquired at a b-value of 1000 s/mm² showing a hyperintense lesion at the base of the prostate with extension into the right seminal vesical (*arrow*) corresponding with a hypointense lesion on the corresponding apparent diffusion coefficient map in (B, *arrow*). (C) Dynamic contrast-enhanced (DCE) MR imaging shows early and focal enhancement of the lesion (*arrow*). (D) Axial T2-weighted (T2w) MR image shows that the lesion in (A–C, *arrow*) corresponds to an extruded circumscribed benign prostatic hyperplasia nodule confirmed on histology after MR/transrectal ultrasound-guided biopsy. This example nicely demonstrates that all sequences have to be taken into account to make the correct diagnosis to avoid the false diagnosis of T3b prostate cancer.

For the evaluation of an infiltration of the seminal vesicles a study on 166 patients (thereof, 30 had a histologically proven tumor infiltration of the vesicles), a combination of T2w imaging with DW-MR imaging significantly improved the specificity (from 87% to 97%) and the accuracy (from 87% to 96%) compared with the use of T2w imaging alone.[84] In a further study on 39 patients with seminal vesicle infiltration, the AUC for T2w imaging combined with DW-MR imaging (0.897) was significantly greater than that for T2w imaging alone (0.779; $P<.05$), leading to a significantly higher accuracy of seminal vesicle infiltration.[85] In 23 patients with seminal vesicle infiltration, Soylu and colleagues[86] found high specificities (93.1% and 93.6 for readers 1 and 2) and high negative predictive values (94.8% and 94%) for 2 readers, but only moderate sensitivities (59% and 52%) and positive predictive values (52% and 50%). In contrast, the addition of DW-MR imaging significantly improved the specificity (to 96.6% for reader 1 and to 98.3% for reader 2; $P = .02$ and .003) and the PPV (to 70% for reader 1 and to 79% for reader 2; $P<.05$ each).

In patients with very low-risk prostate cancer, active surveillance (AS) is a treatment option with regular follow-ups of prostate-specific antigen levels, digital rectal examinations, and repeat prostate biopsies.[87,88] However, AS based on prostate-specific antigen levels and repeat biopsies remains suboptimal because there are doubts that prostate-specific antigen kinetics during follow-up is a reliable trigger for interventions and biopsies owing to an underlying sampling error.[89,90] Giles and colleagues[91] found in 81 patients that suspicious lesions in patients that were upgraded during repeat biopsies were significantly lower than those in histologic stable lesions; therefore, ADC values being a valuable predictor of tumor progression having potential for monitoring patients. A recent study on 287 AS candidates revealed that high ADC values are an independent predictor of organ-confined lesions with a Gleason score of 6 or less disease and insignificant prostate cancer (odds ratio, 2.43 [$P = .011$] and odds ratio, 2.74 [$P = .009$], respectively), concluding that ADC values can be a useful marker for predicting insignificant prostate cancer in candidates for AS.[92]

Besides AS, several studies demonstrated the potential role of DW-MR imaging in follow-up examinations to detect tumor recurrence after radical prostatectomy. A study using 3 T MR imaging to validate the role of DW-MR imaging in the detection of local cancer recurrence showed in 262 patients with radical prostatectomy a sensitivity of 97%, a specificity of 95%, and an accuracy of 9% when T2w imaging was combined with DW-MR imaging (b-value of 3000 s/mm^2).[93] A further study on 43 patients underlined the importance of DWI as sensitivity, specificity, and accuracy were significantly higher for predicting local recurrence when T2w imaging was combined with DWI ($P<.05$).[94]

(Pelvic) Lymph Nodes and Lymph Node Staging

In patients with prostate or muscle-invasive bladder cancer, it is crucial to detect possible lymph node metastases to allow a proper treatment planning and a prognosis assessment of the disease as lymph node metastases correlate with poorer prognosis.[95–97] Lymph node staging is routinely being performed with both CT or MR imaging. However, both cross-sectional imaging techniques rely exclusively on morphologic criteria like size and shape with cutoff values of 8 to 10 mm in the short axis diameter and the internal tissue structure of lymph nodes.[98,99] This was shown to be suboptimal, because there are micrometastases in up to 25% of patients without enlarged lymph nodes in the preoperative cross-sectional imaging.[100,101] In contrast, lymph nodes may also be enlarged, not owing to a metastatic disease, but rather owing to reactive/inflammatory changes leading to false-positive results.[102]

The use of DW-MR imaging to provide a further evaluation of lymph nodes has widely been used in different body regions and has also been used in the pelvic region to evaluate a possible metastatic affection of pelvic lymph nodes by bladder and prostate cancer[103–105] (**Fig. 7**). In a study of 29 patients with prostate cancer using b-values of 50, 300, and 600 s/mm^2, Eiber and colleagues[106] found significantly lower ADC values in lymph nodes that were determined as malignant (n = 16; mean ADC value, $1.11 \pm 0.23 \times 10^{-3}$ mm^2/s) compared with benign lymph nodes (n = 29; mean ADC value, $1.48 \pm 0.23 \times 10^{-3}$ mm^2/s; $P<.0001$). The same result was also true for a subgroup analysis in lymph nodes smaller versus larger than 10 mm, because the mean size of benign and malignant lymph nodes did not differ significantly in size ($P = .3643$). The sensitivity was 86%, specificity 85.3%, and the accuracy 85.6% to differentiate between benign and malignant lymph nodes using a cutoff value of 1.30×10^{-3} mm^2/s. A similar result with significant lower ADC values in metastatic lymph nodes was found in a series of 26 patients with pathologic proven prostate cancer with mean ADC values of $0.79 \pm 0.14 \times 10^{-3}$ mm^2/s in 19 pathologically proven metastatic lymph nodes and of $1.13 \pm 0.29 \times 10^{-3}$ mm^2/s in 85 benign lymph nodes

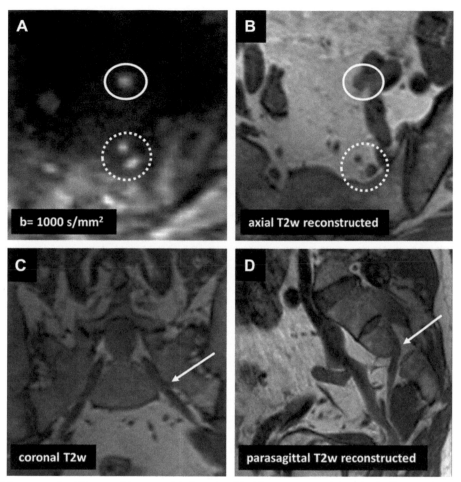

Fig. 7. MR images of a 60-year-old man with invasive bladder cancer and histologically proven lymph node metastasis in the external iliac region on the left. (*A*) Axial diffusion-weighted (DW) MR image acquired at a *b*-value of 1000 s/mm² shows a bight noncontinuous structure (*white circle*) corresponding with a lymph node adjacent to the left external iliac vessels on the axial reconstructed 3-dimensional (3D) T2-weighted (T2w) MR image in (*B*). The *dotted white circle* shows 2 additional bright structures in (*A*) corresponding with sacral nerve roots in (*B, dotted circle; C, arrow*) coronal 3D T2w MR image as well as on the parasagittal reconstructed 3D T2w image in (*D, arrow*). The correlation between the DW-MR images and morphologic images is the prerequisite to make an accurate diagnosis of a suspicious lymph node.

(*P*<.0001, use of multiple *b*-values of 500, 800, 100, and 1500 s/mm²).[107]

With a lesser statistical significance level (*P* = .02), mean ADC values were lower in metastatic lymph nodes than in benign lymph nodes in a study on 36 patients with muscle-invasive bladder cancer (0.85 × 10⁻³ mm²/s vs 1.00 × 10⁻³ mm²/s).[108]

A recent study focused on normal-sized pelvic lymph nodes in 120 patients with prostate and/or bladder cancer (maximum short axis diameter 8 mm for prostate cancer and 10 mm for bladder cancer) who underwent radical cystectomy or radical prostatectomy with extended lymph node dissection of the entire pelvis including histologic workup as gold standard.[109] Of the 120

patients, 33 (27.5%) had metastases in 88 lymph nodes. On a per-patient basis, 3 different radiologists correctly diagnosed positive lymph nodes in 26 (sensitivity of 79%), 21 (64%) and 25 (76%) of the 33 patients with lymph node metastases, whereas the specificity ranged between 79% and 85%, respectively. Diagnostic accuracy could further be improved by correlating DW-MR imaging with meticulous analysis of morphologic criteria. Thus, DW-MR imaging allows noninvasive detection of small metastases in morphologic normal-sized lymph node in a substantial percentage of patients with bladder and prostate cancers who would otherwise not have been diagnosed with conventional cross-sectional imaging.

With the attempt to combine DW-MR imaging with PET with ^{11}C-cholinePET/CT, Beer and colleagues[110] analyzed ADC values and standardized uptake values in PET in the pelvic lymph nodes in a small study population of 14 patients with prostate cancer. Because the authors found ADC values and standardized uptake values highly significant inverse correlated, they concluded that DW-MR imaging provides additional information when combined with standardized uptake values in ^{11}C-choline PET/CT.

Because lymph node staging with conventional cross-sectional imaging is limited, a combination of DW-MR imaging with the use of ultrasmall supraparamagnetic particles of iron oxide (USPIO) revealed an accuracy of 90% to detect lymph node metastases on a per-patient base in a group of 21 patients with bladder and/or prostate cancer.[111] A subsequent study of a larger group of 75 patients revealed a sensitivity of 65% to 75% for the detection of lymph node metastases when combining DW-MR imaging and USPIO, whereas the specificity was 93% to 96%, respectively.[112] Although the results were encouraging and the mean reading time for a combined USPIO–DW-MR imaging was low (9 min), USPIO are currently not in regular clinical use owing to a commercial unavailability.

SUMMARY

As shown, to date DW-MR imaging has been able to address some remaining diagnostic problems of conventional cross-sectional imaging in genitourinary imaging, like a further discrimination between benign and malignant lesions in the kidney, improving the tumor staging in bladder cancer, and the detection of prostate cancer. However, the greatest remaining challenge to allow a further acceptance and widespread use of DW-MR imaging is a standardization of the imaging technique. Attempts for a standardization have been made for DW-MR imaging and especially multiparametric MR imaging for imaging of the prostate.[113,114] A worldwide standardized technique not depending on vendor specifications would allow high-quality multicenter trials to provide a further validation of the technique, which would rapidly distribute the technique to nonacademic institutions.

Furthermore, a wide acceptance of DW-MR imaging with clear cutoff values to differentiate benign from malignant lesions would have a high impact on patient management. This would shorten the diagnostic workup in many patients, might reduce contrast medium administration and may drastically reduce the period of uncertainty through a noninvasive test.

The use of DW-MR imaging has been promising to serve as a noninvasive technique in the early detection of a therapeutic response, for example, in antiangiogenic therapy of metastatic clear cell RCCs.[31,34] In contrast with conventional chemotherapy, many of these new treatment substances do not lead to a regression in tumor size. DW-MR imaging is able to detect early changes in tumor metabolism expressed by microstructural changes that can be visualized by DW-MR imaging. Therefore, DW-MR imaging may not only allow to evaluate if a patient is responding to a therapy, but may also contribute to find the correct dose level in different treatment regimens.

Furthermore, because health care systems in many countries are suffering from increasing costs, DW-MR imaging might contribute to lower costs when imaging protocols are shortened by omitting postcontrast sequences that are being replaced by DW-MR imaging sequences in selected cases.

In conclusion, a further standardization of DW-MR imaging technique and improvements in imaging analysis and interpretation will contribute to a wider distribution, beyond genitourinary imaging of this promising technique.

REFERENCES

1. Le Bihan D, Breton E, Lallemand D, et al. Separation of diffusion and perfusion in intravoxel incoherent motion MR imaging. Radiology 1988; 168(2):497–505.
2. Schaefer PW, Grant PE, Gonzalez RG. Diffusion-weighted MR imaging of the brain. Radiology 2000;217(2):331–45.
3. Merino JG, Warach S. Imaging of acute stroke. Nat Rev Neurol 2010;6(10):560–71.
4. Thoeny HC, De Keyzer F. Extracranial applications of diffusion-weighted magnetic resonance imaging. Eur Radiol 2007;17(6):1385–93.
5. Murtz P, Flacke S, Träber F, et al. Abdomen: diffusion-weighted MR imaging with pulse-triggered single-shot sequences. Radiology 2002; 224(1):258–64.
6. Morani AC, Elsayes KM, Liu PS, et al. Abdominal applications of diffusion-weighted magnetic resonance imaging: where do we stand. World J Radiol 2013;5(3):68–80.
7. Bozgeyik Z, Onur MR, Poyraz AK. The role of diffusion weighted magnetic resonance imaging in oncologic settings. Quant Imaging Med Surg 2013;3(5):269–78.

8. Koh DM, Collins DJ. Diffusion-weighted MRI in the body: applications and challenges in oncology. AJR Am J Roentgenol 2007;188(6):1622–35.

9. Merboldt KD, Hanicke W, Frahm J. Diffusion imaging using stimulated echoes. Magn Reson Med 1991;19(2):233–9.

10. Le Bihan D, Breton E, Lallemand D, et al. MR imaging of intravoxel incoherent motions: application to diffusion and perfusion in neurologic disorders. Radiology 1986;161(2):401–7.

11. Charles-Edwards EM, deSouza NM. Diffusion-weighted magnetic resonance imaging and its application to cancer. Cancer Imaging 2006;6:135–43.

12. Petralia G, Thoeny HC. DW-MRI of the urogenital tract: applications in oncology. Cancer Imaging 2010;10(Spec no A):S112–23.

13. Burdette JH, Elster AD, Ricci PE. Acute cerebral infarction: quantification of spin-density and T2 shine-through phenomena on diffusion-weighted MR images. Radiology 1999;212(2):333–9.

14. Thoeny HC, De Keyzer F, Oyen RH, et al. Diffusion-weighted MR imaging of kidneys in healthy volunteers and patients with parenchymal diseases: initial experience. Radiology 2005;235(3):911–7.

15. Taouli B, Thakur RK, Mannelli L, et al. Renal lesions: characterization with diffusion-weighted imaging versus contrast-enhanced MR imaging. Radiology 2009;251(2):398–407.

16. Kilickesmez O, Inci E, Atilla S, et al. Diffusion-weighted imaging of the renal and adrenal lesions. J Comput Assist Tomogr 2009;33(6):828–33.

17. Razek AA, Farouk A, Mousa A, et al. Role of diffusion-weighted magnetic resonance imaging in characterization of renal tumors. J Comput Assist Tomogr 2011;35(3):332–6.

18. Erbay G, Koc Z, Karadeli E, et al. Evaluation of malignant and benign renal lesions using diffusion-weighted MRI with multiple b values. Acta Radiol 2012;53(3):359–65.

19. Sandrasegaran K, Sundaram CP, Ramaswamy R, et al. Usefulness of diffusion-weighted imaging in the evaluation of renal masses. AJR Am J Roentgenol 2010;194(2):438–45.

20. Zhang J, Tehrani YM, Wang L, et al. Renal masses: characterization with diffusion-weighted MR imaging–a preliminary experience. Radiology 2008;247(2):458–64.

21. Lassel EA, Rao R, Schwenke C, et al. Diffusion-weighted imaging of focal renal lesions: a meta-analysis. Eur Radiol 2014;24(1):241–9.

22. Tanaka H, Yoshida S, Fujii Y, et al. Diffusion-weighted magnetic resonance imaging in the differentiation of angiomyolipoma with minimal fat from clear cell renal cell carcinoma. Int J Urol 2011;18(10):727–30.

23. Reuter VE. The pathology of renal epithelial neoplasms. Semin Oncol 2006;33(5):534–43.

24. Cheville JC, Lohse CM, Zincke H, et al. Comparisons of outcome and prognostic features among histologic subtypes of renal cell carcinoma. Am J Surg Pathol 2003;27(5):612–24.

25. Wang HJ, Pui MH, Guo Y, et al. Diffusion-weighted MRI in bladder carcinoma: the differentiation between tumor recurrence and benign changes after resection. Abdom Imaging 2014;39(1):135–41.

26. Choi YA, Kim CK, Park SY, et al. Subtype differentiation of renal cell carcinoma using diffusion-weighted and blood oxygenation level-dependent MRI. AJR Am J Roentgenol 2014;203(1):W78–84.

27. Rosenkrantz AB, Niver BE, Fitzgerald EF, et al. Utility of the apparent diffusion coefficient for distinguishing clear cell renal cell carcinoma of low and high nuclear grade. AJR Am J Roentgenol 2010;195(5):W344–51.

28. Thomsen HS, Morcos SK, Almén T, et al. Nephrogenic systemic fibrosis and gadolinium-based contrast media: updated ESUR Contrast Medium Safety Committee guidelines. Eur Radiol 2013;23(2):307–18.

29. Kanda T, Ishii K, Kawaguchi H, et al. High signal intensity in the dentate nucleus and globus pallidus on unenhanced T1-weighted MR images: relationship with increasing cumulative dose of a gadolinium-based contrast material. Radiology 2014;270(3):834–41.

30. McDonald RJ, McDonald JS, Kallmes DF, et al. Intracranial Gadolinium Deposition after Contrast-enhanced MR Imaging. Radiology 2015;275(3):772–82.

31. Jeon TY, Kim CK, Kim JH, et al. Assessment of early therapeutic response to sorafenib in renal cell carcinoma xenografts by dynamic contrast-enhanced and diffusion-weighted MR imaging. Br J Radiol 2015;88(1053):20150163.

32. Escudier B, Eisen T, Stadler WM, et al. Sorafenib in advanced clear-cell renal-cell carcinoma. N Engl J Med 2007;356(2):125–34.

33. Kane RC, Farrell AT, Saber H, et al. Sorafenib for the treatment of advanced renal cell carcinoma. Clin Cancer Res 2006;12(24):7271–8.

34. Bharwani N, Miquel ME, Powles T, et al. Diffusion-weighted and multiphase contrast-enhanced MRI as surrogate markers of response to neoadjuvant sunitinib in metastatic renal cell carcinoma. Br J Cancer 2014;110(3):616–24.

35. Montironi R, Mazzucchelli R, Scarpelli M, et al. Update on selected renal cell tumors with clear cell features. With emphasis on multilocular cystic clear cell renal cell carcinoma. Histol Histopathol 2013;28(12):1555–66.

36. Babjuk M, Oosterlinck W, Sylvester R, et al. EAU guidelines on non-muscle-invasive urothelial

carcinoma of the bladder, the 2011 update. Eur Urol 2011;59(6):997–1008.

37. Josephson D, Pasin E, Stein JP. Superficial bladder cancer: part 2. Management. Expert Rev Anticancer Ther 2007;7(4):567–81.

38. Sherif A, Jonsson MN, Wiklund NP. Treatment of muscle-invasive bladder cancer. Expert Rev Anticancer Ther 2007;7(9):1279–83.

39. Ghafoori M, Shakiba M, Ghiasi A, et al. Value of MRI in local staging of bladder cancer. Urol J 2013;10(2):866–72.

40. Tillou X, Grardel E, Fourmarier M, et al. Can MRI be used to distinguish between superficial and invasive transitional cell bladder cancer? Prog Urol 2008;18(7):440–4 [in French].

41. Ng CS. Radiologic diagnosis and staging of renal and bladder cancer. Semin Roentgenol 2006; 41(2):121–38.

42. Watanabe H, Kanematsu M, Kondo H, et al. Preoperative T staging of urinary bladder cancer: does diffusion-weighted MRI have supplementary value? AJR Am J Roentgenol 2009;192(5):1361–6.

43. El-Assmy A, Abou-El-Ghar ME, Mosbah A, et al. Bladder tumour staging: comparison of diffusion- and T2-weighted MR imaging. Eur Radiol 2009; 19(7):1575–81.

44. Takeuchi M, Sasaki S, Ito M, et al. Urinary bladder cancer: diffusion-weighted MR imaging–accuracy for diagnosing T stage and estimating histologic grade. Radiology 2009;251(1):112–21.

45. Ohgiya Y, Suyama J, Sai S, et al. Preoperative T staging of urinary bladder cancer: efficacy of stalk detection and diagnostic performance of diffusion-weighted imaging at 3T. Magn Reson Med Sci 2014;13(3):175–81.

46. Wu LM, Chen XX, Xu JR, et al. Clinical value of T2-weighted imaging combined with diffusion-weighted imaging in preoperative T staging of urinary bladder cancer: a large-scale, multiobserver prospective study on 3.0-T MRI. Acad Radiol 2013;20(8):939–46.

47. Kobayashi S, Koga F, Yoshida S, et al. Diagnostic performance of diffusion-weighted magnetic resonance imaging in bladder cancer: potential utility of apparent diffusion coefficient values as a biomarker to predict clinical aggressiveness. Eur Radiol 2011;21(10):2178–86.

48. Grignon DJ. The current classification of urothelial neoplasms. Mod Pathol 2009;22(Suppl 2):S60–9.

49. Wang Y, Li Z, Meng X, et al. Nonmuscle-invasive and muscle-invasive urinary bladder cancer: image quality and clinical value of reduced field-of-view versus conventional single-shot echo-planar imaging DWI. Medicine (Baltimore) 2016;95(10): e2951.

50. Avcu S, Koseoglu MN, Ceylan K, et al. The value of diffusion-weighted MRI in the diagnosis of malignant and benign urinary bladder lesions. Br J Radiol 2011;84(1006):875–82.

51. Rodel C, Weiss C, Sauer R. Trimodality treatment and selective organ preservation for bladder cancer. J Clin Oncol 2006;24(35):5536–44.

52. Chung PW, Bristow RG, Milosevic MF, et al. Long-term outcome of radiation-based conservation therapy for invasive bladder cancer. Urol Oncol 2007; 25(4):303–9.

53. Yoshida S, Koga F, Kawakami S, et al. Initial experience of diffusion-weighted magnetic resonance imaging to assess therapeutic response to induction chemoradiotherapy against muscle-invasive bladder cancer. Urology 2010;75(2):387–91.

54. Yoshida S, Koga F, Kobayashi S, et al. Role of diffusion-weighted magnetic resonance imaging in predicting sensitivity to chemoradiotherapy in muscle-invasive bladder cancer. Int J Radiat Oncol Biol Phys 2012;83(1):e21–7.

55. Loffroy R, Chevallier O, Moulin M, et al. Current role of multiparametric magnetic resonance imaging for prostate cancer. Quant Imaging Med Surg 2015; 5(5):754–64.

56. Somford DM, Fütterer JJ, Hambrock T, et al. Diffusion and perfusion MR imaging of the prostate. Magn Reson Imaging Clin N Am 2008;16(4): 685–95, ix.

57. Barentsz JO, Weinreb JC, Verma S, et al. Synopsis of the PI-RADS v2 guidelines for multiparametric prostate magnetic resonance imaging and recommendations for use. Eur Urol 2016;69(1):41–9.

58. Miao H, Fukatsu H, Ishigaki T. Prostate cancer detection with 3-T MRI: comparison of diffusion-weighted and T2-weighted imaging. Eur J Radiol 2007;61(2):297–302.

59. Tanimoto A, Nakashima J, Kohno H, et al. Prostate cancer screening: the clinical value of diffusion-weighted imaging and dynamic MR imaging in combination with T2-weighted imaging. J Magn Reson Imaging 2007;25(1):146–52.

60. Haider MA, van der Kwast TH, Tanguay J, et al. Combined T2-weighted and diffusion-weighted MRI for localization of prostate cancer. AJR Am J Roentgenol 2007;189(2):323–8.

61. Lim HK, Kim JK, Kim KA, et al. Prostate cancer: apparent diffusion coefficient map with T2-weighted images for detection–a multireader study. Radiology 2009;250(1):145–51.

62. Kajihara H, Hayashida Y, Murakami R, et al. Usefulness of diffusion-weighted imaging in the localization of prostate cancer. Int J Radiat Oncol Biol Phys 2009;74(2):399–403.

63. Gibbs P, Pickles MD, Turnbull LW. Diffusion imaging of the prostate at 3.0 tesla. Invest Radiol 2006;41(2):185–8.

64. Yoshimitsu K, Kiyoshima K, Irie H, et al. Usefulness of apparent diffusion coefficient map in diagnosing

prostate carcinoma: correlation with stepwise histo-pathology. J Magn Reson Imaging 2008;27(1): 132–9.

65. Wu LM, Xu JR, Ye YQ, et al. The clinical value of diffusion-weighted imaging in combination with T2-weighted imaging in diagnosing prostate carcinoma: a systematic review and meta-analysis. AJR Am J Roentgenol 2012;199(1):103–10.

66. Jie C, Rongbo L, Ping T. The value of diffusion-weighted imaging in the detection of prostate cancer: a meta-analysis. Eur Radiol 2014;24(8): 1929–41.

67. Oto A, Kayhan A, Jiang Y, et al. Prostate cancer: differentiation of central gland cancer from benign prostatic hyperplasia by using diffusion-weighted and dynamic contrast-enhanced MR imaging. Radiology 2010;257(3):715–23.

68. Hoeks CM, Hambrock T, Yakar D, et al. Transition zone prostate cancer: detection and localization with 3-T multiparametric MR imaging. Radiology 2013;266(1):207–17.

69. Rosenkrantz AB, Parikh N, Kierans AS, et al. Prostate cancer detection using computed very high b-value diffusion-weighted imaging: how high should we go? Acad Radiol 2016;23:704–11.

70. Hambrock T, Hoeks C, Hulsbergen-van de Kaa C, et al. Prospective assessment of prostate cancer aggressiveness using 3-T diffusion-weighted magnetic resonance imaging-guided biopsies versus a systematic 10-core transrectal ultrasound prostate biopsy cohort. Eur Urol 2012;61(1):177–84.

71. deSouza NM, Riches SF, Vanas NJ, et al. Diffusion-weighted magnetic resonance imaging: a potential non-invasive marker of tumour aggressiveness in localized prostate cancer. Clin Radiol 2008;63(7): 774–82.

72. Hambrock T, Somford DM, Huisman HJ, et al. Relationship between apparent diffusion coefficients at 3.0-T MR imaging and Gleason grade in peripheral zone prostate cancer. Radiology 2011; 259(2):453–61.

73. Jung SI, Donati OF, Vargas HA, et al. Transition zone prostate cancer: incremental value of diffusion-weighted endorectal MR imaging in tumor detection and assessment of aggressiveness. Radiology 2013;269(2):493–503.

74. Verma S, Rajesh A, Morales H, et al. Assessment of aggressiveness of prostate cancer: correlation of apparent diffusion coefficient with histologic grade after radical prostatectomy. AJR Am J Roentgenol 2011;196(2):374–81.

75. Woodfield CA, Tung GA, Grand DJ, et al. Diffusion-weighted MRI of peripheral zone prostate cancer: comparison of tumor apparent diffusion coefficient with Gleason score and percentage of tumor on core biopsy. AJR Am J Roentgenol 2010;194(4): W316–22.

76. Vargas HA, Akin O, Franiel T, et al. Diffusion-weighted endorectal MR imaging at 3 T for prostate cancer: tumor detection and assessment of aggressiveness. Radiology 2011;259(3):775–84.

77. Turkbey B, Shah VP, Pang Y, et al. Is apparent diffusion coefficient associated with clinical risk scores for prostate cancers that are visible on 3-T MR images? Radiology 2011;258(2):488–95.

78. Lebovici A, Sfrangeu SA, Feier D, et al. Evaluation of the normal-to-diseased apparent diffusion coefficient ratio as an indicator of prostate cancer aggressiveness. BMC Med Imaging 2014;14:15.

79. Donati OF, Jung SI, Vargas HA, et al. Multiparametric prostate MR imaging with T2-weighted, diffusion-weighted, and dynamic contrast-enhanced sequences: are all pulse sequences necessary to detect locally recurrent prostate cancer after radiation therapy? Radiology 2013;268(2):440–50.

80. Eggener SE, Scardino PT, Walsh PC, et al. Predicting 15-year prostate cancer specific mortality after radical prostatectomy. J Urol 2011;185(3):869–75.

81. Pinaquy JB, De Clermont-Galleran H, Pasticier G, et al. Comparative effectiveness of [(18) F]-fluorocholine PET-CT and pelvic MRI with diffusion-weighted imaging for staging in patients with high-risk prostate cancer. Prostate 2015; 75(3):323–31.

82. Lawrence EM, Gallagher FA, Barrett T, et al. Preoperative 3-T diffusion-weighted MRI for the qualitative and quantitative assessment of extracapsular extension in patients with intermediate- or high-risk prostate cancer. AJR Am J Roentgenol 2014; 203(3):W280–6.

83. Giganti F, Coppola A, Ambrosi A, et al. Apparent diffusion coefficient in the evaluation of side-specific extracapsular extension in prostate cancer: development and external validation of a nomogram of clinical use. Urol Oncol 2016;34: 291.e9-17.

84. Kim CK, Choi D, Park BK, et al. Diffusion-weighted MR imaging for the evaluation of seminal vesicle invasion in prostate cancer: initial results. J Magn Reson Imaging 2008;28(4):963–9.

85. Ren J, Huan Y, Wang H, et al. Seminal vesicle invasion in prostate cancer: prediction with combined T2-weighted and diffusion-weighted MR imaging. Eur Radiol 2009;19(10):2481–6.

86. Soylu FN, Peng Y, Jiang Y, et al. Seminal vesicle invasion in prostate cancer: evaluation by using multiparametric endorectal MR imaging. Radiology 2013;267(3):797–806.

87. Heidenreich A, Bastian PJ, Bellmunt J, et al. EAU guidelines on prostate cancer. part 1: screening, diagnosis, and local treatment with curative intent-update 2013. Eur Urol 2014;65(1):124–37.

88. Klotz L, Zhang L, Lam A, et al. Clinical results of long-term follow-up of a large, active surveillance

cohort with localized prostate cancer. J Clin Oncol 2010;28(1):126–31.

89. Ross AE, Loeb S, Landis P, et al. Prostate-specific antigen kinetics during follow-up are an unreliable trigger for intervention in a prostate cancer surveillance program. J Clin Oncol 2010;28(17): 2810–6.

90. Bjurlin MA, Meng X, Le Nobin J, et al. Optimization of prostate biopsy: the role of magnetic resonance imaging targeted biopsy in detection, localization and risk assessment. J Urol 2014; 192(3):648–58.

91. Giles SL, Morgan VA, Riches SF, et al. Apparent diffusion coefficient as a predictive biomarker of prostate cancer progression: value of fast and slow diffusion components. AJR Am J Roentgenol 2011;196(3):586–91.

92. Kim TH, Jeong JY, Lee SW, et al. Diffusion-weighted magnetic resonance imaging for prediction of insignificant prostate cancer in potential candidates for active surveillance. Eur Radiol 2015;25(6):1786–92.

93. Panebianco V, Barchetti F, Sciarra A, et al. Prostate cancer recurrence after radical prostatectomy: the role of 3-T diffusion imaging in multi-parametric magnetic resonance imaging. Eur Radiol 2013; 23(6):1745–52.

94. Cha D, Kim CK, Park SY, et al. Evaluation of suspected soft tissue lesion in the prostate bed after radical prostatectomy using 3T multiparametric magnetic resonance imaging. Magn Reson Imaging 2015;33(4):407–12.

95. Karl A, Carroll PR, Gschwend JE, et al. The impact of lymphadenectomy and lymph node metastasis on the outcomes of radical cystectomy for bladder cancer. Eur Urol 2009;55(4): 826–35.

96. Briganti A, Blute ML, Eastham JH, et al. Pelvic lymph node dissection in prostate cancer. Eur Urol 2009;55(6):1251–65.

97. Tilki D, Brausi M, Colombo R, et al. Lymphadenectomy for bladder cancer at the time of radical cystectomy. Eur Urol 2013;64(2):266–76.

98. McMahon CJ, Rofsky NM, Pedrosa I. Lymphatic metastases from pelvic tumors: anatomic classification, characterization, and staging. Radiology 2010;254(1):31–46.

99. Oyen RH, Van Poppel HP, Ameye FE, et al. Lymph node staging of localized prostatic carcinoma with CT and CT-guided fine-needle aspiration biopsy: prospective study of 285 patients. Radiology 1994;190(2):315–22.

100. Fleischmann A, Thalmann GN, Markwalder R, et al. Prognostic implications of extracapsular extension of pelvic lymph node metastases in urothelial carcinoma of the bladder. Am J Surg Pathol 2005;29(1): 89–95.

101. Schumacher MC, Burkhard FC, Thalmann GN, et al. Good outcome for patients with few lymph node metastases after radical retropubic prostatectomy. Eur Urol 2008;54(2):344–52.

102. Studer UE, Scherz S, Scheidegger J, et al. Enlargement of regional lymph nodes in renal cell carcinoma is often not due to metastases. J Urol 1990;144(2 Pt 1):243–5.

103. Peerlings J, Troost EG, Nelemans PJ, et al. The diagnostic value of MR imaging in determining the lymph node status of patients with non-small cell lung cancer: a meta-analysis. Radiology 2016;281:86–98.

104. Shen G, Zhou H, Jia Z, et al. Diagnostic performance of diffusion-weighted magnetic resonance imaging for detection of pelvic metastatic lymph nodes in patients with cervical cancer: a systematic review and meta-analysis. Br J Radiol 2015. [Epub ahead of print].

105. Wu LM, Xu JR, Hua J, et al. Value of diffusion-weighted MR imaging performed with quantitative apparent diffusion coefficient values for cervical lymphadenopathy. J Magn Reson Imaging 2013; 38(3):663–70.

106. Eiber M, Beer AJ, Holzapfel K, et al. Preliminary results for characterization of pelvic lymph nodes in patients with prostate cancer by diffusion-weighted MR-imaging. Invest Radiol 2010;45(1):15–23.

107. Vallini V, Ortori S, Boraschi P, et al. Staging of pelvic lymph nodes in patients with prostate cancer: usefulness of multiple b value SE-EPI diffusion-weighted imaging on a 3.0 T MR system. Eur J Radiol Open 2016;3:16–21.

108. Papalia R, Simone G, Grasso R, et al. Diffusion-weighted magnetic resonance imaging in patients selected for radical cystectomy: detection rate of pelvic lymph node metastases. BJU Int 2012; 109(7):1031–6.

109. Thoeny HC, Froehlich JM, Triantafyllou M, et al. Metastases in normal-sized pelvic lymph nodes: detection with diffusion-weighted MR imaging. Radiology 2014;273(1):125–35.

110. Beer AJ, Eiber M, Souvatzoglou M, et al. Restricted water diffusibility as measured by diffusion-weighted MR imaging and choline uptake in (11) C-choline PET/CT are correlated in pelvic lymph nodes in patients with prostate cancer. Mol Imaging Biol 2011;13(2):352–61.

111. Thoeny HC, Triantafyllou M, Birkhaeuser FD, et al. Combined ultrasmall superparamagnetic particles of iron oxide-enhanced and diffusion-weighted magnetic resonance imaging reliably detect pelvic lymph node metastases in normal-sized nodes of bladder and prostate cancer patients. Eur Urol 2009;55(4):761–9.

112. Birkhauser FD, Studer UE, Froehlich JM, et al. Combined ultrasmall superparamagnetic particles

of iron oxide-enhanced and diffusion-weighted magnetic resonance imaging facilitates detection of metastases in normal-sized pelvic lymph nodes of patients with bladder and prostate cancer. Eur Urol 2013;64(6):953–60.

113. Dickinson L, Ahmed HU, Allen C, et al. Magnetic resonance imaging for the detection, localisation, and characterisation of prostate cancer: recommendations from a European consensus meeting. Eur Urol 2011;59(4):477–94.

114. Taouli B, Beer AJ, Chenevert T, et al. Diffusion-weighted imaging outside the brain: consensus statement from an ISMRM-sponsored workshop. J Magn Reson Imaging 2016;44:521–40.

Technique of Multiparametric MR Imaging of the Prostate

Andrei S. Purysko, MD[a],*, Andrew B. Rosenkrantz, MD[b]

KEYWORDS

- MR imaging • Prostate cancer • Diffusion-weighted imaging

KEY POINTS

- The prostate imaging reporting and data system version 2 defines minimum acceptable technical parameters for multiparametric MR imaging of the prostate.
- All prostate MR imaging studies should include T2-weighted, T1-weighted, diffusion-weighted, and dynamic contrast-enhanced images.
- Diffusion-weighted images with high b-values ($\geq$1400 s/mm^2) can be calculated from the images with lower b-values (50–1000 s/mm^2) or acquired separately.
- Prostate MR imaging can be adequately performed on 1.5-T or 3-T systems with a pelvic phased array coil and optionally combined with an endorectal coil.
- Eliminating gas and stool from the rectum before the examination is important to minimize artifacts that negatively affect image quality.

 Video content accompanies this article at http://www.urologic.theclinics.com

INTRODUCTION

Since the use of MR imaging of the prostate was first reported in the early 1980s, this imaging modality has become an established noninvasive tool for the assessment of prostate cancer (PCa).[1,2] Advances in hardware and software have since led to faster acquisition of images, improvements in image quality, and the development of pulse sequences that have the ability to probe tissue properties, such as cellularity and perfusion, thus improving the ability of MR imaging to distinguish between benign and malignant tissues. These improvements, coupled with the evolution of MR imaging–targeted biopsy, have facilitated the use of MR imaging in the detection of PCa, assessment of tumor aggressiveness, disease staging, treatment planning, follow-up of patients on active surveillance, and follow-up after treatment in patients with biochemical recurrence.[2]

Despite these advances, significant variations in imaging acquisition, interpretation, and reporting across institutions have resulted in heterogeneous performance of prostate MR imaging and have limited the widespread adoption and acceptance of this method.[3] As a first step toward the standardization of prostate MR imaging, in 2012, the European Society of Urogenital Radiology developed consensus-based guidelines aiming to establish minimum acceptable technical parameters for

This article was previously published in March 2018 *Radiologic Clinics*, Volume 56, Issue 2.
Disclosures: A.S. Purysko has no conflicts of interest to disclose. A.B. Rosenkrantz receives royalties from Thieme Medical Publishers.
[a] Section of Abdominal Imaging, Imaging Institute, Cleveland Clinic, 9500 Euclid Avenue, Mail Code JB-3, Cleveland, OH 44195, USA; [b] Department of Radiology, New York University Langone Medical Center, 660 First Avenue, New York, NY 10016, USA
* Corresponding author:
E-mail address: puryska@ccf.org

Urol Clin N Am 45 (2018) 427–438
https://doi.org/10.1016/j.ucl.2018.03.008

prostate MR imaging, along with a structured category assessment system known as the Prostate Imaging and Reporting and Data System (PI-RADS) version 1 (PI-RADS v1).[4] In collaboration with the American College of Radiology through the PI-RADS Steering Committee, the second iteration of the guidelines (PI-RADS v2) was released in December of 2014, bringing important changes to the system.[5]

This review discusses the techniques that are used in state-of-the-art MR imaging of the prostate, including imaging protocols, hardware considerations, and important aspects of patient preparation, with an emphasis on the recommendations provided in the PI-RADS v2 guidelines.

SEQUENCES

PI-RADS v2 recommends the inclusion of T2-weighted imaging (T2-WI), T1-weighted imaging (T1-WI), diffusion-weighted imaging (DWI), and dynamic contrast-enhanced (DCE) pulse sequences for all prostate MR imaging studies. A set of minimal technical parameters for each of these pulse sequences is provided in the guidelines (**Box 1**). Because sequence acquisition is influenced by equipment availability and capability, centers are encouraged to optimize imaging protocols in order to obtain the best and most consistent image quality.

One change introduced in PI-RADS v2 was the exclusion of findings from magnetic resonance spectroscopic imaging (MRSI) in lesion assessment. This technique requires special expertise and is time consuming; thus, it is considered impractical for widespread use.

T2-Weighted Imaging

T2-WI offers excellent soft tissue contrast and detailed depiction of the zonal anatomy of the prostate, the seminal vesicles, and the neurovascular bundles (NVBs). High-quality T2-WI is considered critical for local staging of PCa, because this method helps to identify the presence of extraprostatic extension (EPE) of tumors and involvement of the seminal vesicles and NVBs.[6,7] According to PI-RADS v2, T2-WI should also be the dominant parameter used to assess lesions in the transition zone (TZ).

Two-dimensional (2D) fast-spin-echo (FSE) or turbo-spin-echo (TSE) T2-WI pulse sequences provide images with high signal-to-noise ratio (SNR) and high spatial resolution. These images are acquired in the true sagittal and oblique axial and oblique coronal planes (**Fig. 1**). Sagittal T2-WI can be obtained first to help define the range of coverage and orientation of the axial

---

Box 1
Summary of technical specifications described in Prostate Imaging Reporting and Data System version 2

T2-weighted images

- Pulse sequence: 2D fast spin-echo or turbo spin-echo (3D can be used as an adjunct to 2D)

- Imaging planes: Sagittal and oblique axial and coronal planes

- Field of view (FOV): 12 to 20 cm (to cover entire prostate gland and seminal vesicles)

- Slice thickness: $\leq$3 mm, no gap

- In-plane dimension: $\leq$0.7 mm (phase) $\times$ $\leq$0.4 mm (frequency)

Diffusion-weighted images (DWI)

- Pulse sequence: Spin-echo echo-planar imaging (EPI) DWI (free-breathing with fat saturation)

- Imaging planes: Same as axial T2-weighted images

- FOV: 16 to 22 cm

- Slice thickness: $\leq$4 mm, no gap

- TE $\leq$90 ms; TR $\leq$3000 ms

- In plane dimension: $\leq$2.5-mm phase and frequency

- b-values: Minimum of 2 for ADC map creation (lower b-value 50–100 s/mm^2, higher value 800–1000 s/mm^2); additional high b-values image ($\geq$1400 s/mm^2) should be acquired separately or calculated from images obtained with b-values <1000 s/mm^2

Dynamic contrast-enhanced images

- Pulse sequence: 2D or 3D T1-weighted gradient echo (3D preferred)

- Fat-suppression technique or subtraction should be considered

- Imaging plane: Same as axial T2-WI

- Contrast injection rate: 2 to 3 mL/s

- FOV: Encompass the entire prostate gland and seminal vesicles

- Slice thickness: $\leq$3 mm, no gap

- TE <5 ms; TR <100 ms

- In plane dimension: $\leq$2.0-mm phase and frequency

- Temporal resolution $\leq$10 s ($\leq$7 s is preferred)

- Acquisition time $\geq$2 min

Abbreviations: TE, echo time; TR, repetition time.

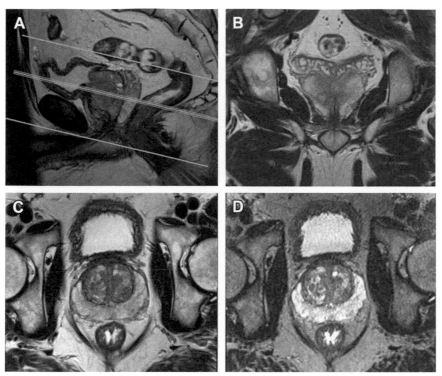

Fig. 1. Multiplanar 2D TSE T2-WI of the prostate obtained in the sagittal (*A*), coronal (*B*), and axial (*C*) planes. The sagittal T2-WI of the prostate can be used to define the scan range (in between the parallel *orange lines, A*) and the orientation of the axial T2-WI, diffusion-weighted, and DCE T1-WI images (*green lines* perpendicular through the long axis of the prostate, *A*). (*D*) Axial high-resolution 3D T2-WI can optionally be obtained in the same plane.

and coronal T2-WI. Axial T2-WI should be obtained in a perpendicular fashion through the long axis of the prostate. Axial T1-WI, DWI, and DCE images should be obtained in the same plane as axial T2-WI to facilitate the precise correlation of findings observed with these pulse sequences.

In PI-RADS v2, high-resolution 3-dimensional (3D) FSE T2-WI is described as an adjunct to 2D acquisitions. Currently available 3D T2-WI pulse sequences use various acceleration techniques that allow for the acquisition of images with isotropic voxels and have 2 main potential advantages.[7] First, by reducing volume-averaging artifacts, these images can be used to help assess certain characteristics of lesions (eg, the presence of a capsule around a nodule in the TZ, which favors a diagnosis of benign prostatic hyperplasia nodule) and to assess the integrity of the prostate capsule (**Fig. 2**). Second, the volumetric data set acquired with isotropic voxels can be used to reconstruct images in all 3 planes, which in turn may shorten the examination time by reducing the number of T2-WI sequences that need to be obtained. However, these images may have lower soft tissue contrast and in-plane resolution compared with 2D images. Furthermore, motion

artifacts during the long 3D acquisition could result in distortion of the entire data set.

T1-Weighted Imaging

T1-WI is useful in detecting postbiopsy changes that can affect the interpretation of other pulse sequences (**Fig. 3**). In general, using spin-echo or gradient-echo sequences with or without fat suppression, T1-WI obtained immediately before intravenous contrast administration can be used to identify such changes. In addition, after DCE images are acquired, T1-WI with a large field of view can be obtained below the level of the aortic bifurcation for evaluation of the lymph nodes and osseous lesions (**Fig. 4**).

Diffusion-Weighted Imaging/Apparent Diffusion Coefficient Maps

DWI assesses the degree of tissue cellularity by measuring the mobility or diffusion of water molecules within tissues. In prostate tissue that has an increased fraction of epithelium in comparison with other tissue compartments, such as in high-grade PCa, water diffusion is impeded or restricted. The first reports of the successful

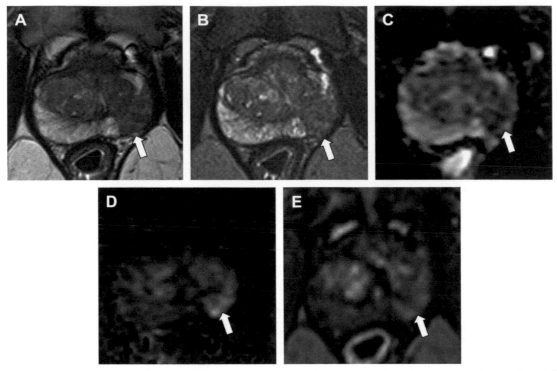

Fig. 2. A 67-year-old man with PCa Gleason score 3 + 4 or grade group 2 undergoing preoperative staging with MR imaging. (*A*) Axial 2D TSE T2-WI shows a 1.6-cm lesion in the right posterolateral PZ with low signal intensity and broad (>1-cm) capsular contact (*arrow, A*), which raises concern for EPE (T2-WI PI-RADS score: 5). (*B*) On axial 3D TSE T2-WI, in addition to broad capsular contact, there is irregularity and discontinuity of the capsule (*arrow, B*). (*C, D*) The lesion demonstrates markedly hypointense signal on the axial ADC map (*arrow, C*) and markedly hyperintense signal on the axial calculated high b-value (1500 s/mm^2) DWI (*arrow, D*) (ADC/DWI PI-RADS score: 5). (*E*) The lesion demonstrates early arterial enhancement on axial DCE T1-WI (*arrow, E*) (DCE: positive). Because the findings are compatible with extraprostatic extension, the lesion's PI-RADS assessment category is 5. The patient underwent radical prostatectomy, which confirmed the presence of extraprostatic extension.

application of DWI echo-planar imaging pulse sequences for evaluation of the prostate occurred in the early 2000s.[8] Since then, numerous studies have demonstrated the value of DWI in detecting and characterizing PCa.[9–11]

DWI plays a key role in the PI-RADS v2 guidelines and is currently considered the dominant parameter for the evaluation of lesions in the peripheral zone (PZ). DWI also plays an important but secondary role in the assessment of lesions in the TZ, because there is significant overlap between cancer and benign prostatic hyperplasia nodules rich in stromal elements.[12]

An important technical parameter for DWI is the selection of b-values. These values are impacted by the magnitude and duration of the gradient applied in the tissue during image acquisition. A monoexponential model of signal decay with increasing b-values is applied to calculate the apparent diffusion coefficient (ADC) values (measured in squared millimeters per second), and the values of each voxel are then displayed in an image that is known as the ADC map. ADC

maps are interpreted in conjunction with DWI to qualitatively determine the presence of diffusion restriction. ADC maps can also be used to obtain a quantitative assessment of lesions by measuring their ADC values. Although an inverse correlation between ADC values and PCa grade has been demonstrated in several studies,[11,13] the clinical adoption of a quantitative assessment is limited by many factors, including a significant overlap between benign and pathologic conditions and the variability in ADC values depending on the selection of different sets of b-values, the magnetic field strength, and MR imaging scanner vendor.

PI-RADS v2 provides specific recommendations regarding the selection of b-values. For the creation of ADC maps, DWI should be acquired with at least 2 b-values, with the lowest b-values set at 50 to 100 s/mm^2 and the highest set at 800 to 1000 s/mm^2. In addition, DWI images with high b-values ($\geq$1400 s/mm^2) are also required. The high b-value images tend to improve tumor conspicuity, distinguishing between PCa and normal tissue or benign conditions (**Fig. 5**).[14] This

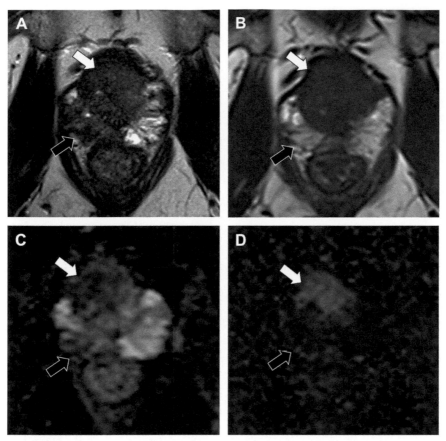

Fig. 3. A 59-year-old man with PCa Gleason score 3 + 4 or grade group 2 diagnosed on TRUS-guided biopsy performed 7 weeks before the staging MR imaging. (*A*) Axial T2-WI shows a focal lesion with low signal intensity in the right posterolateral, posteromedial, and anterior PZ at the midgland associated with capsule irregularity mimicking an aggressive PCa lesion with extraprostatic extension (*black arrow, A*). In addition, there is a 1.6-cm focal lesion in the right anterior TZ with homogenous low signal intensity and ill-defined margins (*white arrow, A*) (T2-WI PI-RADS score 5). (*B*) Axial T1-WI shows diffuse increased signal intensity in the PZ, including in the area with signal abnormality on T2-WI (*black arrow, B*) consistent with postbiopsy hemorrhage. The anterior TZ lesion demonstrates low signal intensity and is spared from the postbiopsy changes (*white arrow, B*). (*C–D*) On the axial ADC map, there is markedly low signal intensity in the right PZ (*black arrow, C*), but without corresponding high signal intensity in the axial calculated high b-value (1500 s/mm²) DWI (*black arrow, D*); conversely, the right anterior TZ lesion demonstrates markedly low signal intensity on the ADC map (*white arrow, C*) and markedly high signal intensity on DWI (*white arrow, D*) (ADC/DWI PI-RADS score: 5). Because there is high signal intensity on T1-WI, the right PZ lesion is highly unlike to represent clinically significant PCa (PI-RADS assessment category 1). Because the T2-WI score is the dominant score for TZ lesions, the PI-RADS assessment category of the right anterior TZ lesion is 5. The patient underwent radical prostatectomy, which confirmed the absence of cancer in the PZ and revealed a Gleason score 4 + 3 or grade group 3 in the TZ.

high b-value DWI can be obtained in 1 of 2 ways.[15] On some MR imaging systems or third-party software, high b-value DWI can be extrapolated or calculated from the DWI data set obtained with lower b-values to generate the ADC map. If this is not possible, the high b-value DWI is advised to be obtained in a separate acquisition from the standard b-values used in ADC map calculation, because the high b-value DWI can affect the appearance of the ADC map. Generating the high b-value DWI from the lower b-value data set is advantageous in that it does not require

additional scanning time and is less prone to artifacts; acquiring the high b-value DWI separately may require longer echo times to accommodate the strong gradient pulses needed.

Diffusion kurtosis imaging (DKI) and restriction spectrum imaging (RSI) are extensions of DWI with additional requirements regarding the DWI acquisition and specialized postprocessing. DKI works on the assumption that water diffusion is non-Gaussian in behavior, a property that may help assess tissue with microstructural complexity.[16] RSI is a multiple b-value, multidirectional diffusion

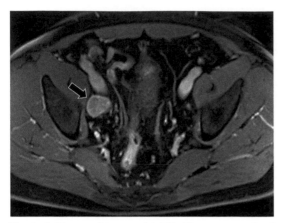

Fig. 4. A 68-year-old man with PCa Gleason score 4 + 5 or grade group 5 detected by TRUS-guided biopsy undergoing preoperative staging with MR imaging. Large field-of-view T1-WI obtained after intravenous administration of gadolinium chelate contrast media demonstrates an enlarged right external iliac lymph node (*black arrow*). Metastatic involvement by PCa was confirmed on pelvic lymph node dissection performed along with radical prostatectomy.

technique. By obtaining an extended spectrum of diffusion images, this technique is able to focus on signal arising from intracellular water and potentially more effectively evaluate tissue cellularity; highly

cellular tumors are thus highlighted by this method.[17] The application of DKI and RSI techniques in prostate imaging has gained attention in recent years because initial studies have shown potential for better distinction of PCa from normal tissue and better discrimination between low-grade and high-grade PCa with these methods.[16,17] RSI and DKI are not included in the PI-RADS v2 recommendations, but these, or other advanced diffusion methods, could be incorporated into future versions if validated in larger and more robust studies.

Dynamic Contrast-Enhanced Imaging

DCE imaging enables noninvasive imaging characterization of tissue vascularity. Angiogenesis in PCa is associated with an increased number or density of poorly organized and poorly formed vessels with increased capillary permeability, which leads to faster and greater enhancement of cancerous lesions relative to the normal surrounding tissues.[18]

DCE consists of a series of T1-WI scans acquired before, during, and after the rapid intravenous administration of a bolus of a low-molecular-weight gadolinium-based contrast agent (Video 1). 3D T1-WI spoiled gradient-recalled echo sequences are used to repeatedly

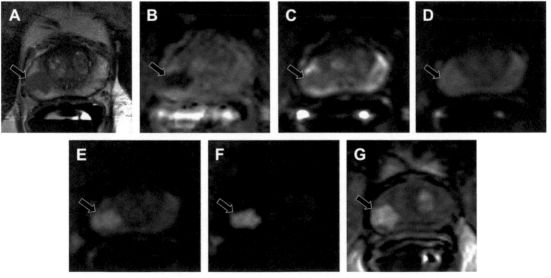

Fig. 5. A 62-year-old man with PCa Gleason score 4 + 3 or grade group 3 undergoing preoperative staging with MR imaging. (*A*) Axial T2-WI shows a well-circumscribed, low-signal-intensity nodule in the right posterolateral and anterior PZ at the midgland and base (*black arrow, A*) (T2-WI PI-RADS score: 5). (*B*) The lesion measures 1.6 cm and shows markedly low signal intensity on the ADC map (*arrow, B*). (*C–F*) Axial DWIs obtained with b-values of 50 (*C*), 400 (*D*), 900 (*E*), and 2000 (*F*) s/mm² demonstrate progressive decrease of the signal intensity of the prostate and surrounding tissues, and progressive increase of the signal intensity of the lesion in the right PZ (*arrows, C–F*) that is most conspicuous and markedly hyperintense on the 2000 s/mm² b-value image (ADC/DWI PI-RADS score: 5). (*G*) Axial DCE T1-WI shows early enhancement by the lesion (*black arrow, G*) that matches the area of signal abnormalities identified on T2-WI and ADC/DWI (DCE: positive). Because ADC/DWI is the dominant parameter for PZ abnormalities, this focal lesion was assigned a PI-RADS assessment category 5. The patient underwent radical prostatectomy that revealed a PCa Gleason score 4 + 4 or grade group 4.

image the prostate over several minutes to assess the enhancement characteristics; a 3D sequence is preferred for this purpose. These images are obtained with a high temporal resolution (faster than at least 10 seconds and preferably than at least 7 seconds, per PI-RADS v2) so as to demonstrate early enhancing lesions. In addition, PI-RADS only requires a DCE acquisition duration of at least 2 minutes. Fat suppression techniques or the creation of imaging data sets from the subtraction of pre-contrast from postcontrast images is recommended to facilitate the visual assessment of these enhancement characteristics.

Because of the significant variability in enhancement patterns of cancerous lesions and the overlap with enhancement patterns of benign conditions (namely prostatitis and benign prostatic hyperplasia), DCE has a relatively limited role in the characterization of PCa lesions when compared with T2-WI and DWI.[19,20] Because of these

limitations, and to simplify the interpretation of DCE images, the assessment of DCE in PI-RADS v2 is based exclusively on qualitative visual assessment of the individual time points of DCE images. A lesion is considered to be DCE "positive" if it demonstrates early arterial enhancement and has a corresponding signal abnormality on DWI or T2-WI (**Fig. 6**). The presence of delayed "washout" is no longer included as a diagnostic imaging feature. PI-RADS v2 does not require the use of a semiquantitative method for the evaluation of enhancement kinetic curves that plot the signal intensity of a lesion as a function of time (as described in PI-RADS v1), nor more sophisticated quantitative methods, because of insufficient evidence to support their use. Furthermore, these methods require specific software for postprocessing of the images that typically is not available in standard picture archiving and communication systems.

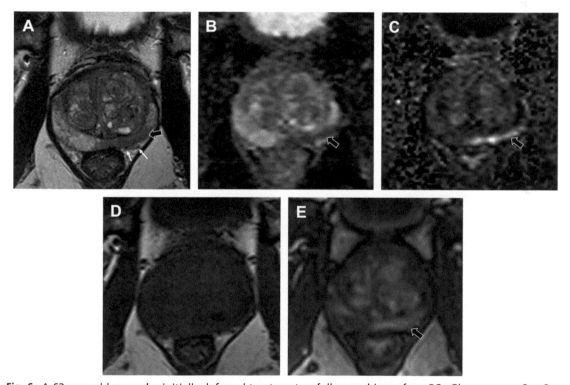

Fig. 6. A 63-year-old man who initially deferred treatment or follow-up biopsy for a PCa Gleason score 3 + 3 or grade group 1 diagnosed 4 years ago and currently presents with increasing prostate-specific antigen (PSA) level (11.4 ng/mL). (*A*) Axial T2-WI shows a lesion with low signal intensity in the left posteromedial and posterolateral PZ (*black arrow, A*) with extraprostatic extension and asymmetric thickening of the ipsilateral NVB fibers (*white arrows, A*) concerning for NVB invasion (T2-WI PI-RADS score 5). (*B–C*) The lesion measures 1.5 cm and demonstrates markedly low signal intensity on axial ADC map (*arrow, B*) and markedly high signal intensity on the axial calculated high b-value (1500 s/mm^2) DWI (*arrow, C*) (ADC/DWI PI-RADS score: 5). (*D–E*) Axial DCE T1-WIs obtained before (*D*) and at the peak arterial enhancement (*E*) show a focal enhancing lesion (*arrow, E*) in the area corresponding to the lesion seen on T2-WI and ADC/DWI (DCE: positive). Because ADC/DWI is the dominant parameter in the PZ, the PI-RADS assessment category is 5. MR/TRUS fusion-guided biopsy of the lesion was performed revealing PCa Gleason score 4 + 3 or grade group 3.

HARDWARE
Magnetic Field Strength

At present, it is generally accepted that multiparametric MR imaging (mpMR imaging) can be adequately performed on 1.5-T or 3-T systems.[5,21] Scanner platforms with field strengths lower than 1.5 T are generally not optimized to obtain pulse sequences with the parameters recommended in the PI-RADS v2 guidelines. Furthermore, the current literature validating the clinical utility of MR imaging in PCa detection and staging is based on images obtained on 1.5-T or 3-T scanners.[9,22]

An increase in magnetic field strength brings certain limitations, such as increased chemical shift and susceptibility artifacts, increased dielectric resonance effects, and increased radiofrequency energy deposition in tissues. Despite these limitations, 3-T MR imaging has clear advantages compared with 1.5-T MR imaging, including a nearly 2-fold increase in SNR, improved spatial resolution, and shortened acquisition times.[23] Thus, although MR imaging examinations can be adequately performed on 1.5-T systems, 3-T systems should be used when available.

Receiver Frequency Coils

MR imaging examinations are performed with a pelvic phased-array coil (PPAC), preferably with a relatively high number of external phased array coil elements and radiofrequency channels (ie, ≥16), with or without an endorectal coil (ERC). The ERC model most commonly used is equipped with a balloon that, when filled, fixes the coil to the rectum. Perfluorocarbon fluid or barium sulfate mixtures are frequently used to fill the balloon; this helps to reduce the susceptibility artifacts and spatial distortions that can affect DWI and MRSI.

The development of an ERC several years after prostate MR imaging was initially introduced represented a major advance that was needed to compensate for the low field strengths available at that time, because the addition of an ERC to MR imaging greatly improves SNR.[24] An ERC was also considered essential to the performance of prostate MRSI.[25] However, using an ERC during MR imaging has significant disadvantages. The addition of an ERC increases the cost and examination time and causes significant patient discomfort. The use of an ERC also leads to deformity of the prostate contour and shape, and this anatomic distortion can potentially hamper the pathology correlation and fusion with other imaging methods that are used for treatment planning.[26,27]

Because of these disadvantages, and because MRSI is no longer recommended in PI-RADS v2,

there is an ongoing debate regarding whether the use of an ERC can be avoided, at least for studies performed on 3-T scanners. In fact, investigators have demonstrated that using 3-T scanners without an ERC may achieve image quality, PCa detection rates, and staging accuracy at least comparable to what is achieved with 1.5-T scanners with an ERC.[22,28] Studies comparing images obtained on 3-T scanners with and without an ERC have demonstrated some advantage for PCa detection with the use of an ERC.[29–31] For example, Costa and colleagues[30] showed that using both an ERC and a PPAC provides superior sensitivity for the detection of PCa when compared with not using an ERC, although in this study, overall accuracy was not significantly different when the images obtained with an ERC were compared with those obtained without an ERC but obtained with an increased number of signal averages. This finding suggests that optimization of the images may help to decrease the performance gap between examinations performed with and without an ERC. For MR imaging studies used to stage PCa, a meta-analysis demonstrated that the addition of an ERC appeared to improve the detection of EPE in scans performed at 1.5 T and in scans that used T2-WI as the only parameter. However, when 3-T field strength or additional functional techniques (eg, DWI and DCE images) were used, scans with an ERC showed lower sensitivity than scans without an ERC.[22]

Based on these results, the use of an ERC is not currently considered by PI-RADS v2 an absolute requirement on 1.5-T or 3-T scanners.[5]

PATIENT PREPARATION

There is no general consensus regarding patient preparation for prostate MR imaging. Several measures are commonly used to address factors that may negatively affect image quality, although scientific evidence to support some of these measures is scarce.

Interval Between Transrectal Ultrasound–Guided Biopsy and mpMR Imaging

MR imaging is commonly performed in men who have previously undergone transrectal ultrasound-guided (TRUS) biopsy. Of note, current statements from major national organizations support the use of MR imaging in men with prior negative TRUS biopsy and in men with biopsy-proven PCa who are undergoing preoperative staging.[32–34] TRUS biopsy causes hemorrhage and inflammation of the prostate gland. The resultant changes on imaging are most evident in the PZ and may persist for many weeks or months. These postbiopsy changes can obscure tumor or misleadingly suggest the presence of EPE of the tumor.[35] Although the optimal time interval between TRUS biopsy and MR imaging to minimize the effect of these changes on imaging interpretation has not been defined, an interval of at least 6 weeks is commonly recommended, especially when MR imaging is performed for disease staging. However, this interval may be modified based on individual circumstances, because studies have shown that mpMR imaging, when properly interpreted, has adequate accuracy for disease detection and staging even in the presence of postbiopsy changes.[35,36] Careful evaluation of DWI and of ADC, in correlation with T1-WI in which postbiopsy changes manifest as areas with intermediate to high signal intensity, may help to prevent confusion.[37]

Bowel Preparation

Patients should be encouraged to evacuate the bowel before the examination to try to eliminate as much stool and gas from the rectum as possible. Stool interferes with the placement of the ERC, and gas can cause distortion of DWI, particularly in examinations performed without an ERC.[38] At some institutions, men are instructed to self-administer a cleansing enema before the examination, although this measure has not been shown to significantly improve image quality or reduce artifacts in prostate MR imaging.[39] If an

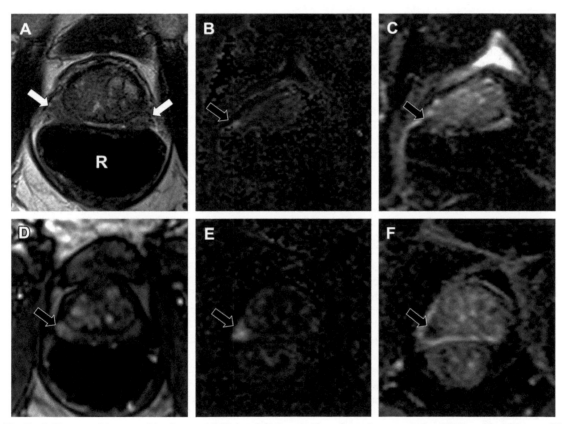

Fig. 7. A 72-year-old man with elevated PSA level (5.5 ng/mL) and previous negative TRUS-guided biopsy. (A) Axial T2-WI shows diffuse decreased signal intensity of the PZ (*white arrows, A*) (PI-RADS score 2). There is also significant distension of the rectum (R) with gas. (B, C) Axial calculated high b-value (1500 s/mm^2) DWI and ADC map shows significant distortion of the prostate due to artifacts from rectal gas. There is an equivocal focal lesion with high signal intensity on DWI (*arrow, B*) and low signal intensity on ADC map (*arrow, C*). (D) Axial DCE T1-WI demonstrates a focal lesion with early arterial enhancement (*black arrow, D*) in the same location with equivocal finding on DWI/ADC map (DCE positive). (E, F) Axial calculated high b-value (1500 s/mm^2) DWI and ADC map obtained after the rectal gas was removed with a tube demonstrate a significant improvement of the image quality and confirmed the presence of a 0.8-cm focal lesion with markedly increased signal intensity on DWI (*black arrow, E*) and markedly low signal intensity on ADC map (*black arrow, F*) in the right posterolateral PZ at the midgland (DWI/ADC score 4). Because DWI/ADC is the dominant sequence in the PZ, the PI-RADS assessment category was 4. MR/ultrasound fusion-guided biopsy of the lesion identified PCa Gleason score 3 + 4 or grade group 2. The patient was treated with radical prostatectomy.

enema is used, it should not be administered immediately before the examination, because doing so may stimulate bowel peristalsis. Alternative methods can be used if gas-related artifacts are encountered during an examination performed without an ERC. These methods include performing the examination with the patient in the prone position, decompressing the rectum using suction through a small catheter, and introducing ultrasound gel into the rectum (**Fig. 7**).[5,38,39]

Antiperistaltic Agents

Patients undergoing MR imaging of the pelvis are often given an antiperistaltic agent such as glucagon or butylscopolamine to reduce artifacts induced by bowel motion, mainly from the small bowel.[40] In prostate MR imaging, the improvement in image quality with an antiperistaltic agent has not been shown to be significant for examinations performed either with or without an ERC.[41,42] The lack of a significant benefit is likely related to the distance between the prostate and the small bowel.[42] Furthermore, the use of these agents increases the cost of the examination and can be associated with side effects.[41] Thus, although the use of an antiperistaltic agent may be helpful in some patients, routine use is not formally recommended.

Abstinence from Ejaculation

The effect of abstinence from ejaculation on PCa detection and staging has not been demonstrated and is therefore not recommended in PI-RADS v2. After ejaculation, T2-WI and ADC values are decreased in the PZ, which in theory could affect PCa detection.[43] In addition, after ejaculation, the seminal vesicles may become collapsed, which can impair assessment. Kabakus and colleagues[44] found that abstinence from ejaculation for 3 or more days before MR imaging improved the assessment of the seminal vesicles in men aged more than 60 years, but this study did not evaluate the effect of this finding on the accuracy of PCa staging.

SUMMARY

MR imaging provides detailed anatomic assessment of the prostate as well as information that allows the detection and characterization of PCa. To obtain high-quality MR imaging of the prostate, radiologists must understand sequence optimization to overcome commonly encountered technical challenges; they must also be aware of the various hardware considerations and important aspects of patient preparation. The use of minimum parameters provided in the PI-RADS v2 guidelines should help to standardize MR imaging protocols. Institutions should strive to optimize imaging protocols in order to obtain the best and most consistent image quality possible with the equipment available.

SUPPLEMENTARY DATA

Supplementary data related to this article can be found online at https://doi.org/10.1016/j.ucl.2018.03.008.

REFERENCES

1. Steyn JH, Smith FW. Nuclear magnetic resonance imaging of the prostate. Br J Urol 1982;54:726–8.
2. Muthigi A, Sidana A, George AK, et al. Current beliefs and practice patterns among urologists regarding prostate magnetic resonance imaging and magnetic resonance-targeted biopsy. Urol Oncol 2017;35:32.e1-7.
3. Heidenreich A. Consensus criteria for the use of magnetic resonance imaging in the diagnosis and staging of prostate cancer: not ready for routine use. Eur Urol 2011;59:495–7.
4. Barentsz JO, Richenberg J, Clements R, et al. European Society of Urogenital Radiology. ESUR prostate MR guidelines 2012. Eur Radiol 2012;22:746–57.
5. Weinreb JC, Barentsz JO, Choyke PL, et al. PI-RADS prostate imaging–reporting and data system: 2015, version 2. Eur Urol 2016;69(1):16–40.
6. Hricak H, Dooms GC, McNeal JE, et al. MR imaging of the prostate gland: normal anatomy. AJR Am J Roentgenol 1987;148:51–8.
7. Rosenkrantz AB, Neil J, Kong X, et al. Prostate cancer: comparison of 3D T2-weighted with conventional 2D T2-weighted imaging for image quality and tumor detection. AJR Am J Roentgenol 2010; 194:446–52.
8. Gibbs P, Tozer DJ, Liney GP, et al. Comparison of quantitative T2 mapping and diffusion-weighted imaging in the normal and pathologic prostate. Magn Reson Med 2001;46:1054–8.
9. de Rooij M, Hamoen EHJ, Futterer JJ, et al. Accuracy of multiparametric MRI for prostate cancer detection: a meta-analysis. AJR Am J Roentgenol 2014;202:343–51.
10. Turkbey B, Shah VP, Pang Y, et al. Is apparent diffusion coefficient associated with clinical risk scores for prostate cancers that are visible on 3-T MR images? Radiology 2011;258(2):488–95.
11. Hambrock T, Somford DM, Huisman HJ, et al. Relationship between apparent diffusion coefficients at 3.0-T MR imaging and Gleason grade in peripheral zone prostate cancer. Radiology 2011;259(2):453–61.

12. Delongchamps NB, Rouanne M, Flam T, et al. Multi-parametric magnetic resonance imaging for the detection and localization of prostate cancer: combination of T2-weighted, dynamic contrast-enhanced and diffusion-weighted imaging. BJU Int 2011;107(9):1411–8.

13. Vargas HA, Akin O, Franiel T, et al. Diffusion-weighted endorectal MR imaging at 3 T for prostate cancer: tumor detection and assessment of aggressiveness. Radiology 2011;259(3):775–84.

14. Godley KC, Syer TJ, Toms AP, et al. Accuracy of high b-value diffusion-weighted MRI for prostate cancer detection: a meta-analysis. Acta Radiol 2017. https://doi.org/10.1177/0284185117702181.

15. Bittencourt LK, Attenberger UI, Lima D, et al. Feasibility study of computed vs measured high b-value (1400 s/mm^2) diffusion-weighted MR images of the prostate. World J Radiol 2014;6(6): 374–80.

16. Rosenkrantz AB, Padhani AR, Chenevert TL, et al. Body diffusion kurtosis imaging: basic principles, applications, and considerations for clinical practice. J Magn Reson Imaging 2015;42: 1190–202.

17. McCammack KC, Kane CJ, Parsons JK, et al. In vivo prostate cancer detection and grading using restriction spectrum imaging-MRI. Prostate Cancer Prostatic Dis 2016;19:168–73.

18. Alonzi R, Padhani AR, Allen C. Dynamic contrast enhanced MRI in prostate cancer. Eur J Radiol 2007;63:335–50.

19. Stanzione A, Imbriaco M, Cocozza S, et al. Biparametric 3T magnetic resonance imaging for prostatic cancer detection in a biopsy-naïve patient population: a further improvement of PI-RADS v2? Eur J Radiol 2016;85(12):2269–74.

20. Hoeks CM, Hambrock T, Yakar D, et al. Transition zone prostate cancer: detection and localization with 3-T multiparametric MR imaging. Radiology 2013;266:207–17.

21. Ullrich T, Quentin M, Oelers C, et al. Magnetic resonance imaging of the prostate at 1.5 versus 3.0 T: a prospective comparison study of image quality. Eur J Radiol 2017;90:192–7.

22. de Rooij M, Hamoen EH, Witjes JA, et al. Accuracy of magnetic resonance imaging for local staging of prostate cancer: a diagnostic meta-analysis. Eur Urol 2016;70:233–45.

23. Rouviere O, Hartman RP, Lyonnet D. Prostate MR imaging at high-field strength: evolution or revolution? Eur Radiol 2006;16:276–84.

24. Schnall MD, Lenkinski RE, Pollack HM, et al. Prostate: MR imaging with an endorectal surface coil. Radiology 1989;172:570–4.

25. Rajesh A, Coakley FV. MR imaging and MR spectroscopic imaging of prostate cancer. Magn Reson Imaging Clin N Am 2004;12:557–79.

26. Heijmink SW, Scheenen TW, van Lin EN, et al. Changes in prostate shape and volume and their implications for radiotherapy after introduction of endorectal balloon as determined by MRI at 3T. Int J Radiat Oncol Biol Phys 2009;73:1446–53.

27. Vilanova JC, Barcelo J. Prostate cancer detection: magnetic resonance (MR) spectroscopic imaging. Abdom Imaging 2007;32:253–61.

28. Shah ZK, Elias SN, Abaza R, et al. Performance comparison of 1.5-T endorectal coil MRI with 3.0-T nonendorectal coil MRI in patients with prostate cancer. Acad Radiol 2015;22:467–74.

29. Turkbey B, Merino MJ, Gallardo EC, et al. Comparison of endorectal coil and nonendorectal coil T2W and diffusion-weighted MRI at 3 Tesla for localizing prostate cancer: correlation with whole-mount histopathology. J Magn Reson Imaging 2014;39: 1443–8.

30. Costa DN, Yuan Q, Xi Y, et al. Comparison of prostate cancer detection at 3-T MRI with and without an endorectal coil: a prospective, paired-patient study. Urol Oncol 2016;34:255.e7-13.

31. Heijmink SW, Futterer JJ, Hambrock T, et al. Prostate cancer: body-array versus endorectal coil MR imaging at 3T – comparison of image quality, localization, and staging performance. Radiology 2007;244:184–95.

32. Eberhardt SC, Carter S, Casalino DD, et al. ACR Appropriateness Criteria prostate cancer-pretreatment detection, staging, and surveillance. J Am Coll Radiol 2013;10:83–92.

33. Carroll PR, Parsons JK, Andriole G, et al. NCCN guidelines insights. Prostate cancer early detection, version 2.2016. Featured updates to the NCCN guidelines. J Natl Compr Canc Netw 2016;14:509–19.

34. Rosenkrantz AB, Verma S, Choyke P, et al. Prostate magnetic resonance imaging and magnetic resonance imaging targeted biopsy in patients with a prior negative biopsy: a consensus statement by AUA and SAR. J Urol 2016;196(6): 1613–8.

35. Tamada T, Sone T, Jo Y, et al. Prostate cancer: relationships between postbiopsy hemorrhage and tumor detectability at MR diagnosis. Radiology 2008; 248:531–9.

36. Sharif-Afshar AR, Feng T, Koopman S, et al. Impact of post prostate biopsy hemorrhage on multiparametric magnetic resonance imaging. Can J Urol 2015;22:7698–702.

37. Barrett T, Vargas HA, Akin O, et al. Value of the hemorrhage exclusion sign on T1-weighted prostate MR images for the detection of prostate cancer. Radiology 2012;263:751–7.

38. Caglic I, Hansen NL, Slough RA, et al. Evaluating the effect of rectal distension on prostate multiparametric MRI image quality. Eur J Radiol 2017;90:174–80.

39. Lim C, Quon J, McInnes M, et al. Does a cleansing enema improve image quality of 3T surface coil

multiparametric prostate MRI? J Magn Reson Imaging 2015;42:689–97.

40. Zand KR, Reinhold C, Haider MA, et al. Artifacts and pitfalls in MR imaging of the pelvis. J Magn Reson Imaging 2007;26:480–97.

41. Wagner M, Rief M, Busch J, et al. Effect of butylscopolamine on image quality in MRI of the prostate. Clin Radiol 2010;65:460–4.

42. Roethke MC, Kuru TH, Radbruch A, et al. Prostate magnetic resonance imaging at 3 Tesla: is

administration of hyoscine-N-butyl-bromide mandatory? World J Radiol 2013;5:259–63.

43. Medved M, Sammet S, Yousuf A, et al. MR imaging of the prostate and adjacent anatomic structures before, during, and after ejaculation: qualitative and quantitative evaluation. Radiology 2014;271:452–60.

44. Kabakus IM, Borofsky S, Mertan FV, et al. Does abstinence from ejaculation before prostate MRI improve evaluation of the seminal vesicles? AJR Am J Roentgenol 2016;207:1205–9.

Multiparametric MR imaging of the Prostate
Interpretation Including Prostate Imaging Reporting and Data System Version 2

Alessandro Furlan, MD[a], Amir A. Borhani, MD[a],
Antonio C. Westphalen, MD, PhD[b,c],*

KEYWORDS

- Prostate cancer • Multiparametric MR imaging • PI-RADS

KEY POINTS

- The key sequences of a prostate mp-MRI scan are high-resolution T2-weighted, high b-value diffusion-weighted, and dynamic contrast-enhanced imaging.
- PI-RADS standardizes interpretation of mp-MRI, resulting in moderate-to-high accuracy for the diagnosis of clinically significant prostate cancer.
- A quantitative approach to functional imaging of the prostate has the potential to further improve diagnostic accuracy of mp-MRI and to provide insights into tumor aggressiveness and prognosis.

INTRODUCTION

Radiologists in the United States are experiencing a significant growth of volume of prostate MR imaging studies.[1] This mirrors an increasing interest from the urology community in the application of this technique for the management of patients with, or at risk for, prostate cancer, particularly for biopsy guidance. The technological developments experienced in the last two decades culminated in a mp-MRI approach that combines anatomic and functional imaging. However, the greater complexity of this technique, along with an increasing demand, brought new challenges to imaging interpretation.

The Prostate Imaging Reporting and Data System (PI-RADS), first proposed in 2011 by the European Society of Uroradiology, is an effort to address these challenges through a standardized approach to the interpretation of prostate mp-MRI.[2] The second version of PI-RADS (PI-RADS v2) was released in 2015 with many simplifications and improvements.[3]

The first part of this article is focused on interpretation of the pulse sequences recommended in the PI-RADS v2 guidelines, including useful tips based on the authors' experiences at two large academic institutions. In the second part, we review advanced quantitative imaging tools and discuss future directions.

This article was previously published in March 2018 Radiologic Clinics, Volume 56, Issue 2.

[a] Department of Radiology, University of Pittsburgh, UPMC Presbyterian Campus, Radiology Suite 200 East Wing, 200 Lothrop Street, Pittsburgh, PA 15213, USA; [b] Department of Radiology and Biomedical Imaging, University of California San Francisco, 505 Parnassus Avenue, M392, Box 0628, San Francisco, CA 94143, USA; [c] Department of Urology, University of California San Francisco, 1825 4th Street, 4th Floor, Box 1711, San Francisco, CA 94143, USA

* Corresponding author. Department of Radiology and Biomedical Imaging, University of California San Francisco, 505 Parnassus Avenue, M392, Box 0628, San Francisco, CA 94143.
E-mail address: AntonioCarlos.Westphalen@ucsf.edu

INTERPRETATION OF MULTIPARAMETRIC MR IMAGING: PULSE SEQUENCES INCLUDED IN PROSTATE IMAGING REPORTING AND DATA SYSTEM VERSION 2

An mp-MRI of the prostate is an examination comprised of multiple pulse sequences, including anatomic and functional images. The key pulse sequences recommended in the PI-RADS v2 guidelines are three-plane high-resolution axial T2-weighted images (T2WI), high b-value axial diffusion-weighted images (DWI), apparent diffusion coefficient (ADC) map, and axial dynamic contrast-enhanced (DCE) images.[3] The high-resolution coronal and sagittal T2WI help to better define the morphology and spatial relationship of a finding already identified on the axial images. A practical approach to review this large data set is to organize the key pulse sequences and display them simultaneously on the viewing monitors, allowing the radiologist to link and quickly correlate the findings detected on anatomic and functional images. According to the PI-RADS v2 guidelines, each prostatic finding should be assigned a score between 1 and 5 based on its appearance on T2WI, DWI, and DCE MR imaging. A score of 5 indicates very high probability of clinically significant prostate cancer, defined as Gleason score greater than or equal to 7, and/or volume greater than or equal to 0.5 mL, and/or extraprostatic extension (EPE).[3]

Anatomic Imaging

T2-weighted images: peripheral zone

Multiplanar high-resolution T2WI is the hallmark sequence for anatomic evaluation of the prostate. In contrast to the normal peripheral zone (PZ), which has high signal intensity (SI) on T2WI because of its large water content, most tumors exhibit low SI.[4] Moreover, tumors with higher Gleason scores tend to have lower SI than less aggressive cancers.[5,6] This is because tumor grade increase represents a progressive loss of the normal glandular anatomy and continuing dedifferentiation and clustering of cancer cells.[7] Three other important anatomic features depicted on T2WI are shape, borders, and size of lesions. Prostate cancer tends to present as a focal round or crescent abnormality on imaging, whereas benign lesions are more often indistinct or have a linear or triangular shape.[8] Although there is an overlap between the features of benign and low-to-intermediate grade prostate cancers, tumors with high Gleason score are usually more noticeable lesions.[6] Lastly, lesion size has been positively correlated with chance of malignancy and Gleason score, that is, larger lesions are more

likely to represent high-grade prostate cancer than smaller ones.[8,9] Furthermore, there is also a positive correlation between tumor size and the probability of EPE and seminal vesicle invasion.[9]

It is not surprising, therefore, that the T2WI PI-RADS v2 categories are based on these four features (**Table 1**).[3] Lesions with high probability of representing a clinically significant prostate cancer are focal masslike, circumscribed, and have homogeneous moderately low SI (score 4 or 5) (**Fig. 1**). The distinction between a score 4 and 5 is based on the presence of definite EPE or size, where the lesions greater than or equal to 1.5 cm are assigned a score 5. On the other end of the spectrum are lesions that are likely benign (score 2). Those lesions are linear, wedge-shaped, or present as areas of mildly low SI with indistinct borders (**Fig. 2**). Lesions that have moderately low SI, but are heterogeneous or noncircumscribed are considered indeterminate and receive a score of 3 (**Fig. 3**). T2WI is only moderately accurate for the detection of cancer, although its performance improves when the goal is to identify high-grade disease. Mucinous adenocarcinomas of the prostate, for example, may have a predominantly high SI resulting in false-negative based on T2WI score.[10] However, many nontumoral lesions, such as inflammation, fibrosis, and hemorrhage, can mimic cancer on T2WI.[11]

T2-weighted images: transition zone

The accurate identification and characterization of prostate cancer within the transition zone (TZ) likely represents the greatest challenge of mp-MRI interpretation. The difficulty arises with the development of benign prostatic hyperplasia (BPH), which affects virtually all middle age or older men, the same population at risk for prostate cancer. BPH affects glandular and stromal tissues and it is characterized by the growth of multiple nodules and intervening hyperplastic stroma, depicted on T2WI as a large, distorted, and markedly heterogeneous TZ, an appearance described as "organized chaos."[12] Differentiating the intertwined hyperplastic stroma or stroma-rich nodule from cancer is problematic because both entities present with low SI on T2WI, and the random appearance of BPH allows prostate cancer to blend within the nodular TZ.[12,13] Hence, detection of these tumors requires a careful analysis of the lesion morphology on high-resolution T2WI (see **Table 1**). Well circumscribed and encapsulated nodules with low or heterogeneous T2 SI are typically benign (PI-RADS v2 score 2) (**Fig. 4**). High-grade tumors, however, characteristically present as lenticular or indistinct foci of homogenous moderately low SI (PI-RADS v2 score 4 or 5)

Table 1
T2 score for peripheral and transition zone according to PI-RADS v2

Score	Signal Intensity	Shape	Size - EPE
Peripheral zone			
1 (normal)	• High • Homogeneous	• N/A	N/A
2	• Low	• Linear/wedge-shaped • Diffuse (homogeneous) • Indistinct	Any size EPE absent
3[a]	• Low (moderate) • Heterogeneous	• Round/noncircumscribed • Diffuse	Any size EPE absent
4	• Moderate-to-low • Homogeneous	• Focus/mass • Circumscribed	<1.5 cm EPE absent
5	• Moderate-to-low • Homogeneous	• Focus/mass • Circumscribed	≥1.5 cm and/or EPE definitely present
Transition zone			
1 (normal)	• Intermediate • Homogeneous	• N/A	N/A
2	• Low/high • Heterogeneous • Homogeneous	• Circumscribed nodule	Any size EPE absent
3[a]	• Heterogeneous	• Obscured margins	Any size EPE absent
4	• Moderate-to-low • Homogeneous	• Lenticular • Noncircumscribed	<1.5 cm EPE absent
5	• Moderate-to-low • Homogeneous	• Lenticular • Noncircumscribed	≥1.5 cm and/or EPE definitely present

Abbreviation: NA, not applicable.
[a] Score 3 also includes lesions that do not fit in categories 2, 3, 4, and 5.

(**Fig. 5**). The identification of a heterogeneous lesion, however, is not as definitive for the diagnosis of cancer; these may represent stromal-rich BPH associated with cystic ectasia and hyperplastic glandular components that are seen on T2WI as foci of high SI.[14] As for lesions in the PZ, the distinction between PI-RADS v2 scores 4 and 5 is based on the lesion size and/or the presence of definite EPE. Lesions that do not meet the criteria for the benign or high-grade lesions are assigned a score 3, denoting an indeterminate finding with equivocal likelihood for clinically significant cancer.

T1-weighted images
Unenhanced T1-weighted images (T1WI) have a limited role in the assessment of prostate cancer and are mainly used for detection of postbiopsy hemorrhage, which appears as focal or diffuse areas of high SI compared with the background gland. Identification of postbiopsy hemorrhage is relevant because it may present as focal or diffuse areas of low SI on T2WI and ADC map, thus mimicking cancer.[15,16] Previous studies, however,

showed that tumors have significantly lower T2 SI and lower ADC values compared with areas of hemorrhage.[16] Additionally, the interpretation of raw DCE images could be confounded by the inherent high T1 SI on baseline precontrast images. Misinterpretation can, however, be avoided with the use of subtraction images. Accordingly, when hemorrhage is detected on T1WI, the additional sequences should be evaluated with higher scrutiny to avoid overestimation of tumor presence or size.

The normal prostatic tissue has a greater concentration of citrate than foci that harbor prostate cancer. Because citrate has an anticoagulant effect, postbiopsy hemorrhage tends to resolve faster within the tumor compared with the surrounding tissue.[17,18] This phenomenon can result in the "hemorrhage exclusion" or "halo" sign, which is defined as presence of a well-defined isointense mass surrounded by hyperintense area on T1WI (**Fig. 6**).[19] When interpreted in conjunction with T2WI and DWI, the sign is highly specific for the detection of cancer and helps to better determine the tumor size.[2]

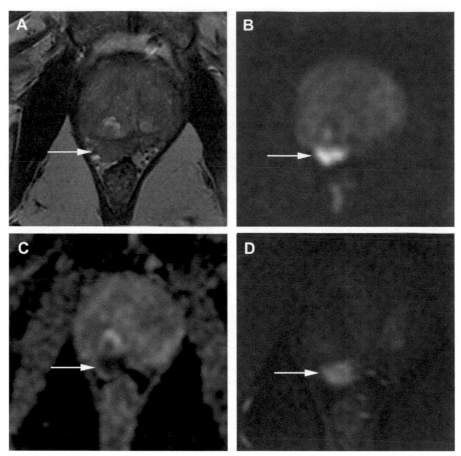

Fig. 1. A 67-year-old man in active surveillance for a Gleason score 6 prostate adenocarcinoma undergoing mp-MRI because of increasing prostate-specific antigen (PSA) value (PSA = 12.6 ng/mL; PSA density = 0.12 ng/mL^2). (*A*) Axial T2WI shows a 1.2-cm hypointense mass in the right peripheral zone of the midgland with extraprostatic extension and invasion of neurovascular bundle (*arrow*). The lesion appears markedly hyperintense on high b-value (b = 1500 s/mm^2) axial DWI (*arrow, B*) and markedly hypointense (mean value = 600 × 10^{-3} mm^2/s) on the ADC map (*arrow, C*) corresponding to a PI-RADS category 5 lesion. The lesion shows avid early enhancement on the axial contrast-enhanced T1WI gradient-recalled echo (GRE) (*arrow, D*).

T1WI can also be used for detection of lymph-adenopathy. The conventional size criteria for characterization of abnormal pelvic lymph nodes have low diagnostic accuracy, however, with a reported pooled sensitivity and specificity of 0.39 and 0.82, respectively.[20] Different thresholds, ranging from 8 mm to 15 mm, have been proposed[21] and PI-RADS v2 classifies lymph nodes larger than 8 mm in short axis as suspicious.[3] Inclusion of lymph node shape, border, enhancement, and ADC values may improve the diagnostic performance of MR imaging.[22]

Functional Imaging

Diffusion-weighted imaging and apparent diffusion coefficient map

Among the functional techniques that comprise a mp-MRI scan of the prostate, DWI plays a key role. Several studies in the last decade have proven that the addition of DWI to T2WI significantly increases the sensitivity and specificity of the technique for the detection of prostate cancer.[23–25] Briefly, DWI depicts the random motion of water molecules within a voxel. The SI on DWI depends on the molecules' motion and the diffusion weighting, which is affected by the imaging acquisition technique (eg, b-value). Generally, the sensitivity of DWI improves when high b-values are used, but this happens at the expense of signal-to-noise ratio. Trace DWI images are, however, diffusion- and T2-weighted. So, lesions with a long T2 value may appear bright on DWI but not restrict diffusion, a phenomenon known as T2 shine-through. Findings on the high-b-value DWI should, therefore, always be correlated with and interpreted in conjunction with the ADC map. Although

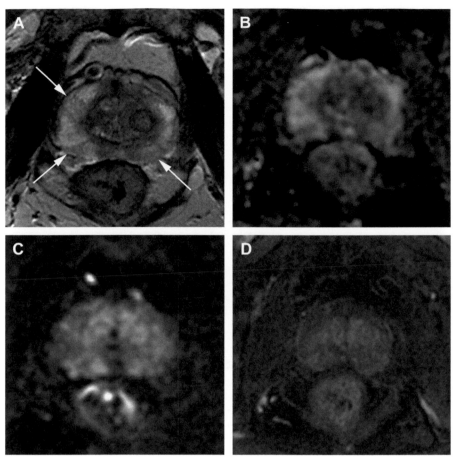

Fig. 2. A 71-year-old man undergoing mp-MRI because of a new diagnosis of prostate adenocarcinoma (Gleason score 3 + 3 = 6) at systematic prostate biopsy. (*A*) Axial T2WI shows multiple and bilateral triangular-shaped areas of mildly low signal intensity (*arrows*) in the peripheral zone of the midgland. (*B*) ADC map at the same level shows indistinct area of low signal intensity. Axial high b-value (b = 1500 s/mm²) DWI (*C*) and axial early contrast-enhanced T1WI GRE (*D*) show no focal abnormality corresponding to a PI-RADS category 2 lesion. The repeated biopsy toward the triangular-shaped foci seen on the images revealed normal prostatic tissue.

the normal PZ demonstrates homogenous low SI on DWI and high SI on ADC map, the more restricted environment of cancer, secondary to the higher cellular density compared with the surrounding glandular tissue, leads to high SI on DWI and low SI on the ADC map.[26,27]

Per PI-RADS v2, each lesion receives a DWI/ADC score that ranges from 1 to 5 based on SI, size, and presence of EPE. The criteria are applicable to lesions located in the PZ or TZ (**Table 2**). A score of 1 denotes normal tissue and absence of abnormalities. A score of 2 is defined as an indistinct area of low SI on the ADC map. A focal abnormality receives a score of 3 or greater, depending on its SI on DWI and ADC map. Lesions highly concerning for prostate cancer (score 4 and 5) show markedly elevated SI on the high b-value DWI and marked low SI on the ADC map (see **Figs. 1** and **5**). A size threshold of 1.5 cm and/or EPE are

again used to assign a score 4 or 5. DWI/ADC is the dominant sequence for characterization of a lesion in the PZ. In the TZ, the sequence plays a secondary role to T2WI because of its lower specificity. Stromal-rich nodules may show restricted diffusion, thus mimicking cancer (**Fig. 7**).[28] Nevertheless, the sensitivity of DWI for detection of cancer in the TZ is high[29] and the technique is used to identify suspicious foci. Once foci with marked restricted diffusion are detected on DWI/ADC, they are characterized based on their appearance on T2WI. DWI/ADC is particularly helpful to detect lesions that are very anterior along the anterior fibromuscular stroma.[30]

Dynamic contrast-enhanced MR imaging
DCE MR imaging consists of multiple series of T1WI, typically three-dimensional gradient-echo images, performed sequentially through the

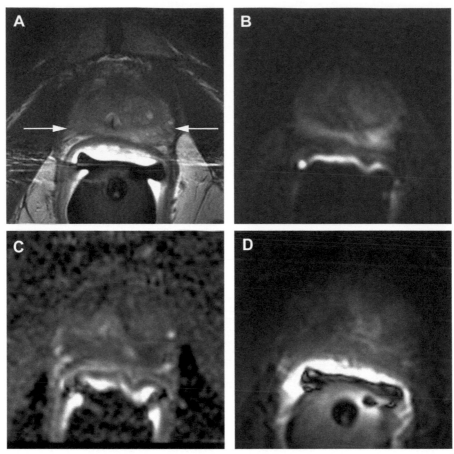

Fig. 3. A 57-year-old man presenting with elevated PSA (PSA = 7.9 ng/mL; PSA density = 0.11 ng/mL^2). (*A*) Axial T2WI shows heterogeneous and moderately low signal intensity in the peripheral zone of the apex (*arrows*). The same area shows heterogeneous mildly high signal intensity on the high b-value (b = 1500 s/mm^2) DWI (*B*) and moderately low (mean = 900 × 10^{-3} mm^2/s) signal intensity on the ADC map (*C*). The DCE study (*D*) is negative for focal early enhancement. The lesion is compatible with a PI-RADS category 3 lesion. Target biopsy of the left posteroapical area showed chronic inflammation.

prostate before, during, and after the intravenous injection of a gadolinium-based contrast agent.[31] The goal of this technique is to assess the tissue perfusion kinetics with high temporal resolution to detect prostate cancer based on the presence of neovascularity and increased vascular permeability.[32] In general, prostate cancer shows earlier and more intense enhancement than the surrounding normal gland.[33]

DCE MR imaging is perhaps the most controversial of all mp-MRI sequences. It has been shown that the technique increases the diagnostic accuracy for cancer detection when added to the anatomic sequences[34,35] and that it is helpful to differentiate tumors located in the anterior gland from the normal anterior fibromuscular stroma because of their earlier enhancement.[30] Unfortunately, DCE MR imaging lacks specificity because multiple other conditions can lead to increased vascularity and early enhancement, including

inflammation in the PZ and some BPH nodules in the TZ.[31] Moreover, lack of standardization of the technique leads to inconsistent results across institutions. Finally, recent publications have documented a limited added value of DCE MR imaging for the detection of prostate cancer when compared with a biparametric approach including T2WI and DWI.[36,37]

Because of these controversies, the role of DCE MR imaging in PI-RADS v2 is limited to the characterization of a PZ lesion considered indeterminate based on DWI. The PI-RADS v2 guidelines recommend a qualitative interpretation of DCE MR imaging, that is, a visual assessment of changes in SI over multiple time points after contrast injection, and a binary description of the pattern of enhancement.[3] If the lesion demonstrates focal and early or contemporaneous enhancement compared with the surrounding normal prostatic parenchyma, DCE MR imaging is considered positive (see

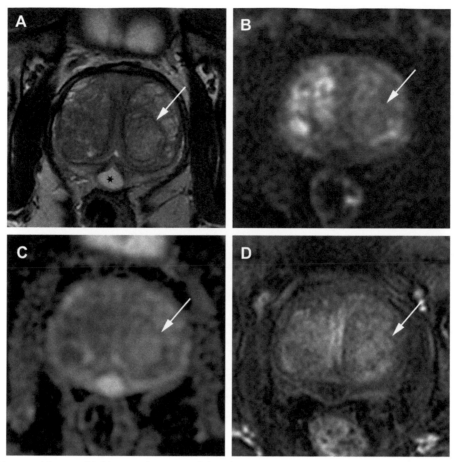

Fig. 4. A 64-year-old man with history of BPH, candidate for transurethral resection of the prostate (PSA = 6.5 ng/mL; prostate volume = 120 mL; PSA density = 0.05 ng/mL^2). (*A*) Axial T2WI shows an enlarged transition zone replaced by innumerable nodules, compatible with BPH. A benign BPH nodule (PI-RADS category 2) is circumscribed with complete hypointense rim on T2WI (*arrow, A*), isointense on high b-value (b = 1500 s/mm^2) DWI (*arrow, B*) and ADC map (*arrow, C*), and shows no early enhancement on the contrast-enhanced T1WI GRE (*arrow, D*). Note a benign utricle cyst (*black star, A*).

Figs. 1 and **5**). Any other finding on DCE MR imaging denotes a negative result.

Prostate Imaging Reporting and Data System Version 2 Overall Assessment

After each lesion (up to four, according to the guidelines) is assigned an individual score based on its T2WI, DWI/ADC, and DCE MR imaging features, a simple algorithm is applied to determine the final PI-RADS category (**Fig. 8**).[3] Lesions are grouped into five categories of risk for clinically significant cancer as follows:

- PI-RADS 1: Very low risk
- PI-RADS 2: Low risk
- PI-RADS 3: Intermediate risk
- PI-RADS 4: High risk
- PI-RADS 5: Very high risk

PI-RADS v2 uses the concept of a dominant sequence, that is, the sequence most affecting the final assessment. Lesions in the PZ are mainly categorized based on their appearance on DWI and ADC map. The indeterminate lesions, that is, score 3, are upgraded to a category 4 if DCE MR imaging is positive. TZ lesions, however, are classified mostly based on their appearance on T2WI. In the TZ, indeterminate lesions are upgraded to a category 4 if their DWI/ADC map score is 5.

Prostate Imaging Reporting and Data System Version 2: Diagnostic Accuracy and Main Limitations

Several retrospective studies reported moderate to high accuracy of PI-RADS v2 for the detection of clinically significant prostate cancer, with areas

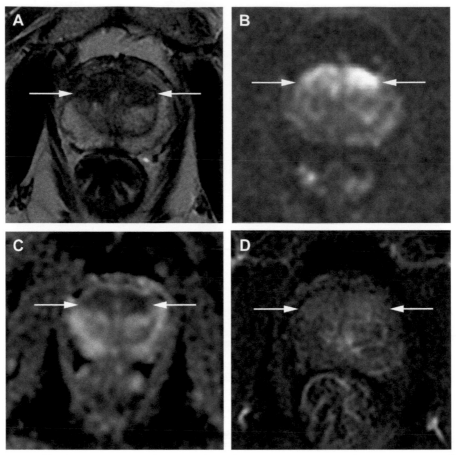

Fig. 5. A 64-year-old man presenting with elevated PSA (PSA = 5.7 ng/mL; PSA density = 0.2 ng/mL^2) and prior negative prostate biopsies. (*A*) Axial T2WI shows a lenticular, noncircumscribed mass with low signal intensity in the anterior midgland (*arrows*) compatible with a PI-RADS category 5 lesion. The mass shows markedly high signal intensity on high b-value (b = 1500 s/mm^2) DWI (*arrows, B*), markedly low signal intensity on ADC map (*arrows, C*), and early enhancement on contrast-enhanced T1WI GRE (*arrows, D*). Target biopsy revealed invasive prostatic adenocarcinoma, Gleason score 3 + 4 = 7.

under the receiver operating characteristic curve ranging from 0.66 to 0.87.[38–40] A recent meta-analysis showed pooled sensitivity and specificity of 89% and 73% for detection of prostate cancer Gleason 3 + 3 or higher using PI-RADS v2 criteria.[41] A recent prospective analysis found that among patients undergoing targeted MR imaging/TRUS fusion biopsy, 78% of lesions categorized as PI-RADS v2 5 represented were cancer.[42] However, PI-RADS v2 scores 4 and 3 were associated with a significantly lower cancer detection rate of 30% and 16%, respectively, suggesting a need for refinement of the current criteria. Another reason for further development of the system comes from interobserver variability studies that report only moderate agreement.[40,43] Additionally, no data are available on the performance of the system by less experienced radiologists in a nonacademic setting. Finally, the current

recommendations are based on qualitative assessment of images, but, as described in the next section, quantitative data from functional images may provide additional information that characterizes tumor biology.

ADVANCED AND QUANTITATIVE IMAGING ANALYSIS OF MULTIPARAMETRIC MR IMAGING OF THE PROSTATE
Diffusion-Weighted Imaging: Apparent Diffusion Coefficient Values

Multiple studies have shown that the measurement of ADC values may improve the characterization of tumor aggressiveness. The ADC values of prostate cancer have an inverse correlation with the Gleason score and the D'Amico clinical risk classification,[26,44–48] and higher degrees of restricted diffusion, characterized by lower ADC

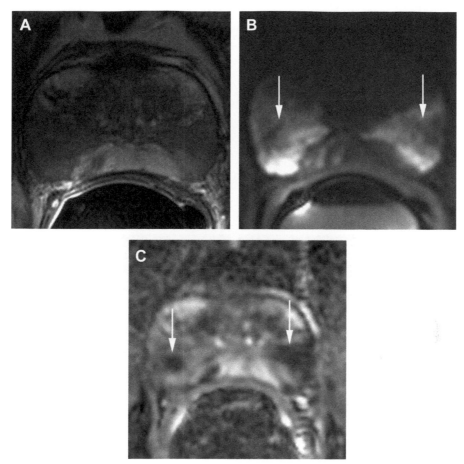

Fig. 6. A 62-year-old man with history of bilateral prostate cancer detected on a systematic biopsy performed 3 weeks before mp-MRI (Gleason score not available; PSA = 4.7 ng/mL). (*A*) Axial T2WI shows extensive areas of hypointensity in posterolateral aspect of midgland peripheral zone on both sides. (*B*) Corresponding precontrast axial T1WI shows diffuse T1 hyperintensity compatible with postbiopsy hemorrhage. Two areas in peripheral zone (*arrows*), however, are spared from hemorrhage (halo sign). (*C*) Corresponding ADC map shows marked restricted diffusion in those areas (*arrows*). Hemorrhage exclusion or halo sign is highly specific for the detection of cancer.

Table 2
DWI score for peripheral and transition zone according to PI-RADS v2

Score	Signal Intensity High b-Value DWI	Signal Intensity ADC Map	Size - EPE
Peripheral and transition zone			
1 (normal)	• Homogeneous • No focal abnormality	• Homogeneous • No focal abnormality	N/A
2	• No focal abnormality	• Indistinct • Low	Any size EPE absent
3	• Focal • Iso-to-mildly high	• Focal • Mildly-to-moderately low	Any size EPE absent
4	• Focal • Markedly high	• Focal • Markedly low	<1.5 cm EPE absent
5	• Focal • Markedly high	• Focal • Markedly low	≥1.5 cm and/or EPE definitely present

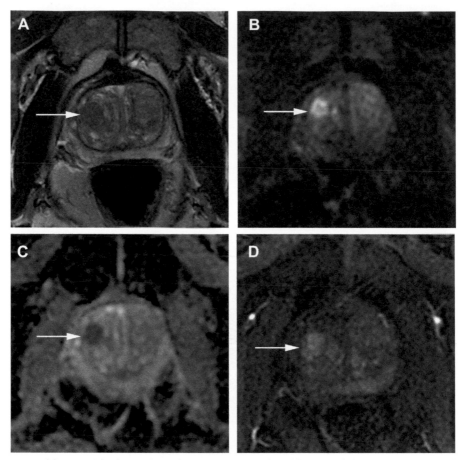

Fig. 7. A 65-year-old man with elevated PSA (PSA = 15.1 ng/mL) and history of chronic prostatitis. (*A*) Axial T2WI of the prostate midgland shows a 1.2-cm circumscribed hypointense nodule (*arrow*) in the enlarged right transition zone. The nodule is hyperintense on high b-value DWI (*arrow*, *B*), hypointense (mean ADC value = 720×10^{-3} mm^2/s) on ADC map (*arrow*, *C*), and shows early enhancement on the axial contrast-enhanced T1WI GRE (*arrow*, *D*). Target biopsy revealed normal prostatic tissue.

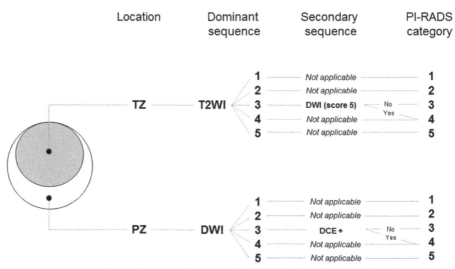

Fig. 8. Diagram is a representation of the algorithm used in PI-RADS v2 to determine the final category of risk for clinically significant risk based on the imaging appearance on mp-MRI.

values, have been associated with a greater probability of EPE.[49] The main limitation of a quantitative interpretation of DWI is the variability of ADC values across institutions, because these are dependent of multiple technical variables and patient features.[45,50] Although a particular threshold cannot be recommended, it is generally accepted that clinically significant tumors have an ADC value lower than approximately 1000×10^{-6} mm^2/s. It is important, however, to determine the range ADC values seen at one's institution, if these will be used to further characterize lesions identified on DWI and ADC maps.

Although the most commonly used method to generate an ADC map from the source DWI is a monoexponential model (based on a Gaussian [ie, random] diffusion behavior), other more sophisticated options are available and promise to capture additional biologic information. These methods are based on the fact that the diffusion signal tends to depart from a monoexponential decay at low (eg, <200) and high (eg, >1000) b-values,[51,52] but to exploit these differences, images need to be obtained with a large number and range of b-values. According to the intravoxel incoherent motion theory, the signal decay is made of perfusion (fast component: water moving within the capillaries) and diffusion (slow component).[53] When low b-value data are acquired, a bi-exponential model is used to take into account these two components.[54] Although the intravoxel incoherent motion–derived parameter molecular diffusion coefficient (D) and perfusion fraction (f) have been shown to be lower in prostate cancer compared with normal parenchyma,[55] the added value of the technique for tumor detection is yet unclear.[56] On the opposite end of the spectrum, when high b-values (>1000) are used, a diffusion kurtosis model can be obtained, based on a non-Gaussian diffusion assumption.[52] The diffusion kurtosis–derived parameter k (apparent diffusional kurtosis) has been shown to be significantly higher in prostate cancer compared with benign tissue.[57] However, the added value of this technique compared with a monoexponential calculation of ADC is also not yet defined.[58,59]

Dynamic Contrast-Enhanced Imaging: Semiquantitative Analysis of Curves of Enhancement and Pharmacokinetic Modeling

Although the current PI-RADS v2 guidelines recommend a qualitative interpretation of the DCE MR imaging, the data can be processed and analyzed semiquantitatively or quantitatively to improve diagnostic accuracy and to extract prognostic imaging biomarkers.[31]

Enhancement curves (semiquantitative analysis)

The SI on DCE MR imaging are plotted against time to create curves of enhancement. Curves are typically classified into three types: type 1, progressive enhancement; type 2, initial upslope followed by plateau; and type 3, decline after initial upslope (wash-in and wash-out) (**Fig. 9**).[31] Type 3 curves are considered the most specific of the curves for the diagnosis of prostate cancer. Although this semiquantitative approach has been advocated by several authors and included in the initial version of PI-RADS,[2] it has been found to have limited effectiveness in differentiating malignant from benign prostatic tissue, particularly in the TZ, and therefore is not included in the updated version of the guidelines.[60] The curves of enhancement can also be processed to extract multiple other parameters, including maximal contrast enhancement, time to peak enhancement, speed of contrast uptake (wash-in), and clearance rate of contrast agent (wash-out).[61] The wash-in parameter has been shown to be the most useful for detecting tumor and discriminating it from benign tissue.[61] Lack of standardization remains the main limitation for a wider application of these semiquantitative tools.

Pharmacokinetic modeling (quantitative analysis)

Changes in concentration of contrast medium over time are quantified using pharmacokinetic modeling.[62] A detailed review of the pharmacokinetic modeling is beyond the purpose of this article. Interested readers are invited to review the excellent papers by Verma and colleagues[31] and Sourbron and Buckley.[62] Commercially available software allows the calculation and display (ie, color-coded parametric maps) of the following parameters, which are particularly relevant for prostate cancer (**Fig. 10**):

- K^{trans} [min^{-1}]: (forward) volume transfer constant or influx (from vascular to extracellular space) rate constant
- k_{ep} [min^{-1}]: reverse reflux rate constant or efflux (from extracellular space to the vascular space) rate constant
- Ve [mL/100 mL]: interstitial volume = K^{trans}/k_{ep}
- Vp [mL/100 mL]: plasma volume

K^{trans} and k_{ep} increase in prostate cancer because of increased cellular and microvascular

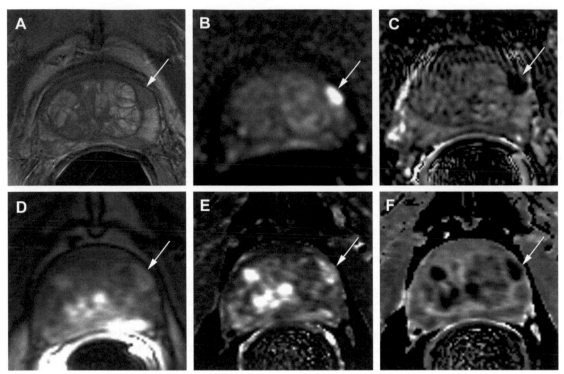

Fig. 9. A 75-year-old man with elevated PSA (8.3 ng/mL) undergoing mp-MRI of the prostate in preparation for fusion biopsy. Axial T2WI (*A*) of the prostate midgland shows a 1.0-cm well-defined T2-hypointense lesion in the left peripheral zone (*arrow*) that appears markedly hyperintense on high b-value (b = 1350 s/mm^2) DWI (*arrow, B*) and markedly hypointense on the ADC map (*arrow, C*) compatible with PI-RADS category 5. The lesion shows focal early enhancement on the axial contrast-enhanced T1WI GRE (*arrow, D*), early wash-in (*arrow on E*, gray-scale wash-in map), and early washout (*arrow on F*, grayscale wash-out map).

density with decreased extracellular space, and correlate with tumor aggressiveness.[63,64] Despite the promising results as prognostic biomarker, the adoption of these metrics in the daily evaluation of mp-MRI of the prostate adds complexity to the examination.

Magnetic Resonance Spectroscopy Imaging

MR spectroscopic imaging provides information that is used to characterize the metabolic profile of the prostatic tissue. Increased cellular density and cell membrane turnover in tumor, along with disruption of the normal glandular tissue, lead to higher levels of choline and lower levels of citrate compared with the normal gland.[65] The results of the postprocessing of data are usually visualized as multiple spectra on a grid that is overlaid on the corresponding axial T2WI. For a quantitative analysis, the choline-plus-creatine-to-citrate ratio is calculated: a choline-plus-creatine-to-citrate ratio of at least three standard deviations greater than the mean normal value (0.22 ± 0.013) is highly suggestive of cancer.[66] Despite the results of several studies showing the usefulness of MR

spectroscopic imaging for cancer detection, assessment of tumor aggressiveness and response to treatment,[67] recent evidence shows no added value of MR spectroscopic imaging for tumor detection when compared with a combination of anatomic and functional (ie, DWI, DCE) imaging.[68,69] In addition, this technique requires a high level of expertise for acquisition and analysis, markedly limiting its widespread use.

FUTURE DIRECTIONS

Preliminary works on texture analysis, a mathematical postprocessing algorithm to quantify the spatial distribution and randomness of pixel intensities, have shown promising results for the assessment of tumor biology. A recent study suggested differences between T2WI MR imaging–derived textural parameters of prostate cancers Gleason score 4 + 3 and 3 + 4.[70] Finally, recent efforts toward the development of dedicated computer-aided diagnostic systems for mp-MRI have the potential of improving interobserver and/or intraobserver variability and diagnostic accuracy.[71]

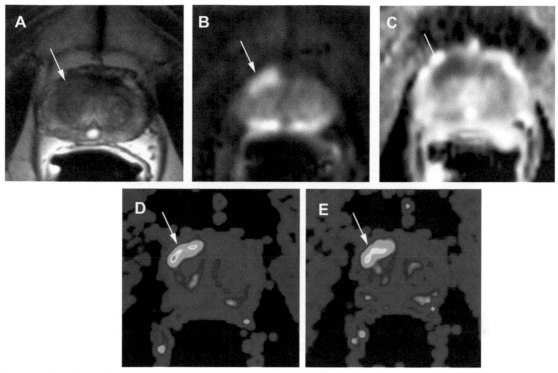

Fig. 10. Role of DCE for the detection of anterior gland prostate cancer. A tumor in the anterior gland shows lenticular shape and ill-defined margins on T2WI (*arrow, A*), markedly high signal intensity on high b-value DWI (*arrow, B*), and markedly low signal intensity on ADC map (*arrow, C*) compatible with a PI-RADS category 5 lesion. Color-encoded K^{trans} forward volume transfer constant (*D*) and k_{ep} reverse reflux rate constant map (*E*) delineate the tumor (*arrow*) against the surrounding gland. (*Courtesy of* Dr Daniel Margolis, Weill Cornell Medicine, New York, NY.)

SUMMARY

mp-MRI of the prostate is a complex imaging study comprising anatomic and functional sequences. The use of the PI-RADS v2 system results in a more standardized interpretation scheme with higher diagnostic accuracy. Further developments, however, are required to overcome the current shortcomings.

REFERENCES

1. Oberlin DT, Casalino DD, Miller FH, et al. Dramatic increase in the utilization of multiparametric magnetic resonance imaging for detection and management of prostate cancer. Abdom Radiol (NY) 2017; 42:1255–8.
2. Barentsz JO, Richenberg J, Clements R, et al. ESUR prostate MR guidelines 2012. Eur Radiol 2012;22: 746–57.
3. Weinreb JC, Barentsz JO, Choyke PL, et al. PI-RADS prostate imaging - reporting and data system: 2015, version 2. Eur Urol 2016;69:16–40.
4. Roethke MC, Lichy MP, Jurgschat L, et al. Tumorsize dependent detection rate of endorectal MRI of prostate cancer: a histopathologic correlation with whole-mount sections in 70 patients with prostate cancer. Eur J Radiol 2011;79:189–95.
5. Ikonen S, Karkkainen P, Kivisaari L, et al. Magnetic resonance imaging of prostatic cancer: does detection vary between high and low Gleason score tumors? Prostate 2000;43:43–8.
6. Wang L, Mazaheri Y, Zhang J, et al. Assessment of biologic aggressiveness of prostate cancer: correlation of MR signal intensity with Gleason grade after radical prostatectomy. Radiology 2008;246:168–76.
7. Gleason DF, Mellinger GT. Prediction of prognosis for prostatic adenocarcinoma by combined histological grading and clinical staging. J Urol 1974;111: 58–64.
8. Cruz M, Tsuda K, Narumi Y, et al. Characterization of low-intensity lesions in the peripheral zone of prostate on pre-biopsy endorectal coil MR imaging. Eur Radiol 2002;12:357–65.
9. Mizuno R, Nakashima J, Mukai M, et al. Maximum tumor diameter is a simple and valuable index associated with the local extent of disease in clinically localized prostate cancer. Int J Urol 2006;13:951–5.
10. Westphalen AC, Coakley FV, Kurhanewicz J, et al. Mucinous adenocarcinoma of the prostate: MRI

and MR spectroscopy features. AJR Am J Roentgenol 2009;193:W238–43.

11. Sciarra A, Barentsz J, Bjartell A, et al. Advances in magnetic resonance imaging: how they are changing the management of prostate cancer. Eur Urol 2011;59:962–77.

12. Ishida J, Sugimura K, Okizuka H, et al. Benign prostatic hyperplasia: value of MR imaging for determining histologic type. Radiology 1994;190:329–31.

13. Moosavi B, Flood TA, Al-Dandan O, et al. Multiparametric MRI of the anterior prostate gland: clinical-radiological-histopathological correlation. Clin Radiol 2016;71:405–17.

14. Guneyli S, Ward E, Thomas S, et al. Magnetic resonance imaging of benign prostatic hyperplasia. Diagn Interv Radiol 2016;22:215–9.

15. White S, Hricak H, Forstner R, et al. Prostate cancer: effect of postbiopsy hemorrhage on interpretation of MR images. Radiology 1995;195:385–90.

16. Rosenkrantz AB, Kopec M, Kong X, et al. Prostate cancer vs. post-biopsy hemorrhage: diagnosis with T2- and diffusion-weighted imaging. J Magn Reson Imaging 2010;31:1387–94.

17. Janssen MJ, Huijgens PC, Bouman AA, et al. Citrate versus heparin anticoagulation in chronic haemodialysis patients. Nephrol Dial Transplant 1993;8:1228–33.

18. Zakian KL, Shukla-Dave A, Ackerstaff E, et al. 1H magnetic resonance spectroscopy of prostate cancer: biomarkers for tumor characterization. Cancer Biomark 2008;4:263–76.

19. Katz S, Rosen M. MR imaging and MR spectroscopy in prostate cancer management. Radiol Clin North Am 2006;44:723–34, viii.

20. Hovels AM, Heesakkers RA, Adang EM, et al. The diagnostic accuracy of CT and MRI in the staging of pelvic lymph nodes in patients with prostate cancer: a meta-analysis. Clin Radiol 2008;63:387–95.

21. Sankineni S, Brown AM, Fascelli M, et al. Lymph node staging in prostate cancer. Curr Urol Rep 2015;16:30.

22. Thoeny HC, Froehlich JM, Triantafyllou M, et al. Metastases in normal-sized pelvic lymph nodes: detection with diffusion-weighted MR imaging. Radiology 2014;273:125–35.

23. Wu LM, Xu JR, Ye YQ, et al. The clinical value of diffusion-weighted imaging in combination with T2-weighted imaging in diagnosing prostate carcinoma: a systematic review and meta-analysis. AJR Am J Roentgenol 2012;199:103–10.

24. Kitajima K, Kaji Y, Fukabori Y, et al. Prostate cancer detection with 3 T MRI: comparison of diffusion-weighted imaging and dynamic contrast-enhanced MRI in combination with T2-weighted imaging. J Magn Reson Imaging 2010;31:625–31.

25. Haider MA, van der Kwast TH, Tanguay J, et al. Combined T2-weighted and diffusion-weighted MRI for localization of prostate cancer. AJR Am J Roentgenol 2007;189:323–8.

26. Gibbs P, Liney GP, Pickles MD, et al. Correlation of ADC and T2 measurements with cell density in prostate cancer at 3.0 Tesla. Invest Radiol 2009;44:572–6.

27. Zelhof B, Pickles M, Liney G, et al. Correlation of diffusion-weighted magnetic resonance data with cellularity in prostate cancer. BJU Int 2009;103:883–8.

28. Oto A, Kayhan A, Jiang Y, et al. Prostate cancer: differentiation of central gland cancer from benign prostatic hyperplasia by using diffusion-weighted and dynamic contrast-enhanced MR imaging. Radiology 2010;257:715–23.

29. Rosenkrantz AB, Kim S, Campbell N, et al. Transition zone prostate cancer: revisiting the role of multiparametric MRI at 3 T. AJR Am J Roentgenol 2015;204:W266–72.

30. Ward E, Baad M, Peng Y, et al. Multi-parametric MR imaging of the anterior fibromuscular stroma and its differentiation from prostate cancer. Abdom Radiol (NY) 2017;42:926–34.

31. Verma S, Turkbey B, Muradyan N, et al. Overview of dynamic contrast-enhanced MRI in prostate cancer diagnosis and management. AJR Am J Roentgenol 2012;198:1277–88.

32. Russo G, Mischi M, Scheepens W, et al. Angiogenesis in prostate cancer: onset, progression and imaging. BJU Int 2012;110:E794–808.

33. Engelbrecht MR, Huisman HJ, Laheij RJ, et al. Discrimination of prostate cancer from normal peripheral zone and central gland tissue by using dynamic contrast-enhanced MR imaging. Radiology 2003;229:248–54.

34. Turkbey B, Pinto PA, Mani H, et al. Prostate cancer: value of multiparametric MR imaging at 3 T for detection–histopathologic correlation. Radiology 2010;255:89–99.

35. Tan CH, Hobbs BP, Wei W, et al. Dynamic contrast-enhanced MRI for the detection of prostate cancer: meta-analysis. AJR Am J Roentgenol 2015;204:W439–48.

36. Vargas HA, Hotker AM, Goldman DA, et al. Updated prostate imaging reporting and data system (PI-RADS v2) recommendations for the detection of clinically significant prostate cancer using multiparametric MRI: critical evaluation using whole-mount pathology as standard of reference. Eur Radiol 2016;26:1606–12.

37. De Visschere P, Lumen N, Ost P, et al. Dynamic contrast-enhanced imaging has limited added value over T2-weighted imaging and diffusion-weighted imaging when using PI-RADSv2 for diagnosis of clinically significant prostate cancer in patients with elevated PSA. Clin Radiol 2017;72:23–32.

38. Lin WC, Muglia VF, Silva GE, et al. Multiparametric MRI of the prostate: diagnostic performance and

interreader agreement of two scoring systems. Br J Radiol 2016;89:20151056.

39. Lin WC, Westphalen AC, Silva GE, et al. Comparison of PI-RADS 2, ADC histogram-derived parameters, and their combination for the diagnosis of peripheral zone prostate cancer. Abdom Radiol (NY) 2016;41:2209–17.

40. Muller BG, Shih JH, Sankineni S, et al. Prostate cancer: interobserver agreement and accuracy with the revised prostate imaging reporting and data system at multiparametric MR imaging. Radiology 2015;277(3):741–50.

41. Woo S, Suh CH, Kim SY, et al. Diagnostic performance of prostate imaging reporting and data system version 2 for detection of prostate cancer: a systematic review and diagnostic meta-analysis. Eur Urol 2017;72(2):177–88.

42. Mertan FV, Greer MD, Shih JH, et al. Prospective evaluation of the prostate imaging reporting and data system version 2 for prostate cancer detection. J Urol 2016;196:690–6.

43. Rosenkrantz AB, Ginocchio LA, Cornfeld D, et al. Interobserver reproducibility of the PI-RADS version 2 lexicon: a multicenter study of six experienced prostate radiologists. Radiology 2016;280:793–804.

44. deSouza NM, Riches SF, Vanas NJ, et al. Diffusion-weighted magnetic resonance imaging: a potential non-invasive marker of tumour aggressiveness in localized prostate cancer. Clin Radiol 2008;63:774–82.

45. Tamada T, Sone T, Jo Y, et al. Apparent diffusion coefficient values in peripheral and transition zones of the prostate: comparison between normal and malignant prostatic tissues and correlation with histologic grade. J Magn Reson Imaging 2008;28:720–6.

46. Nagarajan R, Margolis D, Raman S, et al. Correlation of Gleason scores with diffusion-weighted imaging findings of prostate cancer. Adv Urol 2012;2012:374805.

47. Vargas HA, Akin O, Franiel T, et al. Diffusion-weighted endorectal MR imaging at 3 T for prostate cancer: tumor detection and assessment of aggressiveness. Radiology 2011;259:775–84.

48. Turkbey B, Shah VP, Pang Y, et al. Is apparent diffusion coefficient associated with clinical risk scores for prostate cancers that are visible on 3-T MR images? Radiology 2011;258:488–95.

49. Kim CK, Park SY, Park JJ, et al. Diffusion-weighted MRI as a predictor of extracapsular extension in prostate cancer. AJR Am J Roentgenol 2014;202:W270–6.

50. Kim CK, Park BK, Kim B. Diffusion-weighted MRI at 3 T for the evaluation of prostate cancer. AJR Am J Roentgenol 2010;194:1461–9.

51. Jambor I, Merisaari H, Taimen P, et al. Evaluation of different mathematical models for diffusion-weighted imaging of normal prostate and prostate cancer using high b-values: a repeatability study. Magn Reson Med 2015;73:1988–98.

52. Rosenkrantz AB, Padhani AR, Chenevert TL, et al. Body diffusion kurtosis imaging: basic principles, applications, and considerations for clinical practice. J Magn Reson Imaging 2015;42:1190–202.

53. Le Bihan D, Breton E, Lallemand D, et al. Separation of diffusion and perfusion in intravoxel incoherent motion MR imaging. Radiology 1988;168:497–505.

54. Shinmoto H, Oshio K, Tanimoto A, et al. Biexponential apparent diffusion coefficients in prostate cancer. Magn Reson Imaging 2009;27:355–9.

55. Shinmoto H, Tamura C, Soga S, et al. An intravoxel incoherent motion diffusion-weighted imaging study of prostate cancer. AJR Am J Roentgenol 2012;199:W496–500.

56. Kuru TH, Roethke MC, Stieltjes B, et al. Intravoxel incoherent motion (IVIM) diffusion imaging in prostate cancer: what does it add? J Comput Assist Tomogr 2014;38:558–64.

57. Rosenkrantz AB, Sigmund EE, Johnson G, et al. Prostate cancer: feasibility and preliminary experience of a diffusional kurtosis model for detection and assessment of aggressiveness of peripheral zone cancer. Radiology 2012;264:126–35.

58. Roethke MC, Kuder TA, Kuru TH, et al. Evaluation of diffusion kurtosis imaging versus standard diffusion imaging for detection and grading of peripheral zone prostate cancer. Invest Radiol 2015;50:483–9.

59. Tamada T, Prabhu V, Li J, et al. Prostate cancer: diffusion-weighted MR imaging for detection and assessment of aggressiveness-comparison between conventional and kurtosis models. Radiology 2017;284(1):100–8.

60. Hansford BG, Peng Y, Jiang Y, et al. Dynamic contrast-enhanced MR imaging curve-type analysis: is it helpful in the differentiation of prostate cancer from healthy peripheral zone? Radiology 2015;275:448–57.

61. Isebaert S, De Keyzer F, Haustermans K, et al. Evaluation of semi-quantitative dynamic contrast-enhanced MRI parameters for prostate cancer in correlation to whole-mount histopathology. Eur J Radiol 2012;81:e217–22.

62. Sourbron SP, Buckley DL. Classic models for dynamic contrast-enhanced MRI. NMR Biomed 2013;26:1004–27.

63. Vos EK, Litjens GJ, Kobus T, et al. Assessment of prostate cancer aggressiveness using dynamic contrast-enhanced magnetic resonance imaging at 3 T. Eur Urol 2013;64:448–55.

64. Langer DL, van der Kwast TH, Evans AJ, et al. Prostate tissue composition and MR measurements: investigating the relationships between ADC, T2, K(trans), v(e), and corresponding histologic features. Radiology 2010;255:485–94.

65. Starobinets O, Korn N, Iqbal S, et al. Practical aspects of prostate MRI: hardware and software

considerations, protocols, and patient preparation. Abdom Radiol (NY) 2016;41:817–30.

66. Jung JA, Coakley FV, Vigneron DB, et al. Prostate depiction at endorectal MR spectroscopic imaging: investigation of a standardized evaluation system. Radiology 2004;233:701–8.

67. Kurhanewicz J, Vigneron DB. Advances in MR spectroscopy of the prostate. Magn Reson Imaging Clin N Am 2008;16:697–710, ix–x.

68. Polanec SH, Pinker-Domenig K, Brader P, et al. Multiparametric MRI of the prostate at 3 T: limited value of 3D (1)H-MR spectroscopy as a fourth parameter. World J Urol 2016;34:649–56.

69. Platzek I, Borkowetz A, Toma M, et al. Multiparametric prostate magnetic resonance imaging at 3 T: failure of magnetic resonance spectroscopy to provide added value. J Comput Assist Tomogr 2015;39(5): 674–80.

70. Nketiah G, Elschot M, Kim E, et al. T2-weighted MRI-derived textural features reflect prostate cancer aggressiveness: preliminary results. Eur Radiol 2016;27(7):3050–9.

71. Litjens GJ, Barentsz JO, Karssemeijer N, et al. Clinical evaluation of a computer-aided diagnosis system for determining cancer aggressiveness in prostate MRI. Eur Radiol 2015;25(11):3187–99.

Multiparametric Prostate MR Imaging: Impact on Clinical Staging and Decision Making

Petar Duvnjak, MD[a,b], Ariel A. Schulman, MD[c],
Jamie N. Holtz, MD[a], Jiaoti Huang, MD, PhD[d,e],
Thomas J. Polascik, MD[c,e], Rajan T. Gupta, MD[a,c,e,*]

KEYWORDS

- Prostate cancer • Multiparametric MR imaging (mpMRI) • Staging

KEY POINTS

- The current paradigm for prostate cancer staging is changing with increased incorporation of multiparametric MR imaging (mpMRI) into clinical decision making.
- MpMRI has proved useful in differentiating organ-confined disease (stage ≤T2) from locally advanced (stage ≥T3) disease due to the high sensitivity and specificity for the detection of extraprostatic extension (EPE) and seminal vesicle invasion (SVI).
- Much work on mpMRI is forthcoming regarding the use of mpMRI in preoperative volumetric tumor assessment, improving biopsy targeting of transrectal ultrasound (TRUS)-negative tumors, and selection and follow-up of men on active surveillance.

INTRODUCTION

Prostate cancer is the most common noncutaneous malignancy and second leading cause of cancer-related deaths in men in the United States, with an estimated 180,890 new cases and 26,120 deaths in 2016.[1] The overall 5-year survival rate is relatively high and has increased from 83% in the 1980s to 99% from 2005 to 2011, in part due to earlier detection and earlier aggressive therapy for high-risk disease. Despite the overall high 5-year survival rate, outcomes are variable, ranging

This article was previously published in March 2018 *Radiologic Clinics*, Volume 56, Issue 2.

This project was performed at the Departments of Radiology, Pathology, and Surgery at Duke University Medical Center.

There is no external or internal funding for this project. This article is not under consideration elsewhere.

Financial Disclosures/Conflicts of Interest relevant to this submitted work: Dr R.T. Gupta has no financial disclosures or conflicts of interest related to this work. Dr R.T. Gupta does serve as a consultant to Bayer Pharma AG and Invivo Corp. Dr R.T. Gupta also serves on the Speakers Bureau for Bayer Pharma AG. Dr P. Duvnjak, Dr A.A. Schulman, Dr J.N. Holtz, Dr J. Huang, and Dr T.J. Polascik have no conflicts of interest.

[a] Department of Radiology, Duke University Medical Center, DUMC Box 3808, Durham, NC 27710, USA;
[b] Department of Radiology, Medical College of Wisconsin, 9200 West Wisconsin Avenue, Milwaukee, WI 53226, USA; [c] Division of Urologic Surgery, Department of Surgery, Duke Prostate Center, Duke University Medical Center, DUMC Box 2804, Durham, NC 27710, USA; [d] Department of Pathology, Duke University Medical Center, DUMC Box 3712, Durham, NC 27710, USA; [e] Duke Cancer Institute, DUMC Box 3917, Durham, NC 27710, USA

* Corresponding author. Department of Radiology, Duke University Medical Center, DUMC Box 3808, Durham, NC 27710.

E-mail address: rajan.gupta@duke.edu

Urol Clin N Am 45 (2018) 455–466
https://doi.org/10.1016/j.ucl.2018.03.010

from near 100% survival in organ-confined disease to as low as 28% survival in more advanced stages.[2] Studies have shown that many men with low-risk disease in the United States are over-treated, resulting in significant economic impact and individual morbidity associated with aggressive therapy.[3]

In the past decade, there have been meaningful changes in the approach to the diagnosis, characterization, and management of clinically localized prostate cancer. These have become increasingly defined by more selective population screening, integration of novel diagnostic tools, and increased acceptance of active surveillance and partial ablative strategies as viable management strategies.[4] These trends have driven demand for optimized prostate imaging. The need for accurate pretherapy staging is, therefore, paramount for risk stratification with the ultimate goals of preventing overtreatment of low-risk disease in favor of active surveillance and selection of the optimal early aggressive intervention in high-risk disease. The aim of this article is to review the current and changing paradigm in prostate cancer staging with specific emphasis on the evolving role of multiparametric MR imaging (mpMRI) and how it is being integrated into clinical decision making.

OVERVIEW OF PROSTATE CANCER STAGING AND CLINICAL NOMOGRAMS

Clinical and pathologic staging is most widely performed according to the American Joint Committee on Cancer (AJCC) 2010 TNM classification system, which incorporates clinical T stage (based on digital rectal examination [DRE]) and, if available, serum prostate-specific antigen (PSA) and Gleason score.[5] *The AJCC Cancer Staging Manual*, eighth edition, recently released, incorporates several important changes to the current prostate cancer staging paradigm. Notably, the eighth edition includes the prostate prognostic group grade to histopathologic assessment, which is to be reported along with the Gleason score. Additionally, pathologic staging no longer subcategorizes pT2 due to increased emphasis placed on tumor volume over laterality, because this has been shown to have more practical and prognostic significance.[6]

Numerous clinical nomograms have been developed over the years that take into account various parameters to predict pathologic stage at radical prostatectomy.[7] One of the most widely used clinical nomograms are the Partin tables, which factor in a patient's clinical T stage, serum PSA, and Gleason score.[8,9] The Memorial Sloan Kettering nomogram includes percent positive cores from transrectal ultrasound (TRUS)-guided biopsy and the University of California, San Francisco, Cancer of the Prostate Risk Assessment scoring system also includes the patient age.[10,11]

The current paradigm for prostate cancer diagnosis centers on performing systematic 12-core TRUS-guided biopsy in men with elevated PSA or positive DRE. Aside from issues related to the morbidity of the procedure, there are several well documented limitations to this approach.[12] On one hand, undersampling can occur and has been shown to lead to false-negative biopsy results in up to 30% of cases, particularly in men with larger glands or those with anterior prostate cancers.[13] Undersampling can also lead to inaccurate risk stratification in some men. For example, a 2010 prospective study of 1565 patients showed that 47% of men classified as low-risk (≤Gleason 6) who may have been potential candidates for active surveillance were actually upgraded to Gleason 7 or greater after prostatectomy.[14] Attempts to overcome undersampling errors by increasing the number of core samples by performing serial biopsies have been shown to increase the overall cancer detection rate; however, in 1 study, a majority of these cases were classified as clinically insignificant (75 of 119 cases).[15]

INTEGRATION OF MULTIPARAMETRIC MR IMAGING INTO CLINICAL ALGORITHMS AND STAGING SYSTEMS
Detection and Characterization of Prostate Cancer with Multiparametric MR Imaging

mpMRI has the potential to overcome many of the shortcomings associated with TRUS biopsy systems and has proved valuable for improving the detection of higher-grade disease (histologic Gleason score) and higher-stage disease (extraprostatic extension [EPE] and tumor volume), thereby offering a more complete clinical picture for clinical decision making. In some studies, mpMRI has been shown to increase cancer detection rates and lead to pathologic upgrading in up to 38% of cases in men with persistent clinical suspicion of prostate cancer despite prior negative biopsy.[16] A recent prospective National Institutes of Health study on 1003 men with elevated PSA or positive DRE who underwent mpMRI compared random TRUS biopsy and magnetic resonance (MR) fusion–guided biopsy. They demonstrated a 30% increase in the diagnosis of high-risk disease and a 17% decrease in the detection of low-risk disease in the targeted MR-biopsy group. For men in the series who underwent radical prostatectomy, targeted biopsy alone was the best discriminator between low-risk and intermediate/high-risk disease.[17] Radtke and colleagues[18] also found that integration of MR fusion biopsy decreases the detection of clinically insignificant disease (Gleason score 3 + 3).

mpMRI also has a growing role in the initial evaluation of men without a histologic diagnosis of cancer. Although the utility of mpMRI in men with an elevated PSA but negative TRUS biopsy is well established, there is particular recent interest in mpMRI before biopsy.[19] As noted in the Prostate MR Imaging Study (PROMIS), Ahmed and colleagues[20] demonstrated the potential benefit of mpMRI in the prebiopsy setting with markedly better sensitivity and negative predictive value compared with TRUS biopsy. The investigators found that using mpMRI to select men for biopsy could decrease primary biopsies by 27% and reduce detection of clinically insignificant cancer by 5% and suggested that men with a negative mpMRI can forgo biopsy. It must be recognized, however, that of the 158 nonsuspicious mpMRIs in the study, 17 men (10.8%) harbored clinically significant cancer. Thus, although an increasingly important role of mpMRI before biopsy is recognized, the authors believe that current evidence supports the need for additional systematic TRUS biopsies as well as any targeted biopsies to maximize detection of clinically significant, MR imaging–negative cancers. Yin and colleagues[21] recently proposed a diagnostic algorithm that integrates prebiopsy mpMRI, TRUS biopsy, and targeted biopsy for MR-suspicious lesions and the use of molecular markers to improve risk stratification.

Role of Multiparametric MR Imaging in Clinical Staging

With the emerging role of mpMRI, the current paradigm of prostate cancer staging is shifting, with increased emphasis placed on incorporating mpMRI into clinical staging nomograms. mpMRI-specific staging systems have been developed, one of which is summarized in **Table 1**.[22] There has been a rapidly growing body of literature over the past several years demonstrating the potential utility of mpMRI in prostate cancer staging. For example, a 2012 retrospective study of 388 men with clinically low-risk prostate cancer showed that mpMRI obtained with endorectal coils (ERCs) at 1.5T and 3T could help predict findings on confirmatory biopsy, therefore aiding in stratifying patients eligible for active surveillance versus definitive treatment.[23] There have also been several recent studies that show the benefit of mpMRI compared with clinical staging

Table 1 Multiparametric MR imaging staging for prostate cancer	
MR Imaging Stage	**Stage Description**
T1	No lesions considered suspicious for cancer
T2a	Unilateral lesion(s) highly suspicious for cancer, occupying <50% of the affected side of the gland
T2b	Unilateral lesion(s) highly suspicious for cancer, occupying >50% of the affected side of the gland
T2c	Bilateral lesion(s) highly suspicious for cancer
T3a	High degree of suspicion for extracapsular extension (unilateral or bilateral) without invasion of seminal vesicles
T3b	High degree of suspicion of SVI(s) without involvement of adjacent structures
T4	Tumor invades adjacent structures other than the seminal vesicles, such as the external sphincter, rectum, bladder, levator muscles, and pelvic wall

Adapted from Gupta RT, Faridi KF, Singh AA, et al. Comparing 3-T multiparametric MR Imaging and the Partin tables to predict organ-confined prostate cancer after radical prostatectomy. Urol Oncol 2014;32(8):1293; with permission.

nomograms in predicting organ-confined disease. For example, work done by the authors' group demonstrated that the predictive accuracy of mpMRI was significantly greater than the Partin tables in predicting organ-confined disease, with a positive predictive value of 91.2% and negative predictive value of 89.7%.[22] Similar studies have shown that the addition of preoperative mpMRI to clinical nomograms improves the predictive accuracy for detection of EPE compared with clinical nomograms alone.[24–26] A more recent study of 158 patients by the authors' group validated mpMRI staging as a valuable stand-alone test for predicting organ-confined disease (area under the curve [AUC] 0.88) compared with Partin tables (AUC 0.70).[27]

mpMRI also improves tumor staging with better assessment of the anterior gland, detection of non–organ-confined disease, and estimates of tumor volume. Kongnyuy and colleagues[28] showed the value of mpMRI in detecting anterior lesions classically missed by TRUS biopsy, which in most cases represented the highest-grade tumor in a respective gland (**Fig. 1**). mpMRI also offers a novel way to estimate tumor volume more accurately than conventional staging. Bratan and colleagues[29] examined a cohort of 202 men who underwent mpMRI before prostatectomy and showed that mpMRI volume estimates were most accurate for tumors with the highest Likert suspicion scores and Gleason score greater than or equal to 7.

Multiparametric MR imaging in detecting T3 disease

One of the most important decision points in the management of prostate cancer is the detection of locally advanced (T3) versus organ-confined (T2 or lower) disease. Detection of EPE, seminal vesicle invasion (SVI), and neurovascular bundle involvement not only affects outcome but also can alter the surgical approach. A 2012 prospective study on 104 patients undergoing prostatectomy showed that preoperative mpMRI altered the initial surgical plan with respect to neurovascular bundle sparing 27% of the time, switching to nerve-sparing technique in 17 of 104 patients and to non–nerve-sparing in 11 patients, demonstrating the ability of mpMRI to accurately predict neurovascular bundle involvement prospectively.[30] Similarly, a more recent study of 122 men receiving mpMRI with ERC at 3T showed that management decisions were changed in a risk-dependent manner. In this study, treatment decisions were altered 18% of the time after mpMRI, occurring in 9%, 18%, and 33% of low-risk, intermediate-risk, and high-risk patients, respectively.[31] The data regarding the accuracy of mpMRI for detection of locally advanced disease has been heterogeneous, largely in part due to differences in MR imaging technique (ie, use

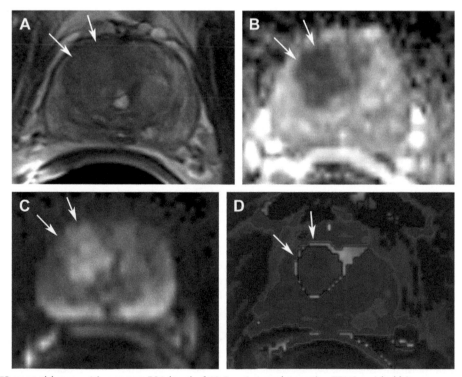

Fig. 1. A 73-year-old man with a serum PSA level of 12.2 ng/mL and negative TRUS-guided biopsy was referred for mpMRI with ERC to assess for prostate cancer due to rising PSA. (*A*) Axial T2WI shows a large region of decreased T2 signal with poorly defined margins in the right anterior midtransition zone (TZ) (*arrows*). This lesion does not demonstrate gross EPE but there is broad-based contact with the anterior fibromuscular stroma and prostate margin. (*B*) Axial apparent diffusion coefficient (ADC) map and (*C*) axial high *b*-value DWIs (*b* = 1400 s/mm²) demonstrate corresponding marked restricted diffusion (*arrows*). (*D*) Colored perfusion map created using post-processing software from dynamic contrast-enhanced MR imaging acquisition demonstrates suspicious perfusion kinetics for prostate cancer (*arrows*), corresponding to the findings seen on T2WI and ADC/DWI. PI-RADS score is 5. The patient underwent radical prostatectomy revealing Gleason 4 + 3 = 7 cancer in right anterior TZ with focal EPE.

of an ERC or varying field strengths) and variable reader experience. A recent meta-analysis of 75 studies, incorporating 9796 patients, reported sensitivities in the high 50% range and specificities in the 90% range for detection of EPE and SVI.[32] Similar results were achieved in a more recent systematic review of 62 studies for the detection of EPE or SVI, although the significant heterogeneity among studies within these analyses potentially limits generalizability.[33]

One of the major hurdles that needs to be addressed as it pertains to mpMRI's role in prostate cancer staging is the great variability between the experienced and nonexperienced prostate MR imaging reader. Although prostate MR imaging has been around for approximately 3 decades, recent advances in research and technology have led to a boom in prostate MR imaging interest, and in turn, a high demand for high-quality mpMRI. There is a substantial learning curve associated with this imaging technique and the lack of experience can lead to some of the discrepancies between dedicated readers who have received training and nonexperienced prostate MR imaging readers. A recent retrospective study of 133 patients at a single community hospital who underwent radical prostatectomy demonstrated sensitivity and specificity for the detection of EPE of 12.5% and 93%, respectively.[34] Similarly, Tay and colleagues[26] showed that the addition of a mpMRI standard read did not significantly improve the detection of EPE over clinical nomograms; however, the addition of a second, subspecialized read improved specificity of organ confined status from 44% to 81%. More recent studies from experienced readers at 3T have demonstrated higher performance for the detection of EPE, with sensitivities and specificities as high as 95% and 100%, respectively.[35–37] A 2014 study by Otto and colleagues[38] showed that mpMRI performed at 3T has an accuracy of 97% and sensitivity/specificity near 100% for the detection of SVI and approximately 80% accuracy for the detection of EPE.

Some of this heterogeneity in reader performance can be mitigated by implementing a standardized reporting system, such as the Prostate Imaging—Reporting and Data System (PI-RADS). This system has proved a helpful tool in standardizing prostate MR imaging interpretations and reducing variability among readers with varying levels of experience. Currently in its second iteration, PI-RADS continues to evolve to facilitate the integration of mpMRI into clinical practice.[39] Another factor that can reduce reader heterogeneity is dedicated training programs. The effect of having a dedicated education program has also been shown to significantly increase the diagnostic accuracy for detection of dominant index cancers, anterior cancers, Gleason grade and reader confidence.[40] To harness the full potential of mpMRI, the continuing need for education is paramount and many additional training resources, in the form of hands-on courses and workshops, among other methods of self-study, are available to those with interest.[41]

Extraprostatic Extension

The International Society of Urological Pathology (ISUP) defines EPE as "the presence of tumor beyond the confines of the prostate."[42] Although a seemingly straightforward definition, EPE can be extremely difficult to diagnose both on mpMRI and on pathologic specimens because the prostate lacks a true "capsule" and determining the border between prostate parenchyma and periprostatic soft tissue is somewhat arbitrary. Pathologically, EPE upstages the tumor to pT3a (EPE or microscopic invasion of the bladder neck) or pT3b (SVI).[5] In comparison to stage pT3b disease, detection of subtle pT3a disease in the form of microscopic invasion/EPE on mpMRI is less reliable, with some reported sensitivities as low as 43% in academic centers and 12.5% in community practice.[34] This is largely due to the fact that SVI occurs in aggressive or advanced-stage tumors whereas less aggressive tumors may only show subtle signs of EPE. For mpMRI to be valuable in staging of disease, it is critical for mpMRI to be able to reliably detect EPE and thereby differentiate non–organ-confined T3 disease from organ-confined disease.

At a 2009 ISUP consensus meeting, the most reliable histologic feature for EPE in the posterior and posterolateral gland is the presence of tumor admixed with periprostatic fat. Diagnosis of EPE in the anterior gland and apex is much more difficult and there is less consensus among pathologists given the lack of periprostatic fat and the fact that prostate stroma blends in with the bladder smooth muscle.[42] Imaging criteria for assessing EPE on mpMRI take advantage of the high anatomic and spatial resolution of T2-weighted MR imaging (T2WI). Detection of EPE on T2WI centers on alterations in morphologic features of the normal prostatic capsule, including asymmetry and contour changes, anatomic narrowing of the rectoprostatic angle, and altered morphology of the neurovascular bundles with loss of surrounding fat planes (**Fig. 2**). Further discussion of the criteria for EPE can be referenced in the latest PI-RADS, Version 2 document.[43] The length of capsular contact on T2WI has recently

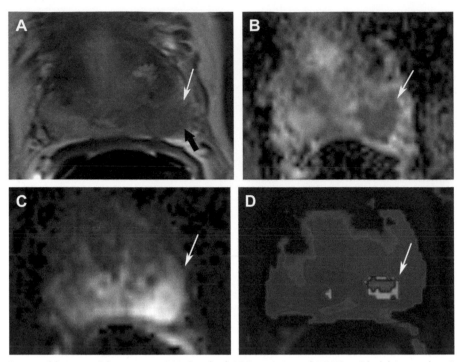

Fig. 2. A 57-year-old man with a serum PSA level of 10.3 ng/mL and TRUS-guided biopsy showing Gleason 4 + 3 = 7 cancer (4/8 cores, 60%–90% each) throughout the left gland. (*A*) Axial T2WI shows a large area of decreased T2 signal intensity in the left base and midlateral peripheral zone (PZ) (*white arrow*). There is associated irregularity and spiculation of the periprostatic fat (*black solid arrow*). (*B*) Axial ADC map and (*C*) axial high *b*-value DWI (b = 1400 s/mm²) demonstrate corresponding marked restricted diffusion (*arrows*). (*D*) Suspicious enhancement kinetics are shown, corresponding to the findings on T2WI and DWI (*arrow*). PI-RADS score is 5 with evidence of gross EPE. The patient underwent radical prostatectomy revealing Gleason 4 + 3 = 7 cancer in the left PZ with EPE at the left base.

been shown one of the most sensitive criteria for detection of EPE with reduced inter-reader variability compared with subjective interpretations using threshold lengths of 10 mm for gross EPE and 6 mm for focal EPE.[44] A similar study showed that tumor contact length (with a threshold value of 12.5 mm) was an independent predictor for EPE (AUC 0.71) (**Fig. 3**).[45]

With regard to EPE detection, a multiparametric MR imaging approach has been shown to increase accuracy. For example, a 2007 study by Bloch and colleagues[46] reported a significant increase in sensitivity (>25%) with an accuracy of 95% for the detection of EPE when using a multiparametric approach compared with T2WI alone. Diffusion-weighted imaging (DWI) has also been shown to be an independent marker for side-specific assessment of EPE with a comparable accuracy to T2WI and better inter-reader agreement and sensitivity for subtle (<2 mm) EPE.[47] More recently, a study of 117 patients by Woo and colleagues[48] demonstrated that DWI adds incremental value in detecting EPE when there is low suspicion on T2WI. Dynamic contrast-enhanced MR imaging

has not been shown as effective in assessing EPE as DWI when combined with T2WI.[49]

Seminal Vesicle Invasion

The detection of SVI on mpMRI is one of the most reliable markers for EPE and easier to diagnose compared with T3a disease given the high spatial resolution of T2WI and aggressive nature of stage T3b tumors. The incidence of SVI in high-risk prostate cancer is relatively low, reported at 7% in some surgical series,[50] but this diagnosis is critical to make on mpMRI because the presence of SVI can preclude surgical intervention in some cases. In general, mpMRI has been shown highly specific for the detection of SVI; however, the data regarding sensitivity of SVI detection are mixed, with some studies reporting sensitivities as low as 44%.[51] A recent meta-analysis by de Rooij and colleagues[32] reported overall sensitivities for SVI of 51% and 59% without and with the use an ERC. Furthermore, they reported increased sensitivity for SVI when using a multiparametric approach compared with T2WI alone, with

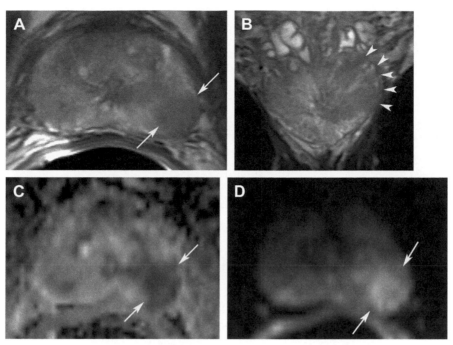

Fig. 3. A 51-year-old man with a serum PSA of 8 ng/nL and TRUS-guided biopsy showing Gleason 4 + 3 = 7 cancer (8/12 cores, 35%–100% each). (*A*) Axial T2WI shows a large area of decreased T2 signal intensity in the left posterolateral peripheral zone at the level of the base to midgland (*arrows*). (*B*) Coronal T2WI shows the large area of decreased T2 signal intensity in the left posterolateral peripheral zone at the level of the base to midgland with broad-based capsular contact (>1 cm) without gross evidence of EPE (*arrowheads*). (*C*) Axial ADC map and (*D*) axial high *b*-value DWI (*b* = 1400 s/mm^2) demonstrate corresponding marked restricted diffusion (*arrows*). PI-RADS score is 5 based on lesion size with no evidence of gross EPE but the presence of broad-based capsular contact is suspicious for microscopic EPE. The patient underwent radical prostatectomy revealing Gleason 3 + 4 = 7 cancer in the left PZ with microscopic EPE in the midgland and base.

sensitivities increasing from 53% to 64%. They also showed that there was no overall significant difference between field strength (1.5T vs 3T); however, sensitivity at 1.5 T was highest with the use of an ERC (62% vs 37%). The reported sensitivity at 3T was higher without the use of an ERC (65% vs 45%), potentially due to the increasing susceptibility effects at higher field strengths. The highest overall sensitivity for SVI detection was found when combing 3T with a multiparametric approach (73% sensitivity and 95% specificity).[32] Criteria for SVI can be found in the latest PI-RADS, Version 2 document and include direct extension of low T2WI signal tumor directly into the seminal vesicles with associated restricted diffusion (**Fig. 4**).[43]

Nodal and Metastatic Staging

The current staging and management algorithms for patients with newly diagnosed prostate cancer are complex, taking into account numerous clinical factors, the T stage, and various nomograms to predict the probability of nodal or distant metastatic disease.[52] Stage N1 disease is defined as involvement of 1 or more regional pelvic nodes, whereas stage M1a is considered involvement of nonregional nodes (ie, common iliac or retroperitoneal nodes). The presence of osseous metastasis denotes stage M1b whereas involvement of other distant sites defines M1c.[5] Nodal staging may be performed with preoperative imaging or at the time of prostatectomy in the form of pelvic lymph node dissection. If performed preoperatively, patients who are high risk (≥T3) or are low risk, with a greater than 10% probability for nodal metastasis based on nomograms, are candidates to undergo pelvic MR imaging or CT to assess for suspicious nodes and receive biopsy if indicated.[52] According to PI-RADS, Version 2, nodes that are enlarged (>8-mm short axis diameter), morphologically abnormal (ie, rounded or spiculated), or hyperenhancing are considered suspicious for metastatic disease.[43] Although the major focus of prostate mpMRI has been on the detection and characterization of disease within and immediately around the prostate, it has been shown that mpMRI may be helpful in the setting

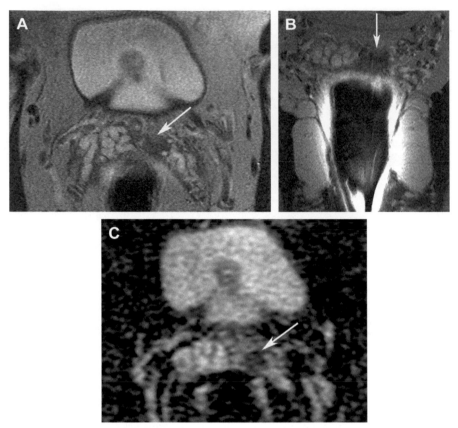

Fig. 4. A 58-year-old man with a serum PSA of 39.1 ng/nL and TRUS-guided biopsy showing Gleason 4 + 3 = 7 throughout the left gland with Gleason 4 + 4 = 8 tumor in the left lateral base. (*A*) Axial and (*B*) coronal T2WIs show a focal region of marked decreased T2 signal in the left seminal vesicles with loss of normal seminal vesicle morphology (*arrows*). (*C*) Axial ADC map demonstrates marked corresponding restricted diffusion at this location (*arrow*). The patient underwent radical prostatectomy revealing Gleason 4 + 3 = 7 cancer in 70% of the gland (left > right) with extensive SVI.

of detection of lymph node involvement as well. For instance, a 2015 study showed a low sensitivity (55%) but a high specificity of mpMRI for nodal metastases (90%) in patients with intermediate or high-risk cancer who underwent preoperative node staging with 3T mpMRI and received subsequent extended pelvic lymph node dissection.[53]

With regard to distant metastatic disease staging, the most common site of disease is the skeleton, specifically, the lumbar spine, pelvis, femoral heads, and ribs. Solid organ metastases, on the other hand, are comparatively rare.[54] The current staging algorithms recommend that high-risk patients receive a bone scan and/or CT of the chest, abdomen, and pelvis to evaluate for distant metastatic disease.[52] Given that the bony pelvis, proximal femurs, and lumbar spine are such frequent sites of osseous metastatic disease and are included in the typical field of view in mpMRI, these findings can be depicted on these

staging mpMRI examinations. Vargas and colleagues[55] recently looked at 3765 patients receiving preoperative mpMRI and showed that although a majority of patients (approximately 70%) had incidental bone lesions, the incidence of osseous metastasis was only 1.5%. Furthermore, there were no cases of bone metastases in any of the low-risk patients. As such, the investigators recommended against expanding standard mpMRI protocols to include larger field of views than currently performed to evaluate for distant sites of osseous metastatic lesions.

IMAGING PITFALLS AND LIMITATIONS OF MULTIPARAMETRIC MR IMAGING STAGING

A variety of imaging pitfalls of mpMRI have been previously described, including normal anatomic structures and benign entities that mimic prostate tumors as well as various technical limitations.[56–58] This topic is discussed in further detail later in this issue; however, it is important to recognize that postbiopsy hemorrhage, susceptibility artifact from hip prostheses, and misinterpretation of the normal periprostatic venous plexus and neurovascular bundles all may lead to overestimation of index tumor size or an incorrect diagnosis of EPE.[56,57] As it pertains to postbiopsy hemorrhage, the presence of blood products may mask underlying tumor, and the "MR imaging exclusion sign" has been described, which aids in detection of tumor in the presence of background hemorrhage.[59]

Although suspicious mpMRI findings improve risk stratification, potential limitations of mpMRI must also be recognized. As it pertains to estimation of tumor volume, Priester and colleagues[60] compared mpMRI visible lesions to whole-mount prostatectomy specimens in 114 men and found that the median tumor had a 13.5-mm maximal extent beyond the MR imaging contour and 80% of cancer volume from matched tumors was outside region of interest boundaries. Le Nobin and colleagues[61] similarly demonstrated MR volumetric underestimation and noted that it was more likely to occur in lesions with an imaging suspicion score greater than or equal to 4 or histologic Gleason score greater than or equal to 7. Truong and colleagues[62] reviewed 22 prostatectomy specimens and found that the architectural variations of Gleason score 4 lesions greater than or equal to 0.5 cm had an impact on MR visibility, specifically that only 5/14 (36%) of Gleason 4 cribriform lesions were seen on mpMRI. Thus, the authors advocate both targeted biopsy of MR suspicious lesions and systematic biopsy of the remaining gland to minimize underdetection, undergrading, or understaging of disease.

It is also important to recognize that the pretest probability of adverse pathology reflected by D'Amico risk has an impact on the predictive utility of mpMRI. Somford and colleagues[63] examined a risk-mixed cohort of 183 men who underwent mpMRI followed by radical prostatectomy and found that the positive predictive value of mpMRI for detecting EPE was highest in high-risk men (88.8%) whereas the negative predictive value was greatest in low-risk men (87.7%).

IMPACT OF MULTIPARAMETRIC MR IMAGING ON CLINICAL DECISION MAKING AND FUTURE DIRECTIONS

In recent years, mpMRI has assumed an increasingly important role in multiple aspects of the initial diagnosis, staging, and management of prostate cancer. As the use of mpMRI expands, communication between the treating physician and interpreting radiologist has become increasingly

important to continually optimize the collaborative process and highlight the most clinically relevant aspects of a particular case. As management of localized prostate cancer has become more nuanced, mpMRI findings have become increasingly useful in initiating and maintaining appropriate men on active surveillance, planning partial gland ablation, and informing surgical decisions. Several recent studies have demonstrated the utility of mpMRI in confirming candidacy for active surveillance, improving biopsy targeting of occult higher-grade disease missed by TRUS biopsy, and follow-up of men on active surveillance.[64–66] mpMRI may also play a central role in the growing practice of partial gland ablation with particular recent growth in focal cryotherapy and high-intensity focused ultrasound.[67,68] For men with higher-risk disease undergoing surgery or radiation therapy, mpMRI improves staging of non–organ-confined disease and may optimize the degree of margin sparing in surgery and modulate radiation therapy.[69,70]

Ultimately, mpMRI provides the highest clinical value when it is used as part of a multidisciplinary collaboration between the treating physician and interpreting radiologist. Distinct clinical scenarios have an impact on both the accuracy of information provided by mpMRI and those areas of the study that require special attention. As the use of mpMRI expands, it is critical that the information that it can provide is used while also continuing to identify and address clinical limitations of mpMRI that are particularly important for men on active surveillance or considering partial gland ablation.

REFERENCES

1. Siegel RL, Miller KD, Jemal A. Cancer statistics, 2016. CA Cancer J Clin 2016;66(1):7–30.
2. Miller KD, Siegel RL, Lin CC, et al. Cancer treatment and survivorship statistics, 2016. CA Cancer J Clin 2016;66(4):271–89.
3. Aizer AA, Gu X, Chen MH, et al. Cost implications and complications of overtreatment of low-risk prostate cancer in the United States. J Natl Compr Canc Netw 2015;13(1):61–8.
4. Lavery HJ, Cooperberg MR. Clinically localized prostate cancer in 2017: a review of comparative effectiveness. Urol Oncol 2017;35(2):40–1.
5. Edge SB, Compton CC. The American Joint Committee on Cancer: the 7th edition of the AJCC cancer staging manual and the future of TNM. Ann Surg Oncol 2010;17(6):1471–4.
6. Buyyounouski MK, Choyke PL, McKenney JK, et al. Prostate cancer - major changes in the American Joint Committee on Cancer eighth edition

cancer staging manual. CA Cancer J Clin 2017; 67(3):245–53.

7. Ross PL, Scardino PT, Kattan MW. A catalog of prostate cancer nomograms. J Urol 2001;165(5):1562–8.

8. Partin AW, Mangold LA, Lamm DM, et al. Contemporary update of prostate cancer staging nomograms (Partin tables) for the new millennium. Urology 2001;58(6):843–8.

9. Eifler JB, Feng Z, Lin BM, et al. An updated prostate cancer staging nomogram (Partin tables) based on cases from 2006 to 2011. BJU Int 2013;111(1):22–9.

10. Cooperberg MR, Pasta DJ, Elkin EP, et al. The University of California, San Francisco Cancer of the Prostate Risk Assessment score: a straightforward and reliable preoperative predictor of disease recurrence after radical prostatectomy. J Urol 2005; 173(6):1938–42.

11. Ohori M, Kattan MW, Koh H, et al. Predicting the presence and side of extracapsular extension: a nomogram for staging prostate cancer. J Urol 2004;171(5):1844–9 [discussion: 1849].

12. Bjurlin MA, Carter HB, Schellhammer P, et al. Optimization of initial prostate biopsy in clinical practice: sampling, labeling and specimen processing. J Urol 2013;189(6):2039–46.

13. Serefoglu EC, Altinova S, Ugras NS, et al. How reliable is 12-core prostate biopsy procedure in the detection of prostate cancer? Can Urol Assoc J 2013;7(5–6):E293–8.

14. Mufarrij P, Sankin A, Godoy G, et al. Pathologic outcomes of candidates for active surveillance undergoing radical prostatectomy. Urology 2010;76(3): 689–92.

15. Zaytoun OM, Stephenson AJ, Fareed K, et al. When serial prostate biopsy is recommended: most cancers detected are clinically insignificant. BJU Int 2012;110(7):987–92.

16. Bjurlin MA, Meng X, Le Nobin J, et al. Optimization of prostate biopsy: the role of magnetic resonance imaging targeted biopsy in detection, localization and risk assessment. J Urol 2014;192(3):648–58.

17. Siddiqui MM, Rais-Bahrami S, Turkbey B, et al. Comparison of MR/ultrasound fusion-guided biopsy with ultrasound-guided biopsy for the diagnosis of prostate cancer. JAMA 2015;313(4):390–7.

18. Radtke JP, Kuru TH, Boxler S, et al. Comparative analysis of transperineal template saturation prostate biopsy versus magnetic resonance imaging targeted biopsy with magnetic resonance imaging-ultrasound fusion guidance. J Urol 2015;193(1): 87–94.

19. Mendhiratta N, Rosenkrantz AB, Meng X, et al. Magnetic resonance imaging-ultrasound fusion targeted prostate biopsy in a consecutive cohort of men with no previous biopsy: reduction of over detection through improved risk stratification. J Urol 2015; 194(6):1601–6.

20. Ahmed HU, El-Shater Bosaily A, Brown LC, et al. Diagnostic accuracy of multi-parametric MRI and TRUS biopsy in prostate cancer (PROMIS): a paired validating confirmatory study. Lancet 2017; 389(10071):815–22.

21. Yin Y, Zhang Q, Zhang H, et al. Molecular signature to risk-stratify prostate cancer of intermediate risk. Clin Cancer Res 2017;23(1):6–8.

22. Gupta RT, Faridi KF, Singh AA, et al. Comparing 3-T multiparametric MRI and the Partin tables to predict organ-confined prostate cancer after radical prostatectomy. Urol Oncol 2014;32(8):1292–9.

23. Vargas HA, Akin O, Afaq A, et al. Magnetic resonance imaging for predicting prostate biopsy findings in patients considered for active surveillance of clinically low risk prostate cancer. J Urol 2012; 188(5):1732–8.

24. Feng TS, Sharif-Afshar AR, Wu J, et al. Multiparametric MRI improves accuracy of clinical nomograms for predicting extracapsular extension of prostate cancer. Urology 2015;86(2):332–7.

25. Morlacco A, Sharma V, Viers BR, et al. The incremental role of magnetic resonance imaging for prostate cancer staging before radical prostatectomy. Eur Urol 2017;71(5):701–4.

26. Tay KJ, Gupta RT, Brown AF, et al. Defining the incremental utility of prostate multiparametric magnetic resonance imaging at standard and specialized read in predicting extracapsular extension of prostate cancer. Eur Urol 2016;70(2):211–3.

27. Gupta RT, Brown AF, Silverman RK, et al. Can Radiologic staging with multiparametric MRI enhance the accuracy of the Partin tables in predicting organ-confined prostate cancer? AJR Am J Roentgenol 2016;207(1):87–95.

28. Kongnyuy M, Sidana A, George AK, et al. The significance of anterior prostate lesions on multiparametric magnetic resonance imaging in African-American men. Urol Oncol 2016;34(6):254.e15-21.

29. Bratan F, Melodelima C, Souchon R, et al. How accurate is multiparametric MR imaging in evaluation of prostate cancer volume? Radiology 2015;275(1): 144–54.

30. McClure TD, Margolis DJ, Reiter RE, et al. Use of MR imaging to determine preservation of the neurovascular bundles at robotic-assisted laparoscopic prostatectomy. Radiology 2012;262(3):874–83.

31. Liauw SL, Kropp LM, Dess RT, et al. Endorectal MRI for risk classification of localized prostate cancer: radiographic findings and influence on treatment decisions. Urol Oncol 2016;34(9):416.e15-21.

32. de Rooij M, Hamoen EH, Witjes JA, et al. Accuracy of magnetic resonance imaging for local staging of prostate cancer: a diagnostic meta-analysis. Eur Urol 2016;70(2):233–45.

33. Salerno J, Finelli A, Morash C, et al. Multiparametric magnetic resonance imaging for pre-treatment local

staging of prostate cancer: a cancer care Ontario clinical practice guideline. Can Urol Assoc J 2016; 10(9–10):E332–9.

34. Davis R, Salmasi A, Koprowski C, et al. Accuracy of multiparametric magnetic resonance imaging for extracapsular extension of prostate cancer in community practice. Clin Genitourin Cancer 2016;14(6): e617–22.

35. Augustin H, Fritz GA, Ehammer T, et al. Accuracy of 3-Tesla magnetic resonance imaging for the staging of prostate cancer in comparison to the Partin tables. Acta Radiol 2009;50(5):562–9.

36. Cerantola Y, Valerio M, Kawkabani Marchini A, et al. Can 3T multiparametric magnetic resonance imaging accurately detect prostate cancer extracapsular extension? Can Urol Assoc J 2013;7(11–12):E699–703.

37. Xylinas E, Yates DR, Renard-Penna R, et al. Role of pelvic phased array magnetic resonance imaging in staging of prostate cancer specifically in patients diagnosed with clinically locally advanced tumours by digital rectal examination. World J Urol 2013; 31(4):881–6.

38. Otto J, Thormer G, Seiwerts M, et al. Value of endorectal magnetic resonance imaging at 3T for the local staging of prostate cancer. Rofo 2014;186(8): 795–802.

39. Rosenkrantz AB, Oto A, Turkbey B, et al. Prostate imaging reporting and data system (PI-RADS), version 2: a critical look. AJR Am J Roentgenol 2016;206(6):1179–83.

40. Garcia-Reyes K, Passoni NM, Palmeri ML, et al. Detection of prostate cancer with multiparametric MRI (mpMRI): effect of dedicated reader education on accuracy and confidence of index and anterior cancer diagnosis. Abdom Imaging 2015;40(1): 134–42.

41. Gupta RT, Spilseth B, Froemming AT. How and why a generation of radiologists must be trained to accurately interpret prostate mpMRI. Abdom Radiol (NY) 2016;41(5):803–4.

42. Magi-Galluzzi C, Evans AJ, Delahunt B, et al. International Society of Urological Pathology (ISUP) consensus conference on handling and staging of radical prostatectomy specimens. Working group 3: extraprostatic extension, lymphovascular invasion and locally advanced disease. Mod Pathol 2011; 24(1):26–38.

43. Weinreb JC, Barentsz JO, Choyke PL, et al. PI-RADS Prostate imaging - reporting and data system: 2015, version 2. Eur Urol 2016;69(1):16–40.

44. Rosenkrantz AB, Shanbhogue AK, Wang A, et al. Length of capsular contact for diagnosing extraprostatic extension on prostate MRI: Assessment at an optimal threshold. J Magn Reson Imaging 2016; 43(4):990–7.

45. Kongnyuy M, Sidana A, George AK, et al. Tumor contact with prostate capsule on magnetic

resonance imaging: a potential biomarker for staging and prognosis. Urol Oncol 2017;35(1). 30.e1–8.

46. Bloch BN, Furman-Haran E, Helbich TH, et al. Prostate cancer: accurate determination of extracapsular extension with high-spatial-resolution dynamic contrast-enhanced and T2-weighted MR imaging–initial results. Radiology 2007;245(1):176–85.

47. Rosenkrantz AB, Chandarana H, Gilet A, et al. Prostate cancer: utility of diffusion-weighted imaging as a marker of side-specific risk of extracapsular extension. J Magn Reson Imaging 2013;38(2):312–9.

48. Woo S, Cho JY, Kim SY, et al. Extracapsular extension in prostate cancer: added value of diffusion-weighted MRI in patients with equivocal findings on T2-weighted imaging. AJR Am J Roentgenol 2015;204(2):W168–75.

49. Tan CH, Wei W, Johnson V, et al. Diffusion-weighted MRI in the detection of prostate cancer: meta-analysis. AJR Am J Roentgenol 2012;199(4):822–9.

50. Meeks JJ, Walker M, Bernstein M, et al. Seminal vesicle involvement at salvage radical prostatectomy. BJU Int 2013;111(8):E342–7.

51. Lee H, Kim CK, Park BK, et al. Accuracy of preoperative multiparametric magnetic resonance imaging for prediction of unfavorable pathology in patients with localized prostate cancer undergoing radical prostatectomy. World J Urol 2017;35(6):929–34.

52. Mohler JL, Armstrong AJ, Bahnson RR, et al. Prostate cancer, version 1.2016. J Natl Compr Canc Netw 2016;14(1):19–30.

53. von Below C, Daouacher G, Wassberg C, et al. Validation of 3 T MRI including diffusion-weighted imaging for nodal staging of newly diagnosed intermediate- and high-risk prostate cancer. Clin Radiol 2016;71(4):328–34.

54. Kundra V, Silverman PM, Matin SF, et al. Imaging in oncology from the University of Texas M. D. Anderson Cancer Center: diagnosis, staging, and surveillance of prostate cancer. AJR Am J Roentgenol 2007;189(4):830–44.

55. Vargas HA, Schor-Bardach R, Long N, et al. Prostate cancer bone metastases on staging prostate MRI: prevalence and clinical features associated with their diagnosis. Abdom Radiol (NY) 2017;42(1): 271–7.

56. Rosenkrantz AB, Taneja SS. Radiologist, be aware: ten pitfalls that confound the interpretation of multiparametric prostate MRI. AJR Am J Roentgenol 2014;202(1):109–20.

57. Panebianco V, Barchetti F, Barentsz J, et al. Pitfalls in interpreting mp-MRI of the prostate: a pictorial review with pathologic correlation. Insights Imaging 2015;6(6):611–30.

58. Kitzing YX, Prando A, Varol C, et al. Benign conditions that mimic prostate carcinoma: MR imaging features with histopathologic correlation. Radiographics 2016;36(1):162–75.

59. Purysko AS, Herts BR. Prostate MRI: the hemorrhage exclusion sign. J Urol 2012;188(5):1946–7.

60. Priester A, Natarajan S, Khoshnoodi P, et al. Magnetic resonance imaging underestimation of prostate cancer geometry: use of patient specific molds to correlate images with whole mount pathology. J Urol 2017;197(2):320–6.

61. Le Nobin J, Rosenkrantz AB, Villers A, et al. Image guided focal therapy for magnetic resonance imaging visible prostate cancer: defining a 3-dimensional treatment margin based on magnetic resonance imaging histology co-registration analysis. J Urol 2015; 194(2):364–70.

62. Truong M, Hollenberg G, Weinberg E, et al. Impact of Gleason subtype on prostate cancer detection using multiparametric Magnetic Resonance Imaging: correlation with final histopathology. J Urol 2017. [Epub ahead of print].

63. Somford DM, Hamoen EH, Futterer JJ, et al. The predictive value of endorectal 3 Tesla multiparametric magnetic resonance imaging for extraprostatic extension in patients with low, intermediate and high risk prostate cancer. J Urol 2013;190(5): 1728–34.

64. Radtke JP, Kuru TH, Bonekamp D, et al. Further reduction of disqualification rates by additional MRI-targeted biopsy with transperineal saturation biopsy compared with standard 12-core systematic biopsies for the selection of prostate cancer patients for active surveillance. Prostate Cancer Prostatic Dis 2016;19(3):283–91.

65. Schoots IG, Petrides N, Giganti F, et al. Magnetic resonance imaging in active surveillance of prostate cancer: a systematic review. Eur Urol 2015;67(4): 627–36.

66. Nassiri N, Margolis DJ, Natarajan S, et al. Targeted biopsy to detect gleason score upgrading during active surveillance for men with low versus intermediate risk prostate cancer. J Urol 2017;197(3 Pt 1): 632–9.

67. Schulman AA, Tay KJ, Robertson CN, et al. High-intensity focused ultrasound for focal therapy: reality or pitfall? Curr Opin Urol 2017;27(2):138–48.

68. Valerio M, Shah TT, Shah P, et al. Magnetic resonance imaging-transrectal ultrasound fusion focal cryotherapy of the prostate: a prospective development study. Urol Oncol 2017;35(4). 150.e1–7.

69. Pullini S, Signor MA, Pancot M, et al. Impact of multiparametric magnetic resonance imaging on risk group assessment of patients with prostate cancer addressed to external beam radiation therapy. Eur J Radiol 2016;85(4):764–70.

70. Radtke JP, Hadaschik BA, Wolf MB, et al. The impact of magnetic resonance imaging on prediction of extraprostatic extension and prostatectomy outcome in patients with low-, intermediate- and high-risk prostate cancer: try to find a standard. J Endourol 2015;29(12):1396–405.

Prostate MR Imaging for Posttreatment Evaluation and Recurrence

Sonia Gaur, BS, Baris Turkbey, MD*

KEYWORDS

- Prostate cancer • Recurrence • mpMRI • Radical prostatectomy • Radiation therapy
- Focal therapy

KEY POINTS

- Multiparametric MR imaging (mpMRI) can help in evaluation of posttreatment changes after diagnosis and treatment of prostate cancer as well as for diagnosis of locally recurrent disease.
- After radical prostatectomy, radiation therapy, or focal therapy, there are certain expected changes in the remaining tissue.
- Many of the mpMRI patterns of recurrent disease are similar to those of primary prostate cancer. In diagnosis of recurrence, however, normal posttreatment changes and possible inflammation must remain considerations in the interpretation of imaging findings.

INTRODUCTION

Prostate cancer (PCa) is the most common solid organ malignancy and second most common cause of cancer-related deaths among men in the United States. Last year, approximately 190,000 men were newly diagnosed with PCa and 26,000 men died of this disease.[1] Increasingly, timely diagnosis of high-grade disease is achieved with use of prostate multiparametric MR imaging (mpMRI), giving patients with localized disease (stages I–III) early options for definitive treatment. Treatment commonly includes radical prostatectomy (RP) or radiation therapy (RT), which can include external-beam RT (EBRT) or brachytherapy. Generally, RP is preferred for younger men with localized tumors and RT is preferred for elder patients or patients who are not ideal surgery candidates.[2] More recently, patients with a certain pattern of disease visualized on mpMRI may also be offered prostate-sparing focal therapy treatment options that utilize laser technology, microwave ablation, cryotherapy, or high-intensity focused ultrasound (HIFU).[3,4] Unfortunately, despite advances in diagnosis and management of PCa, the disease recurs after definitive treatment in up to 40% of patients.[5] Therefore, detection and treatment of recurrent disease has become a relevant focus across multiple disciplines. From an imaging perspective, prostate mpMRI not only can provide insight into primary PCa but also can achieve good anatomic spatial resolution and provide functional data for visualization of recurrent disease.[6]

After treatment, patients are followed closely for biochemical recurrence (BCR), defined based on serum prostate-specific antigen (PSA) criteria specific for each treatment option.[7–9] PSA nadir achieved after each treatment option differs, because in RT and in focal therapy, PSA-

This article was previously published in March 2018 *Radiologic Clinics*, Volume 56, Issue 2.
Disclosure Statement: Authors have nothing to disclose.
Molecular Imaging Program, National Cancer Institute, National Institutes of Health, 10 Center Drive, Building 10, Room B3B85, Bethesda, MD 20814, USA
* Corresponding author.
E-mail address: turkbeyi@mail.nih.gov

Urol Clin N Am 45 (2018) 467–479
https://doi.org/10.1016/j.ucl.2018.03.011
0094-0143/18/Published by Elsevier Inc.

producing prostate parenchyma is not completely eradicated.[9] After RP, PSA nadir of undetectable levels is expected, whereas after RT or focal therapy, a PSA nadir greater than zero is achieved within weeks or months after completion of therapy. Accordingly, in RP patients, recurrence is suspected with an increase in PSA above the threshold greater than or equal to 0.2 ng/mL with a second confirmatory level, whereas in RT patients, an increase in PSA 2.0 ng/mL above the established posttreatment nadir is suspicious.[10] PSA patterns are monitored after focal therapy as well, although consensus about kinetics and a threshold value is still being investigated.[9] In patients who receive definitive therapy, BCR indicates locally recurrent disease in up to two-thirds of patients, and this must be extensively evaluated for appropriate subsequent management.[11–13] Distinction of PSA-producing benign etiologies from local recurrence and distant metastasis is vital. Prostate mpMRI can greatly assist this by aiding visualization of local structures posttreatment, with some considerations.[14–16] This is clinically important because localized recurrence that can be visualized on mpMRI can be offered local salvage treatment, which is drastically different from systemic options offered to patients with distant metastatic disease.

Evaluation and imaging of recurrent disease with mpMRI require certain considerations based on treatment received. Prostate mpMRI's strength lies in combining anatomic data (T1-weighted [T1W] and T2-weighted [T2W] MR imaging) with functional data (diffusion-weighted imaging [DWI] and dynamic contrast-enhanced imaging [DCE]) to provide maximum information about the location and character of possible disease. Established guidelines for characterizing and reporting suspicious areas on prostate mpMRI, such as Prostate Imaging—Reporting and Data System, Version 2, are designed only for characterization of primary cancer.[17] Although baseline pulse sequences (**Box 1**) used are the same for posttreatment evaluation, treatment greatly changes anatomy visualized, can change signal intensity on certain sequences, and can introduce artifact that compromises sequence utility. For example, after RP, a drastically different anatomy is visualized on imaging and image artifact may be introduced with use of surgical clips during the procedure. In contrast, after RT, although the general anatomic structures remain the same, the prostate shrinks greatly in size and has different signal pattern on T2W imaging. The purpose of this article is to discuss general guidelines for identifying normal posttreatment changes and possible recurrence on mpMRI as well as pitfalls

---

Box 1
Pulse sequences used for posttreatment evaluation with multiparametric MR imaging

mpMRI protocol in recurrent PCa work-up

Triplane T2W MR imaging

Diffusion-weighted MR imaging

ADC map

High *b*-value DW MR imaging (>1400) (acquired or calculated)

DCE MR imaging

Pelvic T1W MR imaging

---

of mpMRI interpretation after the various treatments for PCa.

MULTIPARAMETRIC MR IMAGING AFTER RADICAL PROSTATECTOMY

RP is a common active treatment chosen for PCa patients with localized disease, with approximately 40% of patients undergoing definitive therapy choosing this option.[18] RP includes total removal of the prostate and seminal vesicles, along with pelvic lymph node dissection to varying extents for evaluation of local metastasis.[19] Subsequent pathology analysis evaluates surgical margins and lymph nodes for staging. Risk for future BCR is a consideration at this point, because certain characteristics of the original PCa can increase risk of recurrence, such as seminal vesical invasion, positive surgical margins, extraprostatic extension, perineural invasion, lymphovascular invasion, and increased tumor volume.[18] After successful surgery, PSA should drop to undetectable levels within 2 weeks to 3 weeks and patients should be followed with serial serum PSA measurements for early detection of possible BCR. According to the American Urological Association guidelines, BCR after RP is defined as a serum PSA measurement greater than or equal to 0.2 ng/mL, followed by a second confirmatory serum PSA measurement of greater than or equal to 0.2 ng/mL.[7] Post-RP, approximately 35% of patients experience BCR within 10 years, and there are certain parameters that make this recurrence more likely to be found as localized disease.[20–24] These include PSA increase more than 3 years post-RP, PSA doubling time greater than 11 months, original Gleason score less than or equal to 7, and stage less than or equal to pT3a pN0, pTx with negative surgical margins. In contrast, systemic disease can be predicted if PSA increases in less than 1 year post-

RP, PSA doubling time is in 4 months to 6 months, original Gleason score was 8 to 10, and stage pT3b, pTxpN1.[10] Imaging can aid with distinguishing between local and distant metastatic disease, and, if local disease seems likely, mpMRI specifically can play an important subsequent role in evaluation.

After surgery, the male pelvic anatomy is greatly changed, and this is an important consideration when evaluating the area with imaging. Use of mpMRI is ideal for evaluation of the postsurgical bed, because its functional components allow the important differentiation between recurrent cancer, residual prostate tissue, inflammatory tissue, and fibrosis. Presurgical anatomy is relatively consistent between patients—going superior to inferiorly, the bladder neck lies above the prostate base, seminal vesicles appear between the prostate base and bladder neck, and then the prostate is clearly visualized base to apex. Postsurgical anatomy on mpMRI is drastically different due to the open prostatectomy fossa left behind from where the prostate is removed. Imaging should show the bladder neck descended into the prostatectomy fossa with a more conical shape, the vesicourethral anastomosis (VUA) inferior to the bladder neck, and the retrovesical bed posterior to these structures on the sagittal view. Fat stranding may be present around the bladder base on anatomic imaging. In addition to changed anatomy, there are certain expected post-RP signal patterns and artifacts to consider. The VUA should be visualized as a ring of postoperative fibrosis, exhibiting low signal intensity on all sequences of mpMRI. In certain situations, such as if there was extensive hemorrhage at the time of surgery or if there is inflammatory tissue postoperatively, some VUA hyperintense tissue may be seen on T2W imaging. These circumstances are discussed more extensively with other recurrent PCa mimics later. Patterns of fibrosis may differ between patients, based on surgical approach used.[25] If metallic clips were used in the surgery, these can be seen as hyperintense structures on T2W imaging. In up to 20% of cases, seminal vesicles may be left behind in the body, and these can be seen in their presurgical locations with their characteristic tubular structure on T1W or T2W anatomic imaging.[26] They appear as intermediate to high intensity on T2W imaging, may show restricted diffusion on DWI, and often show early enhancement on DCE[27,28] (**Fig. 1**). On postoperative imaging of the wider pelvic field of view, it is possible to see lymphoceles in patients who undergo pelvic lymph node dissection. These form due to the accumulation of lymph from damage to the lymphatic system in the resection.[29]

These are visualized at the locations of former lymph nodes as hyperintense thin-walled cystlike structures on T2Ww imaging and exhibit no enhancement on DCE.

The individual mpMRI sequences vary in utility for post-RP imaging, especially for detection of recurrence. T2W imaging is always used in evaluation postsurgery for anatomy orientation and evaluation of signal patterns. Generally, DWI utility is highly dependent on whether or not surgical clips were used in the surgery. If clips were used, their metallic property introduces susceptibility artifacts to the DWI images, greatly reducing the value of DWI in evaluation.[30] If a patient does not have clips in the postsurgical bed, however, DWI can be useful for distinguishing tumor from mimicking etiologies, such as inflammation or residual benign tissue. Overall, DCE is much more reliable than DWI and has been proved as the most useful sequence for detecting recurrence. If looking at a normal postoperative DCE MR imaging sequence, early enhancement should not be seen in the arterial phase, but there should be some general low-level enhancement of the surgical bed during the venous phase. Changes in early enhancement on DCE MR imaging are very sensitive for being locally recurrent disease.[31]

Locally recurrent PCa in the post-RP patient may occur anywhere in or around the surgical bed but most commonly occurs at the VUA.[19] Recurrence tends to appear nodular and relatively hyperintense in comparison to pelvic muscle signal intensity on T2W imaging.[32] On DCE, these areas readil enhance during the arterial phase with quick washout during the venous phase.[33] This DCE enhancement appears as a focal nodular enhancement that contrasts sharply with the general background low-level venous enhancement at the VUA and has been proved important in the MR imaging evaluation. In 1 study evaluating 46 post-RP BCR patients, Casciani and colleagues[34] found that addition of DCE to T2W for evaluation increased sensitivity from 48% to 88% and increased specificity from 52% to 100%. Cirillo and colleagues[31] reported similar findings with their cohort of 72 post-RP BCR patients, with a sensitivity of 84.1% (compared with 61.4%) and specificity of 89.3% (compared with 82.1%) when DCE was combined with T2W compared with T2W only. Finally, if DWI has not been compromised by use of surgical clips, recurrent disease appears hypointense on the apparent diffusion coefficient (ADC) map and hyperintense on high b-value imaging.[35] Therefore, overall signal patterns are similar to those of in situ primary PCa. Recurrent disease, however, is more difficult to identify due to the changed anatomy

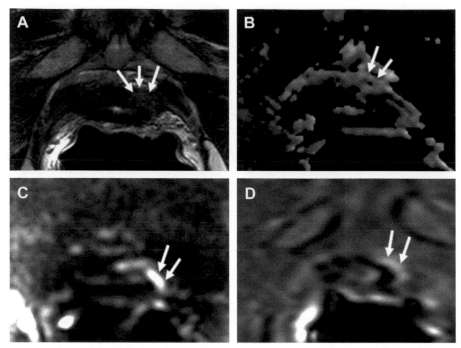

Fig. 1. A 68-year-old man, status post-RP 5 years prior, presenting with PSA = 0.47 ng/mL for mpMRI evaluation. Axial T2W MR imaging (*A*), ADC map (*B*), *b*-2000 DW MR imaging (*C*), and DCE MR imaging (*D*) recurrent lesion (*arrows*). The area suspicious for recurrence appears at the VUA, relatively hyperintense on T2W, corresponding with a hypointense area on the ADC map, hyperintense area on *b*-2000, and early hyperenhancement on DCE MR imaging.

and missing background of normal prostatic tissue. Additionally, unlike in imaging evaluation for primary PCa, DCE serves as the most important sequence in detection.

There are some common mimics and pitfalls that the radiologist should keep in mind when identifying areas suspicious for post-RP recurrent disease. First, there is always a possibility of residual glandular tissue postsurgery, and this is PSA-producing and may mimic recurrent disease on imaging. Residual glandular tissue may take on a nodular appearance on T2W, resembling PCa. The functional data, however, for this area on MR should help differentiate this benign etiology—it should not have any signal abnormality on DWI and should not enhance early in the arterial phase on DCE.[28] PSA kinetics should also help; PSA doubling time for residual benign tissue should be much longer than for recurrent disease.[15] Second, after surgery, it is possible that granulation tissue or hemorrhage is present near the VUA due to the procedure and subsequent natural inflammation. Granulation tissue appears hyperintense on T2W imaging, similar to recurrent tumor, and hyperenhances on an early DCE phase due to hypervascularity. Extensive hemorrhage also hyperenhances early on DCE. These mimics can be best separated from recurrent disease on

DWI, on which they should appear benign with no notable signal abnormalities. Third, the appearance of fibrosis after RP is variable for each patient and may be confused with recurrence. Fibrotic tissue is highly cellular and thus may have restricted diffusion similar to recurrent tumor on DWI sequences.[36] It is also possible that on T2 alone, it may be difficult to distinguish local recurrence from mimicking fibrosis if it occurs in a nodular formation. On T2W and DCE imaging, however, fibrotic tissue should appear as more hypointense than recurrent tumor with a delayed thin layer of enhancement during the venous phase.[19,37]

Various studies have been performed testing the utility of mpMRI in detection of recurrence after prostatectomy. In 84 consecutive post-RP BCR-risk patients, Panebianco and colleagues[38] found that MR imaging had higher diagnostic accuracy (sensitivity 92% and specificity 75%) than the alternative PET/CT modality (sensitivity 62% and specificity 50%) in detection of local recurrence. The same group later verified this with other studies, reporting that mpMRI is the most promising technique for post-RP local recurrence detection.[39] Of all the mpMRI sequences, DCE MR imaging is repeatedly reported as adding exceptional value to detection. In 1 analysis of 80 post-RP patients, different mpMRI combinations were tested for detection value. The combinations of T2W + DCE and T2W + DWI + DCE had significantly higher detection rates (76.5%–82.4%) than T2W alone or T2W + DWI (detection rates 25%–29.4%).[40] This incremental value of DCE is verified in a separate study conducted by Wassberg and colleagues,[41] which showed that detection increases along with inter-reader agreement (58% from 39% agreement) with use of DCE MR imaging. In a different study with 262 high-risk post-RP patients conducted by Panebianco and colleagues,[28] T2W + DCE gave high sensitivity, specificity, and accuracy (98%, 94%, and 93%, respectively). In addition, they found that when DWI is able to be used, it can produce comparable detection in combination with T2W (93% sensitivity, 89% specificity, and 88% accuracy). There is no true consensus, however, on the value of DWI, with other studies reporting T2W + DWI sensitivity as low as 46% to 49%.[30]

In summary, post-RP, there are many considerations when performing local imaging with mpMRI, including changed anatomy, new signal patterns, and abnormalities indicative of recurrent disease. DCE MR imaging provides significantly more value in detection of recurrent disease compared with primary tumors, and optimal imaging may be achieved with use of all 3 sequences. Caution should be used, with radiologists remaining vigilant for disease that is difficult to identify against a reduced prostate background while also keeping common mimics and pitfalls in mind.

MULTIPARAMETRIC MR IMAGING AFTER RADIATION THERAPY

The second most common definitive treatment chosen for stages I to III PCa is RT, given to up to 40% of patients over 65 years old and up to 25% of patients under 65 years old.[42] RT can be offered as EBRT or brachytherapy. EBRT is generally used for earlier-stage disease and may be offered in forms, such as intensity-modulated RT or stereotactic body RT. In this approach, all radiation is delivered externally and focused through beams to the prostate. In contrast, brachytherapy uses radioactive pellets that are implanted into the prostate. The seeds internally give off radiation to treat the prostate, and this is best used for low-grade disease and in smaller prostates. For higher-grade disease, brachytherapy may be combined with EBRT for improved cancer treatment.[43] All RT may be combined with hormonal therapy in an effort to shrink the prostate for maximal treatment efficacy.[11] The method of radiation delivery and the incorporation of hormones in treatment are important considerations for posttreatment imaging.

After RT, PSA nadir is not achieved as quickly because it is post-RP, and the decrement is more variable. Generally, patients take approximately 18 months to reach PSA nadir but may even take up to 3 years.[44–46] Establishment of PSA nadir may be further complicated by an observed PSA bounce that can occur at 9 months to 21 months that lasts for several months and is eventually followed by PSA decrease to nadir.[46–49] Once nadir is established, the patient should be followed with serial serum PSA immunoassays. The American Society for Therapeutic Radiology and Oncology (ASTRO) defines post-RP BCR using the Phoenix criteria, defined as 2 successive measurements showing a rise in serum PSA of at least 2 ng/mL above the nadir.[8] In patients with high-risk disease, up to approximately 30% can have BCR post-RT, and risk factors include higher initial clinical tumor stage, higher pretreatment Gleason score, and a shorter time interval from the end of radiotherapy until the detection of BCR.[50,51] After BCR is first detected, median times to distant metastasis and PCa-specific mortality are 5 years and 10 years, respectively.[52] Unfortunately, when attempting to determine if BCR initially represents localized or metastatic disease, RT has less established risk factors compared with RP. Generally, it has been shown that faster PSA kinetics are associated with more adverse disease; higher initial clinical tumor stage has a worse BCR prognosis; and, if PSA doubles in less than 8 months, especially in the first year after treatment, this can be a predictor for metastatic disease.[13] A majority of post-RT recurrences have been shown to be local, with top site of recurrence the prostate; therefore, evaluation with prostate mpMRI is essential in the follow-up of BCR.[52,53]

If localized disease is present in an RT patient, it most commonly occurs at the site of original tumor. Therefore, a baseline mpMRI study showing the primary tumor site can be helpful for subsequent posttreatment evaluation.[32] Expected posttreatment changes of the prostate on imaging are different based on the mode of radiation delivery used.

Multiparametric MR Imaging After External-Beam Radiation Therapy

EBRT causes overall changes in signal intensity and structure of the prostate. The irradiated prostate appears smaller as a result of gland atrophy and differentiation of the zones is made difficult by effacement of the prostatic tissue.[54] The entire prostate appears hypointense on T2W imaging, further complicating differentiation between zones as well as distinction between benign versus tumor tissue.[55] DWI and DCE appearance of the prostate is impacted as well; postradiation gland fibrosis is less cellular and has diminished vascularity compared with pretreatment prostate tissue. Changes on DWI and DCE, however, are not as drastic as on T2W, and the functional sequences are best for detecting locally recurrent disease.

On anatomic T2 imaging, structures surrounding the prostate appear different as well compared with their pretreatment appearance. Seminal vesicles appear shrunken from effects of radiation and all the muscles appear relatively hyperintense compared with pretreatment.[55,56] Bone marrow visualized around the pelvis are hypointense on T2W imaging as a result of fatty replacement of the bone marrow from the effect of radiation.

Identification of post-EBRT local recurrence is made difficult by the glandular changes that occur from treatment. On T2W imaging, recurrence appears as a nodular structure that often exhibits a capsular bulge. The nodular structure is relatively hypointense compared with normal prostatic tissue and may appear as a bulge due to the rapid growth of tumor relative to the atrophic gland.[35] Recurrence most commonly appears at the original site of the primary tumor, with only 4% to 9% of local recurrent disease appearing elsewhere.[57,58] Unfortunately, due to the changed background signal within the prostate, T2W imaging has marked limitations and is not most important for posttreatment evaluation or recurrence detection. In 1 study with 64 patients with post-EBRT recurrence suspicion, Westphalen and colleagues[59] found an area under the curve (AUC) of only 67%

in correct detection of recurrent disease on T2 alone. This was verified by another study, conducted by Sala and colleagues,[60] analyzing a cohort of 45 patients with BCR post-EBRT. They found that sensitivity for T2W alone ranged from 36% to 75%, and specificity ranged from 65% to 81%. Because T2W seems limited as an independent sequence, the functional sequences of mpMRI play a more dominant role in detection of post-RT recurrence. On DWI, signal characteristics of post-RT recurrence are similar to characteristics of primary PCa, with a focal hypointensity on the ADC map and hyperintensity on high b-value imaging corresponding with a nodular area visualized on T2W imaging. Studies analyzing the utility of DWI combined with T2W compared with T2W alone show great promise for the utility of DWI in post-RT imaging. In 1 study of a cohort of 36 patients with post-RT BCR, T2W + DWI achieved significantly higher AUC compared with T2W alone, at 88% versus 61%.[61] In another study analyzing 16 post-EBRT patients, Hara and colleagues[62] found that patient-based sensitivity and specificity for DWI were 100%, with region-based accuracy of 89%. DCE has been proved important in post-EBRT evaluation as well. Although the vascularity of the overall irradiated prostate decreases with gland atrophy, recurrent tumors retain their highly vascular network.[63,64] Recurrence shows early hyperenhancement on DCE MR imaging relative to the treated prostate, and this is especially powerful if it can be correlated with abnormality on T2 or DWI[65] (**Fig. 2**). In 1 study of 33 post-EBRT patients conducted by Haider and

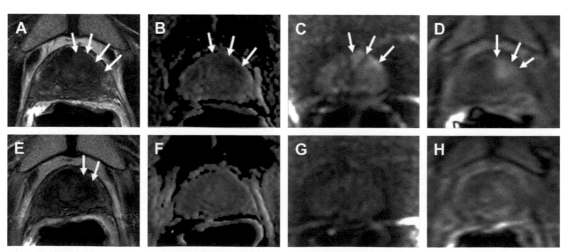

Fig. 2. A 55-year-old man, status post–EBRT, presenting with pretreatment PSA = 7.96 ng/mL. Axial T2W (*A*), ADC map (*B*), *b*-2000 DW MR imaging (*C*), and DCE MR imaging (*D*) show the original tumor in the left midanterior transition zone (*arrows*). On 1 year posttreatment follow-up, patient presented with PSA = 0.76 ng/mL. Posttreatment axial T2W MR imaging (*E*), ADC map (*F*), *b*-2000 DW MR imaging (*G*), and DCE MR imaging (*H*) show the prostate decreased in size and overall gland intensity changes. The tumor (*arrows*) is smaller and appears less concerning with indistinct DWI signal intensity and no focal enhancement on DCE MR imaging.

colleagues,[66] significantly higher sensitivity (72% vs 38%), positive predictive value (49% vs 24%), and negative predictive value (95% vs 88%) were found for DCE compared with T2W imaging. Finally, Kim and colleagues[67] tested utility of both functional sequences and found that DWI and DCE are both important for detection of recurrent disease. In their cohort of 24 patients, DWI + DCE was able to achieve significantly higher AUC (86%) than T2W, DWI, or DCE alone (P<.05).

Multiparametric MR Imaging After Brachytherapy

Posttreatment changes to the prostate gland are similar in brachytherapy to EBRT, however, with the addition of visualization of the radioactive seeds used. Brachytherapy seeds are radioactive material contained in small nonradioactive metallic capsules. These metallic capsules introduce magnetic resonance (MR) susceptibility artifacts, which can distort DWI the most and make interpretation difficult. On T2W imaging, the brachytherapy seeds appear as small hypointense ellipsoid structures scattered throughout the prostate gland. The gland itself is hypointense compared with pretreatment imaging, and, as seen in post-EBRT imaging, zonal and tissue differentiation are made difficult by the signal change. As a patient completes a brachytherapy course, the prostate gland becomes progressively more atrophic and the seeds gradually migrate peripherally within the gland as it shrinks in size.

Fortunately, recurrence is less of a concern after brachytherapy than it is after EBRT, due to a majority of the patients having very-low-risk primary disease. If BCR is detected and local recurrence is present, the recurrence appears as a hypointense nodule on T2W imaging that shows rapid hyperenhancement on DCE MR imaging. If DWI is not too limited, recurrent tumor appears hypointense on the ADC map and hyperintense on high b-value imaging. Just as with EBRT, T2W interpretation should be performed with caution due to the changed glandular background. The general signal properties remain the same between EBRT and brachytherapy; however, fewer studies have been performed to support the use of mpMRI postbrachytherapy, likely because BCR rates are so low. It is suggested that DCE is more important postbrachytherapy than it is post-EBRT due to the seed artifact on DWI.[37] Similar to EBRT, however, the most common site of recurrence postbrachytherapy is at the location of the original tumor.

Thus far, the traditional low-dose rate (LDR) brachytherapy has been described, but a new form of brachytherapy is offered in temporary

high-dose rate (HDR) form. The advantage of HDR is that the source dwell time and position can be modulated, allowing more exact dosimetry.[68] Post-brachytherapy imaging differs with HDR, because the seeds are removed, so the quality does not suffer from susceptibility artifacts. Because HDR is so new and BCR postbrachytherapy occurs less frequently, data validating the use of mpMRI post-HDR are limited. In a study of 16 HDR patients conducted by Tamada and colleagues,[69] DWI shows high sensitivity for detection of recurrence and remains noncompromised with the removal of seeds, and DCE shows early hyperenhancement in recurrent disease. T2W sensitivity is limited due to the limitation of gland background (Fig. 3).

Many of the pitfalls encountered when performing post-RT imaging overlap with usual pitfalls encountered in mpMRI evaluation for primary tumor detection.[70] False-positive results seen on the mpMRI sequences often correspond with prostatitis, hemorrhage, dysplasia, or benign prostatic hyperplasia, even in the irradiated prostate.[71] Specific to post-RT imaging, however, a focal hypointensity on T2 may actually be treated tumor. Mimics like this are most unclear if there is no pretreatment imaging available. Finally, it is important to make note of whether a patient received hormonal therapy in conjunction with RT. Hormonal therapy can cause additional changes to the gland, which can make interpretation even more difficult. Post–androgen deprivation, the prostate shrinks in size, overall ADC values significantly increase, and gland vascularity decreases.[72,73]

In summary, post-RT, there are various factors to consider in local imaging evaluation. If a patient is post-EBRT, overall gland changes must be accounted for. Similar changes must be accounted for in postbrachytherapy patients, with the addition of imaging artifact from the brachytherapy seeds used. Generally, the functional sequences of mpMRI remain best for detecting local disease post-RT.

MULTIPARAMETRIC MR IMAGING AFTER FOCAL THERAPY

Focal therapy is a newly emerging treatment option for patients with localized PCa that falls within a certain criteria that allows the index tumor to be directly targeted. Focal therapy relies on use of various energies for local destruction of cancer cells in the gland, such as microwave, focal laser ablation (FLA), cryotherapy, and HIFU. Regardless of which energy is used, there are numerous posttreatment changes seen on follow-up MR imaging that are important to consider for success of treatment as well as for

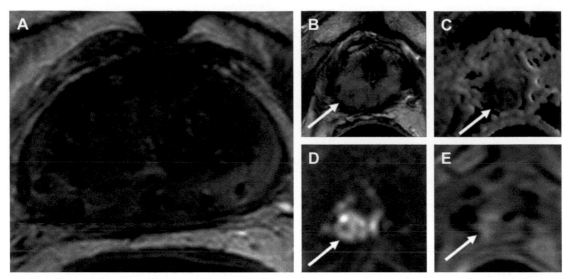

Fig. 3. A 77-year-old man, status post-LDR brachytherapy 8 years ago for Gleason 4 + 4 PCa, presenting with PSA = 11.97 ng/mL. He underwent endorectal coil 3T MR imaging after treatment, and then 8 years later for recurrence suspicion. Axial T2W image shows normal posttreatment changes of the gland, with brachytherapy seeds visible as hypointense structures and the background of the gland hypointense with zonal differentiation made difficult (*A*). Axial T2W (*B*), ADC map (*C*), *b*-2000 DW MR imaging (*D*), and DCE MR imaging (*E*) at distal apex of the prostate shows the recurrent lesion (*arrows*).

evaluation of possible recurrence. After a patient receives focal therapy, a good treatment response is defined as a negative control biopsy, absence of a persistent lesion on posttreatment imaging, and a decrease in PSA of at least 50%.[9] Focal therapy is still greatly in its investigative stages and seems to demonstrate reasonable efficacy. PSA, however, is not very reliable in postfocal therapy follow-up because there is preservation of a large amount of prostate tissue postablation and thus no agreement on a definition for BCR.[4] The consensus is that postablation PSA surveillance should be judged based on PSA kinetics. Many institutions use the Phoenix or ASTRO (increase in 3 successive PSA measurements) criteria for monitoring BCR after focal therapy, but these were both designed for surveillance of whole-gland disease.[74–78] Therefore, an integrated approach, incorporating mpMRI for imaging surveillance, has been recommended for postfocal therapy follow-up.[9]

In postfocal therapy follow-up, it is important to establish posttreatment changes very soon after the energy is applied to the prostate and to pay attention to the PSA nadir that is established after treatment. In 2014, attempt at standardization of postfocal therapy follow-up was made using the Delphi consensus method, by Muller and colleagues.[79] Right after treatment, it is prudent to establish a baseline with regular follow-up: a post-ablation control biopsy that includes targeting of the treated area should be performed, and

follow-up should be done with mpMRI for a minimum of 5 years (**Fig. 4**). mpMRI should include the standard sequences T1W, T2W, DWI (ADC map and high *b*-value >1000), and DCE, optimized at 3T with endorectal coil. It is also suggested by some that an mpMRI be obtained within 2 days to 7 days after treatment to capture early posttreatment findings.[80] Generally, the appearance that focal therapy has on mpMRI can make it difficult to assess for recurrence, because the changes that the therapy induces in the prostatic architecture overlap greatly with tumor appearance.[32]

Posttreatment appearance of the prostate varies somewhat based on energy used in the therapy. Cryotherapy alternates freeze-thaw cycles, producing coagulative necrosis within the prostate gland. The visualized area affected by the cycles is often larger than the actual area of cells killed, and imaging can underestimate true effect of the cryotherapy. The treatment area shows drastically changed architecture and hypointensity on T2.[81] HIFU, which uses focused ultrasound for heating, shows similar heterogenous hypointensity on T2 but may also show DCE perfusion at the periphery of the treatment area.[81,82] Finally, FLA shows the heterogenous T2 hypointensity along with restricted diffusion on DWI.[6] Generally, all treatments eventually result in atrophy of the treated area, causing decreased T2 signal, lower signal on DWI, and lower perfusion on DCE[35] (**Fig. 5**).

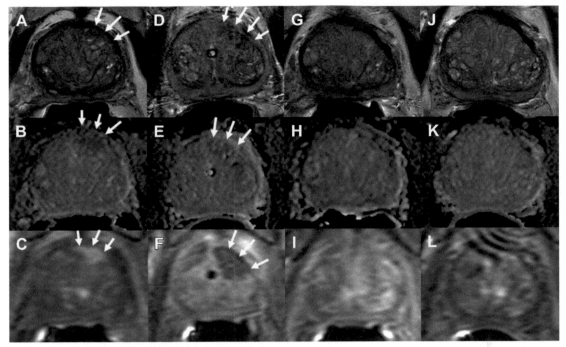

Fig. 4. A 74-year-old man, initially presenting with PSA = 7.33 ng/mL. Axial T2W (*A*), ADC map (*B*), and DCE MR imaging (*C*) show the site of original tumor in the left mid anterior transition zone (*arrows*), found positive for Gleason 3 + 4 PCa on targeted biopsy. The patient was offered FLA, and 1 day posttreatment axial T2W (*D*) shows a hypointensity within the treated area (*arrows*) with some focal changes in prostatic architecture, ADC map (*E*) shows corresponding restricted diffusion in the treated area (*arrows*), and DCE MR imaging (*F*) shows low perfusion of this region (*arrows*). On follow-up 1 year later, patient presented with PSA = 2.59 ng/mL and axial T2W (*G*), ADC map (*H*), and DCE MR imaging (*I*) show shrinkage of the original tumor area with less distinct findings on all sequences. Targeted biopsy of the treated area was negative for disease. At 2-year posttreatment follow-up, patient presented with PSA = 5.58 ng/mL with axial T2W (*J*), ADC map (*K*), and DCE MR imaging (*L*) showing overall slightly changed architecture in the left midanterior transition zone compared with baseline but no signal findings indicative of disease. A 2-year follow-up targeted biopsy of the treated area was negative for disease.

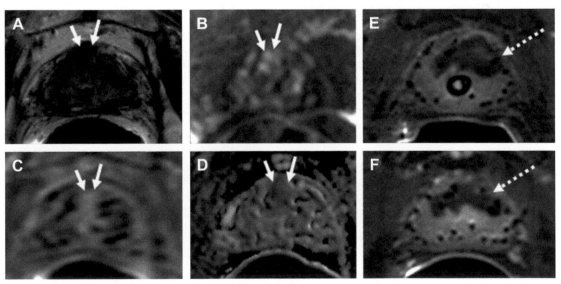

Fig. 5. A 62-year-old man, status post–LDR brachytherapy presenting with PSA = 1.98 ng/mL. Axial T2W (*A*), b2000 DW MR imaging (*B*), DCE MR imaging (*C*), and ADC map (*D*) show recurrent lesion in the midline anterior transition zone (*arrows*). This area was subsequently biopsied and came back positive for PCa. After diagnosis of postbrachytherapy focal recurrence, patient was offered FLA. The 1-day postablation DWI image is shown (*E*), with the treatment area (*dotted arrows*) shrinking in size 1 year postablation, as shown in (*F*). Postablation, biopsy of the area was benign, and PSA = 0.21 ng/mL.

Most focal therapy methods do not have long follow-up times reported, but there are some data about recurrent disease in current studies. Postcryotherapy, 20% to 40% of treated patients have can have BCR, reported up to 10 years from treatment.[83,84] For post-HIFU follow-up, a 160-patient study conducted by Mearini and colleagues[85] found that BCR-free rate in 72 months was 70% for low-risk disease and 41% for intermediate-risk disease. Finally, in a phase II study of FLA in 27 patients, Eggener and colleagues[86] found cancer in 10 patients at 12-month follow-up, with 27% tumors found in the ablation zone and 73% found outside the ablation zone. Appearance of recurrence itself after all treatments takes on signal properties similar to primary disease. Recurrence may be most difficult to differentiate from normal posttreatment on T2, however, making the functional sequences more important for identification.[35]

SUMMARY

Prostate mpMRI offers promising potential for visualization of posttreatment changes and for evaluation of local recurrent disease in the context of BCR. Because the mpMRI evaluation is so important in detection of localized recurrence, it is vital that radiologists be communicative with the multidisciplinary team. The referring urologist, radiation oncologist, or medical oncologist should be aware that the radiologist will be acquiring and interpreting a dedicated MR imaging for posttreatment follow-up and recurrence detection. Therefore, referring physicians should provide all the information that they can about a patient, including entire PCa history, PSA measurements, past treatments, and any past imaging (**Box 2**). Referring physicians should also advise their patients that for optimal imaging, they will receive a full mpMRI with endorectal coil, acquired at 3T with contrast injection.

Box 2
What the referring physician needs to know for local imaging evaluation after treatment of prostate cancer

- This is a dedicated high-resolution MR imaging for posttreatment follow-up
- Essential to provide
  - Complete PCa history
  - PSA measurements
  - All past treatments
  - Any past imaging

Radiologists can make an important difference in the care of a posttreatment PCa patient. They should be comfortable not only with interpretation of mpMRI for detection of primary PCa but also with the evaluation of posttreatment local imaging. Diagnosis and timely treatment of recurrent PCa are vital because care of primary cancer improves and course of disease is followed more closely. In cases of a rising PSA, it is important for any radiologist reading prostate images to be familiar with treatment types, with posttreatment anatomy, with appearance of recurrent disease, and with common pitfalls.

REFERENCES

1. Siegel RL, Miller KD, Jemal A. Cancer statistics, 2016. CA Cancer J Clin 2016;66(1):7–30.
2. Lu-Yao GL, Yao SL. Population-based study of long-term survival in patients with clinically localised prostate cancer. Lancet 1997;349(9056):906–10.
3. Trewartha D, Carter K. Advances in prostate cancer treatment. Nat Rev Drug Discov 2013;12(11):823–4.
4. Bozzini G, Colin P, Nevoux P, et al. Focal therapy of prostate cancer: energies and procedures. Urol Oncol 2013;31(2):155–67.
5. Babaian RJ, Troncoso P, Bhadkamkar VA, et al. Analysis of clinicopathologic factors predicting outcome after radical prostatectomy. Cancer 2001;91(8):1414–22.
6. Mertan FV, Greer MD, Borofsky S, et al. Multiparametric magnetic resonance imaging of recurrent prostate cancer. Top Magn Reson Imaging 2016;25(3):139–47.
7. Stephenson AJ, Kattan MW, Eastham JA, et al. Defining biochemical recurrence of prostate cancer after radical prostatectomy: a proposal for a standardized definition. J Clin Oncol 2006;24(24):3973–8.
8. Roach M 3rd, Hanks G, Thames H Jr, et al. Defining biochemical failure following radiotherapy with or without hormonal therapy in men with clinically localized prostate cancer: recommendations of the RTOG-ASTRO Phoenix consensus conference. Int J Radiat Oncol Biol Phys 2006;65(4):965–74.
9. Barret E, Harvey-Bryan KA, Sanchez-Salas R, et al. How to diagnose and treat focal therapy failure and recurrence? Curr Opin Urol 2014;24(3):241–6.
10. Heidenreich A, Bastian PJ, Bellmunt J, et al. EAU guidelines on prostate cancer. Part II: treatment of advanced, relapsing, and castration-resistant prostate cancer. Eur Urol 2014;65(2):467–79.
11. Bolla M, Van Tienhoven G, Warde P, et al. External irradiation with or without long-term androgen suppression for prostate cancer with high metastatic risk: 10-year results of an EORTC randomised study. Lancet Oncol 2010;11(11):1066–73.

12. Siegel R, Ward E, Brawley O, et al. Cancer statistics, 2011: the impact of eliminating socioeconomic and racial disparities on premature cancer deaths. CA Cancer J Clin 2011;61(4):212–36.

13. Zagars GK, Pollack A. Kinetics of serum prostate-specific antigen after external beam radiation for clinically localized prostate cancer. Radiother Oncol 1997;44(3):213–21.

14. Panebianco V, Barchetti F, Sciarra A, et al. Multiparametric magnetic resonance imaging vs. standard care in men being evaluated for prostate cancer: a randomized study. Urol Oncol 2015;33(1):17.e1-e7.

15. Notley M, Yu J, Fulcher AS, et al. Pictorial review. Diagnosis of recurrent prostate cancer and its mimics at multiparametric prostate MRI. Br J Radiol 2015;88(1054):20150362.

16. Abd-Alazeez M, Ramachandran N, Dikaios N, et al. Multiparametric MRI for detection of radiorecurrent prostate cancer: added value of apparent diffusion coefficient maps and dynamic contrast-enhanced images. Prostate Cancer Prostatic Dis 2015;18(2):128–36.

17. Weinreb JC, Barentsz JO, Choyke PL, et al. PI-RADS prostate imaging - reporting and data system: 2015, version 2. Eur Urol 2016;69(1):16–40.

18. Adamis S, Varkarakis IM. Defining prostate cancer risk after radical prostatectomy. Eur J Surg Oncol 2014;40(5):496–504.

19. Lopes Dias J, Lucas R, Magalhaes Pina J, et al. Post-treated prostate cancer: normal findings and signs of local relapse on multiparametric magnetic resonance imaging. Abdom Imaging 2015;40(7):2814–38.

20. Freedland SJ, Humphreys EB, Mangold LA, et al. Risk of prostate cancer-specific mortality following biochemical recurrence after radical prostatectomy. JAMA 2005;294(4):433–9.

21. Han M, Partin AW, Pound CR, et al. Long-term biochemical disease-free and cancer-specific survival following anatomic radical retropubic prostatectomy. The 15-year Johns Hopkins experience. Urol Clin North Am 2001;28(3):555–65.

22. Roehl KA, Han M, Ramos CG, et al. Cancer progression and survival rates following anatomical radical retropubic prostatectomy in 3,478 consecutive patients: long-term results. J Urol 2004;172(3):910–4.

23. Hull GW, Rabbani F, Abbas F, et al. Cancer control with radical prostatectomy alone in 1,000 consecutive patients. J Urol 2002;167(2 Pt 1):528–34.

24. Amling CL, Blute ML, Bergstralh EJ, et al. Long-term hazard of progression after radical prostatectomy for clinically localized prostate cancer: continued risk of biochemical failure after 5 years. J Urol 2000;164(1):101–5.

25. Allen SD, Thompson A, Sohaib SA. The normal post-surgical anatomy of the male pelvis following radical prostatectomy as assessed by magnetic resonance imaging. Eur Radiol 2008;18(6):1281–91.

26. Sella T, Schwartz LH, Hricak H. Retained seminal vesicles after radical prostatectomy: frequency, MRI characteristics, and clinical relevance. AJR Am J Roentgenol 2006;186(2):539–46.

27. Vargas HA, Wassberg C, Akin O, et al. MR imaging of treated prostate cancer. Radiology 2012;262(1):26–42.

28. Panebianco V, Barchetti F, Sciarra A, et al. Prostate cancer recurrence after radical prostatectomy: the role of 3-T diffusion imaging in multi-parametric magnetic resonance imaging. Eur Radiol 2013;23(6):1745–52.

29. Keskin MS, Argun OB, Obek C, et al. The incidence and sequela of lymphocele formation after robot-assisted extended pelvic lymph node dissection. BJU Int 2016;118(1):127–31.

30. Cha D, Kim CK, Park SY, et al. Evaluation of suspected soft tissue lesion in the prostate bed after radical prostatectomy using 3T multiparametric magnetic resonance imaging. Magn Reson Imaging 2015;33(4):407–12.

31. Cirillo S, Petracchini M, Scotti L, et al. Endorectal magnetic resonance imaging at 1.5 Tesla to assess local recurrence following radical prostatectomy using T2-weighted and contrast-enhanced imaging. Eur Radiol 2009;19(3):761–9.

32. Grant K, Lindenberg ML, Shebel H, et al. Functional and molecular imaging of localized and recurrent prostate cancer. Eur J Nucl Med Mol Imaging 2013;40(Suppl 1):S48–59.

33. Sella T, Schwartz LH, Swindle PW, et al. Suspected local recurrence after radical prostatectomy: endorectal coil MR imaging. Radiology 2004;231(2):379–85.

34. Casciani E, Polettini E, Carmenini E, et al. Endorectal and dynamic contrast-enhanced MRI for detection of local recurrence after radical prostatectomy. AJR Am J Roentgenol 2008;190(5):1187–92.

35. McCammack KC, Raman SS, Margolis DJ. Imaging of local recurrence in prostate cancer. Future Oncol 2016;12(21):2401–15.

36. De Visschere PJ, De Meerleer GO, Futterer JJ, et al. Role of MRI in follow-up after focal therapy for prostate carcinoma. AJR Am J Roentgenol 2010;194(6):1427–33.

37. Rouviere O, Vitry T, Lyonnet D. Imaging of prostate cancer local recurrences: why and how? Eur Radiol 2010;20(5):1254–66.

38. Panebianco V, Sciarra A, Lisi D, et al. Prostate cancer: 1HMRS-DCEMR at 3T versus [(18)F]choline PET/CT in the detection of local prostate cancer recurrence in men with biochemical progression after radical retropubic prostatectomy (RRP). Eur J Radiol 2012;81(4):700–8.

39. Alfarone A, Panebianco V, Schillaci O, et al. Comparative analysis of multiparametric magnetic resonance and PET-CT in the management of local recurrence after radical prostatectomy for prostate cancer. Crit Rev Oncol Hematol 2012;84(1):109–21.

40. Kitajima K, Hartman RP, Froemming AT, et al. Detection of local recurrence of prostate cancer after radical prostatectomy using endorectal coil MRI at 3 T: addition of DWI and dynamic contrast enhancement to T2-Weighted MRI. AJR Am J Roentgenol 2015;205(4):807–16.

41. Wassberg C, Akin O, Vargas HA, et al. The incremental value of contrast-enhanced MRI in the detection of biopsy-proven local recurrence of prostate cancer after radical prostatectomy: effect of reader experience. AJR Am J Roentgenol 2012;199(2):360–6.

42. Siegel R, DeSantis C, Virgo K, et al. Cancer treatment and survivorship statistics, 2012. CA Cancer J Clin 2012;62(4):220–41.

43. Moon DH, Efstathiou JA, Chen RC. What is the best way to radiate the prostate in 2016? Urol Oncol 2017;35(2):59–68.

44. Kuban DA, Thames HD, Levy LB, et al. Long-term multi-institutional analysis of stage T1-T2 prostate cancer treated with radiotherapy in the PSA era. Int J Radiat Oncol Biol Phys 2003;57(4):915–28.

45. Shipley WU, Thames HD, Sandler HM, et al. Radiation therapy for clinically localized prostate cancer: a multi-institutional pooled analysis. JAMA 1999; 281(17):1598–604.

46. Pickles T, British Columbia Cancer Agency Prostate Cohort Outcomes Initiative. Prostate-specific antigen (PSA) bounce and other fluctuations: which biochemical relapse definition is least prone to PSA false calls? An analysis of 2030 men treated for prostate cancer with external beam or brachytherapy with or without adjuvant androgen deprivation therapy. Int J Radiat Oncol Biol Phys 2006; 64(5):1355–9.

47. Kim DN, Straka C, Cho LC, et al. Early and multiple PSA bounces can occur following high-dose prostate stereotactic body radiation therapy: subset analysis of a phase 1/2 trial. Pract Radiat Oncol 2017;7(1):e43–9.

48. Horwitz EM, Levy LB, Thames HD, et al. Biochemical and clinical significance of the posttreatment prostate-specific antigen bounce for prostate cancer patients treated with external beam radiation therapy alone: a multiinstitutional pooled analysis. Cancer 2006;107(7):1496–502.

49. Caloglu M, Ciezki JP, Reddy CA, et al. PSA bounce and biochemical failure after brachytherapy for prostate cancer: a study of 820 patients with a minimum of 3 years of follow-up. Int J Radiat Oncol Biol Phys 2011;80(3):735–41.

50. Rosenbaum E, Partin A, Eisenberger MA. Biochemical relapse after primary treatment for prostate cancer: studies on natural history and therapeutic considerations. J Natl Compr Canc Netw 2004; 2(3):249–56.

51. Spratt DE, Pei X, Yamada J, et al. Long-term survival and toxicity in patients treated with high-dose intensity modulated radiation therapy for localized prostate cancer. Int J Radiat Oncol Biol Phys 2013; 85(3):686–92.

52. Zumsteg ZS, Spratt DE, Romesser PB, et al. The natural history and predictors of outcome following biochemical relapse in the dose escalation era for prostate cancer patients undergoing definitive external beam radiotherapy. Eur Urol 2015;67(6): 1009–16.

53. Zumsteg ZS, Spratt DE, Romesser PB, et al. Anatomical patterns of recurrence following biochemical relapse in the dose escalation era of external beam radiotherapy for prostate cancer. J Urol 2015;194(6):1624–30.

54. Sugimura K, Carrington BM, Quivey JM, et al. Post-irradiation changes in the pelvis: assessment with MR imaging. Radiology 1990;175(3):805–13.

55. Chan TW, Kressel HY. Prostate and seminal vesicles after irradiation: MR appearance. J Magn Reson Imaging 1991;1(5):503–11.

56. Coakley FV, Teh HS, Qayyum A, et al. Endorectal MR imaging and MR spectroscopic imaging for locally recurrent prostate cancer after external beam radiation therapy: preliminary experience. Radiology 2004;233(2):441–8.

57. Arrayeh E, Westphalen AC, Kurhanewicz J, et al. Does local recurrence of prostate cancer after radiation therapy occur at the site of primary tumor? Results of a longitudinal MRI and MRSI study. Int J Radiat Oncol Biol Phys 2012;82(5):e787–93.

58. Jalloh M, Leapman MS, Cowan JE, et al. Patterns of local failure following radiation therapy for prostate cancer. J Urol 2015;194(4):977–82.

59. Westphalen AC, Kurhanewicz J, Cunha RM, et al. T2-Weighted endorectal magnetic resonance imaging of prostate cancer after external beam radiation therapy. Int Braz J Urol 2009;35(2):171–80 [discussion: 181–2].

60. Sala E, Eberhardt SC, Akin O, et al. Endorectal MR imaging before salvage prostatectomy: tumor localization and staging. Radiology 2006;238(1):176–83.

61. Kim CK, Park BK, Lee HM. Prediction of locally recurrent prostate cancer after radiation therapy: incremental value of 3T diffusion-weighted MRI. J Magn Reson Imaging 2009;29(2):391–7.

62. Hara T, Inoue Y, Satoh T, et al. Diffusion-weighted imaging of local recurrent prostate cancer after radiation therapy: comparison with 22-core three-dimensional prostate mapping biopsy. Magn Reson Imaging 2012;30(8):1091–8.

63. Rouviere O, Valette O, Grivolat S, et al. Recurrent prostate cancer after external beam radiotherapy:

value of contrast-enhanced dynamic MRI in local-izing intraprostatic tumor–correlation with biopsy findings. Urology 2004;63(5):922–7.

64. Franiel T, Ludemann L, Taupitz M, et al. MRI before and after external beam intensity-modulated radio-therapy of patients with prostate cancer: the feasi-bility of monitoring of radiation-induced tissue changes using a dynamic contrast-enhanced inver-sion-prepared dual-contrast gradient echo sequence. Radiother Oncol 2009;93(2):241–5.

65. Barchetti F, Panebianco V. Multiparametric MRI for recurrent prostate cancer post radical prostatec-tomy and postradiation therapy. Biomed Res Int 2014;2014:316272.

66. Haider MA, Chung P, Sweet J, et al. Dynamic contrast-enhanced magnetic resonance imaging for localization of recurrent prostate cancer after external beam radiotherapy. Int J Radiat Oncol Biol Phys 2008;70(2):425–30.

67. Kim CK, Park BK, Park W, et al. Prostate MR imaging at 3T using a phased-arrayed coil in predicting locally recurrent prostate cancer after radiation ther-apy: preliminary experience. Abdom Imaging 2010; 35(2):246–52.

68. Skowronek J. Low-dose-rate or high-dose-rate brachytherapy in treatment of prostate cancer - be-tween options. J Contemp Brachytherapy 2013; 5(1):33–41.

69. Tamada T, Sone T, Jo Y, et al. Locally recurrent pros-tate cancer after high-dose-rate brachytherapy: the value of diffusion-weighted imaging, dynamic contrast-enhanced MRI, and T2-weighted imaging in localizing tumors. AJR Am J Roentgenol 2011; 197(2):408–14.

70. Hamstra DA, Rehemtulla A, Ross BD. Diffusion mag-netic resonance imaging: a biomarker for treatment response in oncology. J Clin Oncol 2007;25(26): 4104–9.

71. Venkatesan AM, Stafford RJ, Duran C, et al. Prostate magnetic resonance imaging for brachytherapists: anatomy and technique. Brachytherapy 2017; 16(4):679–87.

72. Hotker AM, Mazaheri Y, Zheng J, et al. Prostate can-cer: assessing the effects of androgen-deprivation therapy using quantitative diffusion-weighted and dynamic contrast-enhanced MRI. Eur Radiol 2015; 25(9):2665–72.

73. Kim AY, Kim CK, Park SY, et al. Diffusion-weighted imaging to evaluate for changes from androgen deprivation therapy in prostate cancer. AJR Am J Roentgenol 2014;203(6):W645–50.

74. Ellis DS, Manny TB Jr, Rewcastle JC. Focal cryosur-gery followed by penile rehabilitation as primary treatment for localized prostate cancer: initial re-sults. Urology 2007;70(6 Suppl):9–15.

75. Lindner U, Weersink RA, Haider MA, et al. Image guided photothermal focal therapy for localized prostate cancer: phase I trial. J Urol 2009;182(4): 1371–7.

76. Truesdale MD, Cheetham PJ, Hruby GW, et al. An eval-uation of patient selection criteria on predicting progression-free survival after primary focal unilateral nerve-sparing cryoablation for prostate cancer: recom-mendations for follow up. Cancer J 2010;16(5):544–9.

77. Ward JF, Jones JS. Focal cryotherapy for localized prostate cancer: a report from the national Cryo On-Line Database (COLD) Registry. BJU Int 2012; 109(11):1648–54.

78. Ahmed HU, Hindley RG, Dickinson L, et al. Focal therapy for localised unifocal and multifocal prostate cancer: a prospective development study. Lancet Oncol 2012;13(6):622–32.

79. Muller BG, van den Bos W, Brausi M, et al. Follow-up modalities in focal therapy for prostate cancer: re-sults from a Delphi consensus project. World J Urol 2015;33(10):1503–9.

80. Ahmed HU, Moore C, Lecornet E, et al. Focal ther-apy in prostate cancer: determinants of success and failure. J Endourol 2010;24(5):819–25.

81. Martino P, Scattoni V, Galosi AB, et al. Role of imag-ing and biopsy to assess local recurrence after definitive treatment for prostate carcinoma (surgery, radiotherapy, cryotherapy, HIFU). World J Urol 2011; 29(5):595–605.

82. Kirkham AP, Emberton M, Hoh IM, et al. MR imaging of prostate after treatment with high-intensity focused ultrasound. Radiology 2008;246(3):833–44.

83. Levy DA, Ross AE, ElShafei A, et al. Definition of biochemical success following primary whole gland prostate cryoablation. J Urol 2014;192(5):1380–4.

84. Long JP, Bahn D, Lee F, et al. Five-year retrospec-tive, multi-institutional pooled analysis of cancer-related outcomes after cryosurgical ablation of the prostate. Urology 2001;57(3):518–23.

85. Mearini L, D'Urso L, Collura D, et al. High-intensity focused ultrasound for the treatment of prostate cancer: a prospective trial with long-term follow-up. Scand J Urol 2015;49(4):267–74.

86. Eggener SE, Yousuf A, Watson S, et al. Phase II eval-uation of magnetic resonance imaging guided focal laser ablation of prostate cancer. J Urol 2016;196(6): 1670–5.

Imaging of Prostate Cancer Using ¹¹C-Choline PET/Computed Tomography

Paolo Castellucci, MD, Francesco Ceci, MD*,
Stefano Fanti, MD

KEYWORDS

- Prostate cancer • Choline PET/CT • Diagnosis • Staging

KEY POINTS

- ¹¹C-Choline PET/CT has a limited role in the diagnosis of prostate cancer, whereas for nodal staging, choline PET/CT showed low sensitivity but a high specificity.
- The main application of this imaging procedure is the restaging of the disease in case of biochemical recurrence.
- ¹¹C-Choline-PET/CT proved its value for metastases-directed salvage therapies and for monitoring therapy response in castration-resistant patients.
- PSA and PSA kinetics values confirmed their correlation with ¹¹C-choline PET/CT sensitivity.

INTRODUCTION

Prostate cancer (PCa) is the most common solid cancer in men.[1] The evidence of PCa is generally assessed by digital rectal examination, serum levels of prostate-specific antigen (PSA), and transrectal ultrasound.[1] Many different imaging procedures, such as transrectal ultrasound, MR imaging, computerized tomography (CT), and bone scintigraphy, are used for local staging (to evaluate the tumor extension) and to assess the presence of distant metastasis.[1] Although primary treatment with radical intent (radical prostatectomy associated with lymph node dissection or radiation therapy) is associated with excellent oncologic results, many patients experience relapse after primary treatment.

This article reviews the role of ¹¹C-choline PET/CT in patients with PCa for staging and restaging the disease in case of biochemical recurrence (BCR) after primary treatment and for therapy monitoring in patients with castration-resistant PCa (CRPC) treated with systemic therapy.

¹¹C-CHOLINE PET/COMPUTED TOMOGRAPHY IN PROSTATE CANCER DIAGNOSIS

Multiparametric MR imaging represents the standard of reference for the detection of intraprostatic cancer.[2] The role of ¹¹C-choline PET/CT for the initial diagnosis of PCa has been extensively evaluated over the last decade. The first study performed on a sextant-basis in comparison with histology was by Farsad and colleagues.[3] The authors investigated 36 patients scheduled for surgery. ¹¹C-Choline PET/CT showed a sensitivity of 66%, a specificity of 81%, an accuracy of 71%, a positive predictive value (PPV) of 87%, and a low negative predictive value of 55%. In the following years other authors confirmed these findings.[4–6] Other results confirming the lack of accuracy for ¹¹C-choline PET/CT in this field were recently published. Bundschuh and colleagues[7] correlated the uptake of ¹¹C-choline PET/CT in the prostate gland with histopathology. The assessed sensitivity was poor because only 46%

This article was previously published in April 2017 *PET Clinics*, Volume 12, Issue 2.
The authors have nothing to disclose.
Service of Nuclear Medicine, S. Orsola-Malpighi University Hospital, University of Bologna, Bologna, Italy
* Corresponding author: UO Medicina Nucleare PAD. 30, Azienda Ospedaliero-Universitaria di Bologna, Policlinico S. Orsola-Malpighi, Via Massarenti 9, Bologna 40138, Italy.
E-mail address: francesco.ceci@studio.unibo.it

Urol Clin N Am 45 (2018) 481–487
https://doi.org/10.1016/j.ucl.2018.03.007
0094-0143/18/© 2016 Elsevier Inc. All rights reserved.

of lesions evaluated by histology showed an increased choline uptake. In a study proposed by Grosu and colleagues,[8] ^{11}C-choline-increased uptake has been found in neoplastic and nonneoplastic tissue. Moreover in some cases the intensity of the uptake was even higher in nonneoplastic tissue. Van den Bergh and colleagues[9] compared ^{11}C-choline PET/CT and MR imaging, showing that sensitivity increased, but specificity decreased combining both modalities. In conclusion, the suboptimal sensitivity of ^{11}C-choline PET/CT is mainly caused by the presence of small foci of cancer, whereas the suboptimal specificity is mainly caused by the frequent presence of nonneoplastic conditions within the prostate gland that may show increased choline uptake, such as benign prostatic hyperplasia or prostatitis.

PET/COMPUTED TOMOGRAPHY IN PROSTATE CANCER STAGING

Over the last decade many authors have evaluated the role of ^{11}C-choline PET/CT for lymph nodal or bone staging before primary treatment. The detection of nodal or distant metastases assessed by ^{11}C-choline PET/CT should help clinicians provide patients a tailored treatment strategy.[1] Schiavina and colleagues[10] showed that ^{11}C-choline PET/CT has low sensitivity (60%) but high specificity (98%) in a population of 57 with intermediate and high risk PCa. Contractor and colleagues[11] showed a sensitivity of 40% and a specificity of 98% in nodal staging using ^{11}C-choline PET/CT before surgery in 28 patients with PCa. Van Den Bergh and colleagues[12] prospectively used ^{11}C-choline PET/CT and diffusion weighted (DW)-MR imaging for nodal staging in patients with high risk for nodal involvement. Seventy-five patients N0 at CT were enrolled. A total of 37 of 75 patients (49%) were positive at histology. On a patient-based analysis ^{11}C-choline PET/CT showed a sensitivity of 18.9% and a PPV of 63.6%, whereas DW-MR imaging showed a sensitivity of 36.1% and a PPV of 86.7%. On a region-based analysis, ^{11}C-choline PET/CT showed a sensitivity of 8.2% and a PPV of 50.0%, whereas DW-MR imaging showed a sensitivity of 9.5% and a PPV of 40.0%. The poor results obtained by both these imaging modalities should remind clinicians that even in patients at high risk for positive lymph nodes at presentation and even in highly selected patient populations, poor sensitivity and poor PPV may occur either on a patient or lymph node based analysis. Finally, Evangelista and colleagues[13] evaluated by a systematic review the role of ^{18}F or ^{11}C-choline PET/CT for staging PCa. Most of the papers analyzed confirmed preliminary findings showing a lack of sensitivity but high specificity for nodal staging. Pooled sensitivity and specificity were, respectively, 49% and 95% on a patient basis. ^{11}C-Choline PET/CT low sensitivity could be explained by the presence of micrometastasis and thus by the size of nodal metastatic deposit, because it is unlikely that ^{11}C-choline PET/CT may detect lesions smaller than 5 mm. On the contrary, the main reason for false-positive findings is the presence of reactive lymph nodes that may show increased choline uptake.

In conclusion, the use of ^{11}C-choline PET/CT for lymph nodal staging should be reserved to high-risk and very-high-risk patients (according to the most accepted nomograms) to reduce the incidence of false-negative scans and to optimize the number of positive ^{11}C-choline PET/CT.

PET/COMPUTED TOMOGRAPHY IN PROSTATE CANCER RESTAGING

BCR after radical treatment is a frequent event, involving up to 50% of patients treated.[14] The role of any imaging procedure is to differentiate between the presence of a local and/or distant relapse.[14] Imaging should select patients with single or oligometastatic disease (potentially treatable with salvage treatments) from patients affected by metastatic disease treatable with systemic therapies. In the last years ^{11}C-choline-PET/CT demonstrated a significant clinical impact on patient management. In three papers recently published from three different patient series, ^{11}C-choline PET/CT demonstrated a change in the decision-making process in approximately 50% of cases.[15–17]

Prostate-Specific Antigen Values and ^{11}C-Choline PET/Computed Tomography

[11]C-Choline PET/CT has been widely used in case of BCR. Nevertheless, despite the large number of data available, there is still no consensus about the optimal timing to perform the scan. Recently, the European Association of Urology guidelines[14] suggested the use of choline PET/CT in patients with BCR and PSA levels greater than 1 ng/mL, preferably with PSA values between 1 and 2 ng/mL. At this stage of the disease, differentiating between the presence of single, oligo, or multi metastatic disease would have a major impact on clinical management. In a recent meta-analysis Fanti and colleagues[18] analyzed 29 studies with a total of 2686 patients enrolled. The authors reported for ^{11}C-choline PET/CT a detection rate for any site of relapse of 62% (95% confidence interval, 53%–71%). In a single-institution patient series, analyzing 4426 scans in 3203 patients with BCR,

Graziani and colleagues[19] assessed overall sensitivity for ^{11}C-choline PET/CT of 52.8%. It is interesting to point out that in 995 scans that were performed in patients with PSA levels between 1 and 2 ng/mL the sensitivity for ^{11}C-choline PET/CT was not as low (44.7%) if compared with the sensitivity assessed in the whole population. In the receiver operating characteristic curve analysis, PSA value of 1.16 ng/mL was the optimal cutoff value able to predict a positive scan.

Sites of Relapse and Choline PET

MR imaging is the standard of reference for the detection of prostate bed recurrence.[20] ^{11}C-Choline PET/CT showed low sensitivity in the detection of local relapse in comparison with MR imaging.[20–22] The assessed sensitivity for local recurrence (either using ^{18}F or ^{11}C-choline PET/CT)[20–22] was 50% to 60%. Kitajima and colleagues[23] confirmed these data in a population of 115 patients showing a sensitivity, specificity, and accuracy of 54%, 92%, and 65% for ^{11}C-choline PET/CT in the detection of local relapse, in comparison with a sensitivity, specificity, and accuracy of 88%, 84%, and 87% showed by MR imaging. However, in the same study, the authors showed a better accuracy for ^{11}C-choline PET/CT compared with MR imaging (92% vs 70%) in pelvic lymph node metastasis detection, regardless of PSA values.[23] The performance of ^{11}C-choline PET/CT in the detection of bone lesions has been compared with bone scan by Picchio and colleagues[24] in 78 patients with BCR. The authors showed lower sensitivity values for ^{11}C-choline PET/CT compared with bone scan (89% vs 100%), but a significant higher specificity (98% vs 75%). Fuccio and colleagues[25] showed the presence of multiple sites of relapse at ^{11}C-choline PET/CT in almost half of the 25 patients who showed only one single lesion at bone scan. The authors confirmed the high sensitivity and the high specificity for ^{11}C-choline PET/CT (86% and 100%, respectively) in the detection of bone metastatic lesions. Choline uptake in bone lesions changes and may vary in the different type of bone lesions. Ceci and colleagues[26] analyzed 304 bone lesions (184 osteoblastic, 99 osteolytic, and 21 bone marrow lesions) in a cohort of 140 patients with PCa with BCR. They demonstrated a significant difference for SUVmax values between osteoblastic (lower values) and osteolytic (higher values) lesions.

Salvage Therapies and Choline PET

One of the most promising applications for PET/CT imaging is to select and differentiate those patients who can benefit from tailored PET-guided treatment from patients who should be addressed by systemic therapies. However, before performing aggressive treatment, such as metastasis-directed salvage radiation therapy (S-RT) or salvage lymph node dissection (S-LND), all efforts should made to exclude the presence of metastasis already present at the time of salvage treatments and not included in the planned target volume or that could not be removed by an S-LND. In this regard, Castellucci and colleagues[27] studied with ^{11}C-choline PET/CT a cohort 605 recurrent patients showing low PSA values (PSA range, 0.2–2 ng/mL) after radical prostatectomy (RP) and listed for S-RT in the prostatic bed. ^{11}C-Choline PET/CT detected a disease limited to the pelvis in 13.7% of patients, whereas the presence of an extrapelvic disease was observed in 14.7%. The authors observed that ^{11}C-choline PET/CT detection rate increased dramatically in patients with fast PSA doubling time (^{11}C-choline PET/CT detection rate 47% with PSA doubling time <6 months). The authors concluded that ^{11}C-choline PET/CT should be performed before salvage therapies especially in those patients showing fast PSA kinetics to exclude the presence of distant lesions that could not be removed with SLND or included in the planned target volume.

The first prospective study aimed to assess the role of ^{11}C-choline PET/CT in guiding aggressive treatments has been published by Rigatti and colleagues.[28] The authors studied a cohort of 79 patients showing BCR after RP. Patients who showed no more than two positive lymph nodes on ^{11}C-choline PET/CT received S-PLND. Biochemical relapse-free survival rates at 3 years of 27.5% and at 5 years of 10.3% were reported. Five-year clinical recurrence-free survival was lower for patients with positive retroperitoneal lymph nodes at ^{11}C-choline PET/CT versus patients with only pelvic ^{11}C-choline PET/CT-positive nodes (11% vs 53%; $P < .001$). Karnes and colleagues[29] enrolled a group of 52 patients treated with S-LND according to ^{11}C-choline PET/CT results. After a median follow-up of 20 months, 30 out of 52 patients (57.7%) were biochemical relapse-free and 50 of 52 patients (96.2%) were alive. Suardi and colleagues[30] studied 56 patients and demonstrated clinical relapse-free and cancer-specific mortality-free survival rates at 8 years of 38% and 81%, respectively. Multivariate analysis showed that PSA higher than 2 ng/mL at the time of ^{11}C-choline PET/CT and the presence of retroperitoneal positive lymph nodes on ^{11}C-choline PET/CT were predictors of clinical relapse. PET/CT-guided S-RT can be performed in patients showing single or

484

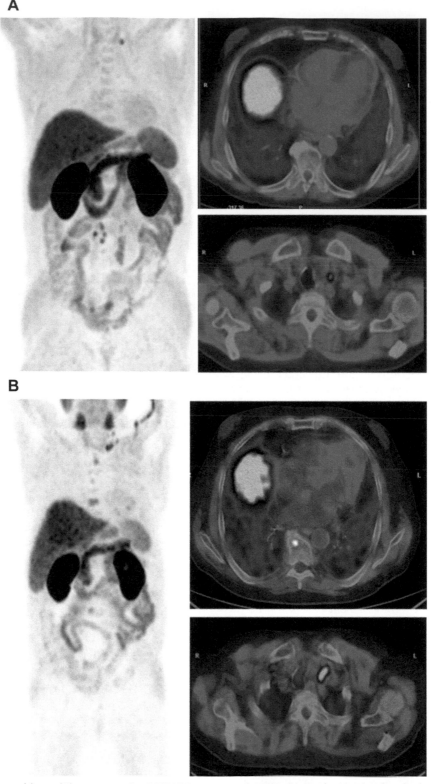

Fig. 1. A 64-year-old man (Gleason score 4 + 4; T3N1Mx; presentation PSA, 9 ng/mL) treated with radical prostatectomy and pelvic lymph node dissection as primary treatment. BCR occurred 20 months after surgery. Patient was subsequently treated continuously with androgen-deprivation therapy for 27 months with good PSA response, once showed resistance to androgen-deprivation therapy. (*A*) With increasing PSA levels (PSA, 8.73 ng/mL) ^{11}C-choline PET/CT has been performed assessing the presence of multiple sites of disease. The patient was addressed with abiraterone acetate + prednisone. The PSA levels decreased up to 5.35 ng/mL after 4 months of treatment and the patient was referred to a further ^{11}C-choline PET/CT to restage the disease. (*B*) ^{11}C-Choline PET/CT demonstrated progression of the disease with the appearance of new active lesions. Progression of the disease was confirmed with clinical follow-up.

oligometastatic disease.[31,32] Würschmidt and colleagues[33] performed ^{11}C-choline PET/CT-guided S-RT in 19 patients showing BCR. Almost half of the patients were biochemical relapse-free after 28 months of follow-up. Picchio and colleagues[34] used ^{11}C-choline PET/CT to guide helical tomotherapy in 83 patients showing lymph node relapse after primary treatment. The authors achieved an early biochemical response in 70% of cases. The same research group published a study[35] in which 68 patients showing ^{11}C-choline PET/CT-positive lymph nodes were enrolled. After PET-guided helical tomotherapy 2-year overall survival, locoregional relapse-free survival, clinical relapse-free survival, and biochemical-free survival were 87%, 91%, 51%, and 40%, respectively.

Early detection of the site relapse in patients with PCa with BCR is crucial, because it leads to a more favorable patient outcome. The detection of oligometastatic disease on ^{11}C-choline PET/CT gives clinicians the chance to plan a dedicated and personalized treatment strategy.

PET/COMPUTED TOMOGRAPHY IN CASTRATION-RESISTANT PROSTATE CANCER

CRPC is a frequent condition in advanced disease and is related to a high mortality rate, with an overall survival of 2 to 3 years. In this condition, palliation is the goal of treatment.[14] Many different therapies can be used, such as docetaxel and cabazitaxel, or new novel androgen receptor targeted therapies, such as abiraterone and enzalutamide.[14] The assessment of PSA levels over time is routinely used to evaluate therapy response and outcome prediction. However, this is not a reliable marker because it can be impaired by flare phenomena, tumor cells heterogeneity, and active visceral metastases not producing PSA. Conventional imaging methods, including CT, MR imaging, and bone scan, are late indicators of treatment efficacy, whereas PET/CT has the potential to identify the response to therapy early. The evaluation of changes provided by PET/CT, rather than morphologic changes during therapy, may be an early and reliable alternative to other indicators of treatment benefit, such as radiologic progression-free survival and PSA.

In a few preliminary studies[9,10] the role of choline-PET/CT was investigated. De Giorgi and colleagues[36] used ^{18}F-choline PET/CT for evaluating the early response to treatment with abiraterone in 43 patients with metastatic CRPC (mCRPC). The authors confirmed that the response assessed with ^{18}F-choline PET/CT was associated with a more favorable overall survival than a PSA response of greater than or equal to

50%. Maines and colleagues[37] confirmed these data in 30 patients with mCRPC treated with enzalutamide. The authors observed that SUVmax values measured at ^{18}F-choline PET/CT performed before enzalutamide were significantly related with biochemical, radiologic, and overall survival. Ceci and colleagues[38] studied a cohort of 61 patients with mCRPC with ^{11}C-choline PET/CT performed before and after treatment with docetaxel. A comparison between the response to docetaxel assessed by ^{11}C-choline PET/CT and the PSA response has been performed. ^{11}C-Choline PET/CT showed progression of the disease in the 44% of patients who showed a PSA response after docetaxel. The tumor burden, expressed as more than 10 PET-positive bone lesions measured before docetaxel, was also significantly associated with an increased probability of progression after treatment.

Prospective future trials should better investigate this potential application of choline PET/CT. It could be interesting to assess if PET/CT imaging could identify progression versus nonprogression of the disease earlier and more accurately than PSA and conventional imaging (**Fig. 1**). In particular, the more relevant clinical contribution of PET/CT will occur when decreasing PSA is associated with radiologic progression. The availability of a procedure to accurately and early assess the response to systemic therapies will have an important impact on CRPC management. It could lead to a more tailored therapy, especially for those patients presenting with decreasing PSA levels during treatment, whereas imaging could show progression. These patients could switch to a second line of chemotherapy and/or new antiandorgen therapies and radiotherapy on the not-responding lesions or [223]radium. As a consequence, besides an improvement in life expectancy, the collateral effects/toxicity and costs of futile therapy will be reduced.

REFERENCES

1. Heidenreich A, Bastian PJ, Bellmunt J, et al. EAU guidelines on prostate cancer. Part 1: screening, diagnosis, and local treatment with curative intent-update 2013. Eur Urol 2014;65(1):124–37.
2. Metzger GJ, Kalavagunta C, Spilseth B, et al. Detection of prostate cancer: quantitative multiparametric MR imaging models developed using registered correlative histopathology. Radiology 2016;279(3): 805–16.
3. Farsad M, Schiavina R, Castellucci P, et al. Detection and localization of prostate cancer: correlation of (11)C-choline PET/CT with histopathologic step-section analysis. J Nucl Med 2005;46:1642–9.

4. Giovacchini G, Picchio M, Coradeschi E, et al. [(11)C]Choline uptake with PET/CT for the initial diagnosis of prostate cancer: relation to PSA levels, tumour stage and anti-androgenic therapy. Eur J Nucl Med Mol Imaging 2008;35:1065–73.

5. Martorana G, Schiavina R, Corti B, et al. 11C-Choline positron emission tomography/computerized tomography for tumor localization of primary prostate cancer in comparison with 12-core biopsy. J Urol 2006;176:954–60.

6. Testa C, Schiavina R, Lodi R, et al. Prostate cancer: sextant localization with MR imaging, MR spectroscopy, and 11C-choline PET/CT. Radiology 2007; 244(3):797–806.

7. Bundschuh RA, Wendl CM, Weirich G, et al. Tumour volume delineation in prostate cancer assessed by [11C]choline PET/CT: validation with surgical specimens. Eur J Nucl Med Mol Imaging 2013;40:824–31.

8. Grosu AL, Weirich G, Wendl C, et al. 11C-Choline PET/pathology image coregistration in primary localized prostate cancer. Eur J Nucl Med Mol Imaging 2014;41:2242–8.

9. Van den Bergh L, Koole M, Isebaert S, et al. Is there an additional value of (11)C choline PET-CT to T2-weighted MRI images in the localization of intraprostatic tumor nodules? Int J Radiat Oncol Biol Phys 2012;83:1486–92.

10. Schiavina R, Scattoni V, Castellucci P, et al. 11C-Choline positron emission tomography/computerized tomography for preoperative lymph-node staging in intermediate-risk and high-risk prostate cancer: comparison with clinical staging nomograms. Eur Urol 2008;54:392–401.

11. Contractor K, Challapalli A, Barwick T, et al. Use of [11C]choline PET-CT as a noninvasive method for detecting pelvic lymph node status from prostate cancer and relationship with choline kinase expression. Clin Cancer Res 2011;17:7673–83.

12. Van den Bergh L, Lerut E, Haustermans K, et al. Final analysis of a prospective trial on functional imaging for nodal staging in patients with prostate cancer at high risk for lymph node involvement. Urol Oncol 2015;33(3):109.e23-31.

13. Evangelista L, Guttilla A, Zattoni F, et al. Utility of choline positron emission tomography/computed tomography for lymph node involvement identification in intermediate- to high-risk prostate cancer: a systematic literature review and metaanalysis. Eur Urol 2013;63:1040–8.

14. Heidenreich A, Bastian PJ, Bellmunt J, et al. EAU guidelines on prostate cancer. Part II: treatment of advanced, relapsing, and castration-resistant prostate cancer. European Association of Urology. Eur Urol 2014;65(2):467–79.

15. Ceci F, Herrmann K, Castellucci P, et al. Impact of 11C-choline PET/CT on clinical decision making in recurrent prostate cancer: results from a retrospective two-centre trial. Eur J Nucl Med Mol Imaging 2014;41(12):2222–31 [Erratum in Eur J Nucl Med Mol Imaging 2014;41(12):2359].

16. Soyka JD, Muster MA, Schmid DT, et al. Clinical impact of 18F-choline PET/CT in patients with recurrent prostate cancer. Eur J Nucl Med Mol Imaging 2012;39(6):936–43.

17. Goldstein J, Even-Sapir E, Ben-Haim S, et al. Does choline PET/CT change the management of prostate cancer patients with biochemical failure? Am J Clin Oncol 2014. [Epub ahead of print].

18. Fanti S, Minozzi S, Castellucci P, et al. PET/CT with (11)C-choline for evaluation of prostate cancer patients with biochemical recurrence: meta-analysis and critical review of available data. Eur J Nucl Med Mol Imaging 2016;43(1):55–69.

19. Graziani T, Ceci F, Castellucci P, et al. (11)C-Choline PET/CT for restaging prostate cancer. Results from 4,426 scans in a single-centre patient series. Eur J Nucl Med Mol Imaging 2016;43(11):1971–9.

20. Panebianco V, Sciarra A, Lisi D, et al. Prostate cancer: 1HMRS-DCEMR at 3T versus [(18)F]choline PET/CT in the detection of local prostate cancer recurrence in men with biochemical progression after radical retropubic prostatectomy (RRP). Eur J Radiol 2012;81(4):700–8.

21. Castellucci P, Fuccio C, Rubello D, et al. Is there a role for 11C-choline PET/CT in the early detection of metastatic disease in surgically treated prostate cancer patients with a mild PSA increase of 1.5 ng/ml? Eur J Nucl Med Mol Imaging 2011;38(1):55–63.

22. Mamede M, Ceci F, Castellucci P, et al. The role of 11C-choline PET imaging in the early detection of recurrence in surgically treated prostate cancer patients with very low PSA level <0.5 ng/mL. Clin Nucl Med 2013;38(9):e342–5.

23. Kitajima K, Murphy RC, Nathan MA, et al. Detection of recurrent prostate cancer after radical prostatectomy: comparison of 11C-choline PET/CT with pelvic multiparametric MR imaging with endorectal coil. J Nucl Med 2014;55(2):223–32.

24. Picchio M, Spinapolice EG, Fallanca F, et al. [11C]Choline PET/CT detection of bone metastases in patients with PSA progression after primary treatment for prostate cancer: comparison with bone scintigraphy. Eur J Nucl Med Mol Imaging 2012 Jan; 39(1):13–26.

25. Fuccio C, Castellucci P, Schiavina R, et al. Role of 11C-choline PET/CT in the re-staging of prostate cancer patients with biochemical relapse and negative results at bone scintigraphy. Eur J Radiol 2012; 81(8):e893–6.

26. Ceci F, Castellucci P, Graziani T, et al. 11C-Choline PET/CT identifies osteoblastic and osteolytic lesions in patients with metastatic prostate cancer. Clin Nucl Med 2015;40(5):e265–70.

27. Castellucci P, Ceci F, Graziani T, et al. Early biochemical relapse after radical prostatectomy: which prostate cancer patients may benefit from a restaging 11C-choline PET/CT scan before salvage radiation therapy? J Nucl Med 2014;55(9):1424–9.

28. Rigatti P, Suardi N, Briganti A, et al. Pelvic/retroperitoneal salvage lymph node dissection for patients treated with radical prostatectomy with biochemical recurrence and nodal recurrence detected by [11C] choline positron emission tomography/computed tomography. Eur Urol 2011;60(5):935–43.

29. Karnes RJ, Murphy CR, Bergstralh EJ, et al. Salvage lymph node dissection for prostate cancer nodal recurrence detected by 11C-choline positron emission tomography/computerized tomography. J Urol 2015;193(1):111–6.

30. Suardi N, Gandaglia G, Gallina A, et al. Long-term outcomes of salvage lymph node dissection for clinically recurrent prostate cancer: results of a single-institution series with a minimum follow-up of 5 years. Eur Urol 2015;67(2):299–309.

31. Bolla M, Van Tienhoven G, Warde P, et al. External irradiation with or without long-term androgen suppression for prostate cancer with high metastatic risk: 10-year results of an EORTC randomised study. Lancet Oncol 2010;11:1066–73.

32. Stephenson AJ, Bolla M, Briganti A, et al. Postoperative radiation therapy for pathologically advanced prostate cancer after radical prostatectomy. Eur Urol 2012;61(3):443–51.

33. Wurschmidt F, Petersen C, Wahl A, et al. [18F]Fluoroethylcholine-PET/CT imaging for radiation treatment planning of recurrent and primary prostate cancer with dose escalation to PET/CT-positive lymph nodes. Radiat Oncol 2011;6:44.

34. Picchio M, Berardi G, Fodor A, et al. 11C-Choline PET/CT as a guide to radiation treatment planning of lymph-node relapses in prostate cancer patients. Eur J Nucl Med Mol Imaging 2014;41(7):1270–9.

35. Incerti E, Fodor A, Mapelli P, et al. Radiation treatment of lymph node recurrence from prostate cancer: is 11C-choline PET/CT predictive of survival outcomes? J Nucl Med 2015;56(12):1836–42.

36. De Giorgi U, Caroli P, Burgio SL, et al. Early outcome prediction on 18F-fluorocholine PET/CT in metastatic castration-resistant prostate cancer patients treated with abiraterone. Oncotarget 2014;5(23):12448–58.

37. Maines F, Caffo O, Donner D, et al. Serial (18)F-choline-PET imaging in patients receiving enzalutamide for metastatic castration-resistant prostate cancer: response assessment and imaging biomarkers. Future Oncol 2016;12(3):333–42.

38. Ceci F, Castellucci P, Graziani T, et al. 11C-Choline PET/CT in castration-resistant prostate cancer patients treated with docetaxel. Eur J Nucl Med Mol Imaging 2016;43(1):84–91.

Imaging of Prostate Cancer Using Fluciclovine

Bital Savir-Baruch, MD[a],*, Lucia Zanoni, MD[b], David M. Schuster, MD[c]

KEYWORDS

• FACBC • Fluciclovine • Axumin • CT • PET • Prostate

KEY POINTS

- Functional molecular imaging with PET improved the ability to detect prostate cancer.
- Fluciclovine is beneficial for the localization of recurrent prostate disease when other conventional images are negative.
- When interpreted with knowledge of radiotracer biodistribution and normal variants, fluciclovine PET is highly specific for extraprostatic metastasis but has lower specificity for disease within intact or treated prostate.
- Fewer data are available on the performance of fluciclovine in bone metastases; therefore, skeletal-specific imaging is recommended for suspected bone involvement if fluciclovine PET is unrevealing.

RADIOLABELED AMINO ACIDS AS PET RADIOTRACERS FOR PROSTATE CANCER IMAGING

Amino acids play a central role in cell metabolism and are the building blocks of proteins. Transmembrane amino acid transporters are upregulated in cancer cells to provide nutrients for tumor cell growth.[1,2] Certain amino acids such as leucine and glutamine are key components in the mammalian target of rapamycin cancer signaling pathway.[3] Because this upregulation of amino acid transport also occurs in prostate cancer cells, using an amino acid–based radiotracer can localize prostate cancer as well.[4]

Many amino acid transporter systems are overexpressed in prostate cancer, predominantly large neutral amino acid transporters (systems L: LAT1, LAT3, and LAT4) and alanine-serine-cysteine transporters (systems ASC: ASCT1, ASCT2).[1,3,5–14] Of these transporters, LAT1 and ASCT2 are particularly associated with more aggressive tumor behavior.[7,15–17] Both ASCT2 and LAT3 expression are stimulated by androgen signaling in androgen-dependent prostate cancer cells.[18]

Prostate cancer may be imaged using both radiolabeled natural and synthetic amino acids. Naturally occurring amino acids such as C-11-methionine are not optimal for imaging because of the accumulation of metabolites in nontarget organs, whereas radiolabeled synthetic, nonmetabolized amino acid analogues are preferred owing to simpler kinetics and the ability to radiolabel with longer-lived radionuclides.[1]

Anti–1-amino-3-F-18-fluorocyclobutane-1-carboxylic acid (FACBC or fluciclovine) is a

Portions of this article was previously published in April 2017 *PET Clinics*, Volume 12, Issue 2.

Disclosure Statement: B. Savir-Baruch has a scientific relationship with the company Blue Earth Diagnostics, Ltd, as principle investigator of a sponsored study BED003 (LOCATE). L. Zanoni has a scientific relationship with the company Blue Earth Diagnostics, Ltd, as Medical Staff of the Sponsored Study BED001 (118/2014/O/Oss). D.M. Schuster has participated in sponsored research involving fluciclovine through the Emory University Office of Sponsored Projects, including funding from Blue Earth Diagnostics, Ltd and Nihon Medi-Physics Co., Ltd. Emory University and Dr Mark Goodman are eligible to receive royalties from fluciclovine.

a Department of Radiology, Loyola University Medical Center, 2160 South 1st Avenue, Maywood, IL 60153, USA; b Department of Nuclear Medicine, Azienda Ospedaliero-Universitaria di Bologna, Policlinico Sant'Orsola-Malpighi, via Massarenti 9, Bologna 40138, Italy; c Department of Radiology and Imaging Sciences, Emory University Hospital, Emory University, 1364 Clifton Road, Atlanta, GA 30322, USA

* Corresponding author.

E-mail address: biatl.savir-baruch@lumc.edu

https://doi.org/10.1016/j.ucl.2018.03.015
0094-0143/18/

nonnaturally occurring amino acid analogue for which the most comprehensive clinical studies for prostate cancer have been performed to date.[10,17,19–26] Fluciclovine is predominantly transported via ASCT2 and LAT1. Because these transporters mediate both influx and efflux of amino acids, peak uptake in tumors occurs at 5 to 20 minutes after injection with variable washout.[17,22,27]

FLUCICLOVINE FROM DEVELOPMENT TO UNITED STATES FOOD AND DRUG ADMINISTRATION APPROVAL

The development of C-11 aminocyclobutane arboxylic acid (ACBC) was first described in 1978 by Washburn and colleagues.[28] ACBC was structurally modified from 1-aminocyclopentanecarboxylic acid. Subsequently, ACBC was radiolabeled with carbon-11 (C-11) and found to have potential for imaging soft tissue tumors in humans.[29] However, C-11 has a half-life of 20 minutes, which requires an on-site cyclotron for production. In 1995, Dr Mark Goodman and coworkers described the synthesis of fluorine-18 (half-life 109.8 minutes) labeled anti-1-amino-3-fluorocyclobutane-1-carboxylic acid, or 3-FACBC. In 1999, they reported the evaluation of 3-FACBC in gliomas.[30] In 2002, the synthesis of the 3-FACBC labeling precursor and 3-FACBC were improved for routine production for clinical use.[31,32]

Early work suggested that fluciclovine was transported into the cell most like leucine via system L, especially LAT1.[31,33] Subsequent in vitro studies found that the ASC transporter system, specifically ASCT2, plays the largest role in fluciclovine transport, whereas LAT1 transport may become elevated in an acidic tumor environment or with castration-resistant cells.[10,16–18] Thus, it is currently thought that fluciclovine transport more closely mirrors that of glutamine rather than leucine.[34] When compared with methionine, glutamine, choline, and acetate, the uptake of fluciclovine in prostate cancer cell lines has also been noted to be higher.[17] Experiments with a rat orthotopic prostate cancer model compared the uptake of fluciclovine with that of fludeoxyglucose (FDG). It was found that the target-to-background ratio was higher for fluciclovine, with only minimal bladder accumulation.[33]

In human clinical studies, fluciclovine was initially developed for the evaluation of cerebral gliomas.[30] Further evaluation in human dosimetry studies demonstrated physiologic highest tracer uptake by the liver and pancreas, with less intense heterogeneous uptake within the marrow, salivary glands, lymphoid tissue, and pituitary gland, and only minimal brain and kidney uptake. Variable activity was noted in the bowel[27] (**Fig. 1**). When compared with FDG, fluciclovine is only minimally eliminated by the kidneys during the typical imaging time course. Hence, the evaluation of fluciclovine for the imaging of renal and pelvic malignancies seemed promising.

Fluciclovine was next evaluated for the staging of patients with renal cancer. Although no highly promising data from renal mass evaluation were observed, an important incidental finding was reported in a patient with intense uptake within retroperitoneal lymphadenopathy and subsequent biopsy-proven metastatic prostate cancer.[35] The evaluation of fluciclovine for prostate cancer imaging took priority, and in 2007, Schuster and colleagues[22] described the first experience with fluciclovine for the evaluation of 9 patients with primary and 6 patients with recurrent prostate cancer. Early results reported promising correlation between biopsy-proven disease and fluciclovine uptake. Further human studies with fluciclovine, which will be detailed in elsewhere in this discussion, demonstrated the potential to detect local and distant recurrent prostate cancer.

A New Drug Application was subsequently accepted in December 2015 by the US Food and Drug Administration (FDA) as filed by Blue Earth Diagnostics, Ltd, for priority review based on data collected from 877 subjects, including 797 patients with prostate cancer in the United States and Europe, and approval was granted to fluciclovine (trade name Axumin) in May 2016 for the clinical indication of suspected prostate cancer recurrence based on elevated prostate-specific antigen (PSA) levels after prior treatment.[36]

FLUCICLOVINE IN THE EVALUATION OF PATIENTS WITH SUSPECTED RECURRENCE OF PROSTATE CANCER

Fluciclovine has been most extensively studied in relation to recurrent prostate cancer. Fluciclovine diagnostic performance has been reported to be significantly higher than that of In-111-capromab pendetide and computed tomography (CT) in the diagnosis of patients with suspected disease relapse.[21,24,37] A single-center study of 115 patients who underwent definitive treatment of prostate cancer and presented with biochemical failure by the American Urologic Association and American Society of Radiation Oncology criteria was completed.[38] In a subset analysis of 93 patients with negative bone scan and In-111-capromab pendetide, single-photon emission CT (SPECT)–CT within 90 days of the fluciclovine PET/CT, overall positive scans (positivity rate) was 82.8%. Biopsy was the primary reference standard. One hundred percent of true-positive prostate/prostate bed lesions and

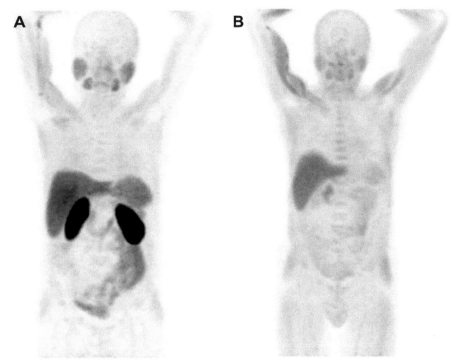

Fig. 1. Comparison of 11C choline and 18F fluciclovine physiologic biodistribution. 18F fluciclovine (*B*, maximum intensity projection [MIP]) is physiologically found in pancreas, liver, bone marrow, and muscle, with negligible uptake in kidneys, bowel, and delayed urinary excretion, thus, leading to a more favorable distribution in the abdomen and pelvis, compared with 11C choline (*A*, MIP), for evaluating prostate cancer. (*Courtesy of* Dr Cristina Nanni, Programma di ricerca Regione-Università 2010–2012 Regione Emilia Romagna-Bando Giovani Ricercatori, Bologna, Italy.)

86.4% of true-positive extraprostatic lesions were confirmed histologically. For prostate/prostate bed recurrence, fluciclovine had 90.2% sensitivity, 40.0% specificity, 73.6% accuracy, 75.3% positive predictive value (PPV), and 66.7% negative predictive value (NPV); the respective values for In-111-capromab pendetide were 67.2%, 56.7%, 63.7%, 75.9%, and 45.9%. For extraprostatic recurrence, fluciclovine had 55.0% sensitivity, 96.7% specificity, 72.9% accuracy, 95.7% PPV, and 61.7% NPV; the respective values for In-111-capromab pendetide were10.0%, 86.7%, 42.9%, 50.0%, and 41.9%. Fluciclovine identified 14 more positive prostate/prostate bed recurrences (55 vs 41) and 18 more patients with extraprostatic involvement (22 vs 4), and a 25.7% change in stage was reported by use of fluciclovine PET.

Similar patterns were reported when fluciclovine imaging was compared with the performance of CT (n = 53) in another subanalysis from this trial.[21] For the prostate/prostate bed, fluciclovine had 88.6% sensitivity, 56.3% specificity, 78.4% accuracy, 81.6% PPV, and 69.2% NPV; the respective values for CT were 11.4%, 87.5%, 35.3%, 66.7%, and 31.1%. For extraprostatic regions, fluciclovine had 46.2% sensitivity, 100% specificity, 65.9%

accuracy, 100% PPV, and 51.7% NPV; the respective values for CT were 11.5%, 100%, 43.9%, 100%, and 39.5%. Positivity rates with fluciclovine PET/CT varied with PSA levels, PSA doubling times, and original Gleason scores, but were higher than positivity rates for CT. For PSA levels of less than 1, 1 to 2, greater than 2 to 5, and greater than 5 ng/mL, 37.5%, 77.8%, 91.7%, and 83.3% fluciclovine scans were positive, respectively.

Although fluciclovine demonstrates high PPV for extraprostatic disease, the usefulness of fluciclovine for the evaluation of local recurrence within the prostate may be challenging with relatively higher false-positive results compared with extraprostatic locations. In particular, patients who underwent prostate-sparing initial therapies may demonstrate nonspecific uptake patterns, which are likely confounded by prostatic hypertrophy and chronic inflammation. Savir-Baruch and colleagues[39] reported that the fluciclovine pattern of heterogeneous tracer distribution exhibits lower maximum standard uptake value (SUV_{max}) and lower PPV and also is associated with the presence of brachytherapy seeds when compared with focal or multifocal distribution patterns.

The evaluation of potential skeletal lesions is essential for proper staging and treatment of patients with suspected prostate cancer recurrence. Because patients with known bone metastasis were excluded from the initial studies via negative bone scan, there are few data concerning accuracy of fluciclovine for skeletal metastasis. Nevertheless, patients with fluciclovine-positive bone lesions have been reported.[20,21,37,40] Nanni and colleagues[20] reported 7 of 89 patients in their study with bone lesions in which 5 were positive with fluciclovine (**Fig. 2**). Schuster and colleagues[37] reported 3 of 93 patients with uptake within skeletal lesions enrolled after negative bone scan. A phase IIa clinical trial by Inoue and colleagues[41] of 10 patients reported 7 patients with abnormal increased fluciclovine uptake within metastatic bone lesions, similar to that of conventional imaging. In these authors' experience, fluciclovine demonstrates intense focal uptake in lytic prostate cancer lesions, and moderate uptake within mixed sclerotic lesions, but there may be absent uptake in dense sclerotic lesions. Thus, it is recommended that fluciclovine should not replace the use of dedicated bone scintigraphy when clinically indicated.

For clinical practice use of fluciclovine, Gill and colleagues[42] reported overall positivity rate of 86% in the first 32 patients who underwent fluciclovine PET/CT scans for biochemical recurrence in a single institution. For the prostate bed, 37.5% of patients had positive findings and 62.5% of the patients had extraprostatic lesions. Multiple larger cohorts evaluating the performance of fluciclovine in clinical practice are being performed.

Fluciclovine Performance Compared with Other PET Radiotracers

Other reported molecular imaging PET radiotracers have demonstrated promising results in the detection of prostate cancer, including C-11 choline, F-18 choline, C-11 acetate (**Fig. 3**), and Ga-68 or F-18–labeled prostate-specific membrane antigen ligands (PSMA).[40,43–50] For C-11 choline, a recent metaanalysis of 1270 patients reported a pooled sensitivity and specificity of 89% and 89%, respectively.[40] For F-8 choline, a cohort of 1000 patients recently reported a sensitivity of 97.6% and specificity of 79.7%.[51] Although these results suggest that the diagnostic performance of choline is superior to that of fluciclovine, cautioned must be exercised because differences in study design, interpretative criteria, and reference standards may bias results. In fact, a single-center study by Nanni and colleagues[20] found fluciclovine to be slightly superior to the performance of C-11 choline for patients radically treated for prostate

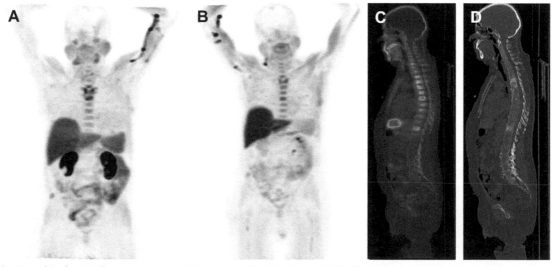

Fig. 2. In biochemically recurrent prostate cancer, 11C choline and 18F fluciclovine PET/CT detects multiple bone metastases. Patient with prostate cancer treated with radical surgery and hormonal therapy, now presenting with high and rapidly increasing prostate-specific antigen (PSA) (PSA trigger = 14.80 ng/mL; PSA doubling time, 2.8 months; A velocity, 33.5 ng/mL/y) underwent PET imaging. Both 11C choline (*A*, maximum intensity projection [MIP]) and 18F fluciclovine PET/computed tomography (CT) (*B*, MIP; *C*, sagittal fused) identified multiple avid bone lesions in right femur, right iliac bone, left pubis, multiple vertebra, sternum, and left scapula, corresponding with small osteosclerotic lesions on low-dose CT images (*D*, sagittal). Positive findings were concordant with the 2 tracers, although showing different uptake patterns. (*Courtesy of* Dr Cristina Nanni, Programma di ricerca Regione-Università 2010–2012 Regione Emilia Romagna-Bando Giovani Ricercatori, Bologna, Italy.)

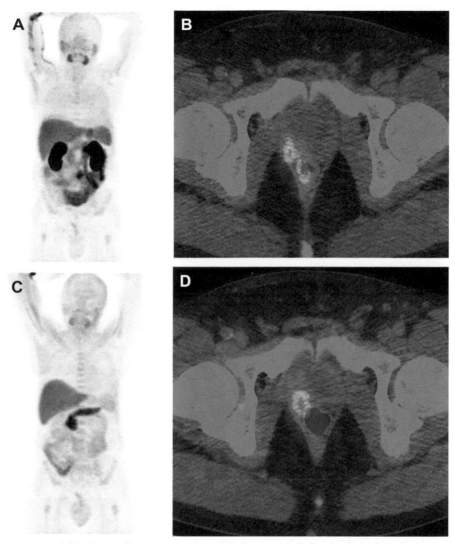

Fig. 3. In a patient with biochemically recurrent prostate cancer, 11C choline and 18F fluciclovine PET/computed tomography (CT) detect local relapse. A patient with prostate cancer treated with radical surgery, salvage radiation, and hormonal therapy, now presenting with rapidly increasing prostate-specific antigen (PSA) (PSA trigger, 4.8 ng/mL; PSA doubling time, 0.8 months; PSA velocity, 24.8 ng/mL/y) and inconclusive findings at conventional 18F choline PET/CT and MRI. Performed within 1 week, 11C choline PET/CT (*A, B,* maximum intensity projection and transaxial fused) and 18F fluciclovine (*C, D*) demonstrated focal uptake in the right prostate bed, more evident with the amino acidic compound. A subsequent transrectal ultrasound biopsy reported a 7- to 10-mm nodule of adenocarcinoma GS 4 + 4, confirming local relapse. (*Courtesy of* Dr Cristina Nanni, Programma di ricerca Regione-Università 2010–2012 Regione Emilia Romagna-Bando Giovani Ricercatori, Bologna, Italy.)

cancer with biochemical relapse when a single patient underwent both scans within 1 week (n = 89). With C-11 choline versus fluciclovine, sensitivity was 32% and 37%, specificity was 40% and 67%, PPV was 90% and 97%, NPV was 3% and 4%, and accuracy was 32% and 38%, respectively.[20] Overall, it was concluded that fluciclovine as an imaging radiotracer also demonstrates other advantages, including ease of production, longer half-life, and lower physiologic background activity.

Ga-68 PSMA also has demonstrated promising results for the imaging of patients with suspected prostate cancer relapse.[47–49,52] PSMA is overexpressed in prostate cancer cells. Targeting of PSMA expression was previously used in imaging with In-111-capromab pendetide directed to the intracellular epitope of the PSMA receptor, which significantly limits its diagnostic performance. Ga-68–labeled PSMA ligands have been structured to attach to the extracellular domain, significantly increasing sensitivity.[53,54] When Ga-68

PSMA performance was compared with F-18 choline within the same patients, Ga-68 PSMA was found to be superior to choline with significantly higher SUV_{max}. Ga-68 PSMA detected 56 lesions versus 26 with F-18 choline.[46] Similar results were published when Ga68-PSMA-11 was compared with C-11-choline.[55] The same pattern may well occur with fluciclovine in comparison to PSMA-based radiotracers. Direct comparison may be the subject of future research. As of today, Ga-68 production from each Ge-68/Ga-68 generator is limited. A recent publication by Bluemel and colleagues[56] suggests offering Ga-68-PSMA scans to those patients with negative choline images. Of 32 patients with negative F18 choline, 14 patients (43.8%) had positive Ga68-PSMA I&T scans. F-18–based PSMA tracers such as F-18 PSMA-1007 and [(18)F] DCFPyL are also being investigated, which may result in more widespread availability of PSMA PET.[57,58]

FLUCICLOVINE EVALUATION OF PRIMARY PROSTATE CANCER

Multiparametric MRI (MP-MRI) is considered the most useful single modality for the characterization of primary prostate cancer, although there are limitations including that of specificity.[44,59] Turkbey and colleagues[60] investigated the use of fluciclovine PET with MP-MRI for 22 patients with primary prostate cancer scheduled to undergo prostatectomy and whole mount histologic analysis. Although the mean SUV_{max} of the tumor was significantly higher than that of normal prostate tissue, there was a significant overlap of fluciclovine uptake between tumor foci and benign prostate hyperplasia. Adding the information from fluciclovine PET to MP-MRI increased the PPV from 50% for fluciclovine alone and 76% for MP-MRI alone to 82% for a combination of all methods. The limitations of fluciclovine for primary prostate cancer had also been reported previously by Schuster and colleagues[25] in a 10-patient study correlating fluciclovine uptake with MRI and histologic sextant analysis.[25] Although the study reported a correlation between SUV_{max} and Gleason score, and statistically significant differences in SUV_{max} between malignant and benign sextants, overlap was noted. No correlation was found between uptake (SUV_{max}) and Ki-67. Both studies concluded that fluciclovine imaging for the evaluation of primary prostate cancers was limited, although there may be some usefulness as an adjunct to MP-MRI and to help guide biopsy as well as possibly staging of high-risk disease. In addition, both studies suggested that delayed imaging, 15 to 20 minutes in the first study and 28 minutes in the second study, could improve diagnostic performance for the characterization of primary lesions (**Figs. 4** and **5**).

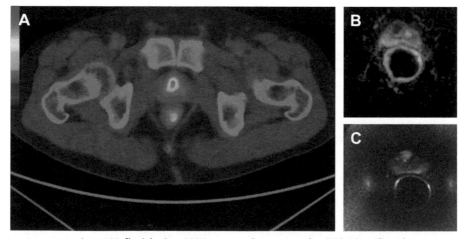

Fig. 4. Pretreatment staging 18F fluciclovine PET/computed tomography (CT) identifies the most predominant aggressive intraprostatic lesion in primary prostate cancer (in agreement with 11C choline and MP-MRI). A 71-year-old patient affected by high-risk prostate cancer (prostate-specific antigen, 8 ng/mL; GS 4 + 4; cT2) underwent multiparametric-MRI (*B*, axial T2-weighted image; *C*, axial diffusion-weighted imaging) and 11C choline PET/CT, as part of the normal staging workflow before radical surgery, and an additional 18F fluciclovine scan (*A*, transaxial fused), as part of an ongoing clinical trial. The procedures detected a focal right intermediate prostate lesion, corresponding to with 19-mm, GS 4 + 5 nodule of acinar adenocarcinoma. A smaller and less aggressive focus of GS 3 + 3 was under the limit of lesion detectability in all cases. (*Courtesy of* Dr Lucia Zanoni, Programma di ricerca Regione-Università Area 1-Bando Giovani ricercatori "Alessandro Liberati" 2013, Bologna, Italy.)

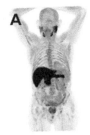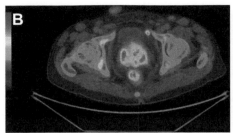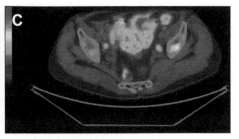

Fig. 5. Pretreatment staging 18F fluciclovine PET/computed tomography (CT) in a patient with primary prostate cancer, scheduled for radical surgery, detects multiple nodal and bone metastases leading to a change in treatment management. A patient with high-risk prostate cancer (prostate-specific antigen; 18.65; GS 4 + 5; 50% positive core biopsy) was scheduled for radical surgery and lymphadenectomy according to pelvic MRI and 11C choline PET/CT standard staging. The experimental tracer 18F fluciclovine detected multiple avid pelvic lymphadenopathies (*B* and *C*, transaxial fused) and inhomogeneous and diffuse uptake throughout the skeleton (*A*, maximum intensity projection). Considering the disease extent, the patient was finally excluded from surgery. (*Courtesy of* Dr Lucia Zanoni, Programma di ricerca Regione-Università Area 1-Bando Giovani ricercatori "Alessandro Liberati" 2013, Bologna, Italy.)

IMAGING PROTOCOL AND INTERPRETATIVE CRITERIA FOR SUSPECTED RECURRENT PROSTATE CANCER

Differing protocols of fluciclovine imaging have been reported.[19,22,24,25,35,37,40,61] During early clinical investigation, triple time point imaging of the abdomen and pelvis was used, and uptake was defined as mild, moderate, or intense when activity in the region of interest was visually below that of the bone marrow (typically at L3), equal to or greater than that of the bone marrow, and equal to or greater than that in the liver, respectively. Positive lesions were defined as persistent moderate or intense uptake based on early to delayed sequences.[24,37] Nevertheless, it was recognized that triple time point imaging is not clinically practical. A subsequent retrospective analysis compared results from early single time point imaging with multiple time point interpretation. It was concluded that early imaging with fluciclovine is feasible with modestly increased sensitivity and decreased specificity.[62] Other centers have also used whole body single time point imaging with success.[20] With the knowledge of efflux of radiotracer with a generally downsloping time activity curve, early imaging within the first 30 minutes after injection is therefore recommended. A protocol for imaging and study interpretation as adapted from the FDA package insert and the Axumin (fluciclovine F18) Imaging and Interpretation Manual is provided in **Table 1**, and it is recommended that the full documents be reviewed by the reader.[63]

As with other radiotracers, knowledge of normal physiologic distribution and variants as well as typical patterns of cancer recurrence is important for proper interpretation of fluciclovine PET. A comprehensive review paper describing radiotracer uptake patterns, incidental findings, and variants that may simulate disease is available.[23] Uptake may not only occur in prostate cancer, but also in other malignancies (**Fig. 6**). Gill and colleagues[64] reported abnormal fluciclovine uptake in male breast cancer incidentally found in a patient with suspected prostate cancer recurrence. It was noticed that liver metastatic lesions demonstrated decreased uptake compared with intense uptake of FDG on an intrapatient analysis. Hence, careful attention is required for evaluation of potential lesions in liver parenchyma. Fluciclovine uptake may also be present in benign conditions, such as inflammation and infection, and in other metabolically active benign lesions, such as meningioma and osteoid osteoma (**Fig. 7**).

For patients who have undergone nonprostatectomy therapy, nonspecific elevation of fluciclovine uptake in remaining prostate likely owing to underlying hyperplastic prostate tissue or inflammation may be present.[60] Moderate focal asymmetric uptake, visually equal to or greater than bone marrow, is considered suspicious for cancer recurrence. Ongoing studies are exploring the use of fluciclovine for biopsy planning for recurrent disease.[65] For patients with a history of prostatectomy, any focal uptake within the prostate bed or seminal vesicles may be considered abnormal especially if greater than bone marrow, although small lesions (<1 cm) subject to the partial volume effect may be suspicious if visually greater than blood pool. A review of sagittal images is especially useful for evaluation of the urethral anastomosis. Uptake within lymph nodes at sites of typical prostate cancer spread is highly specific for neoplastic involvement with a low false-positives rate, and understanding the common patterns of lymph node metastasis in prostate

Table 1
Axumin (fluciclovine F18) imaging and interpretation manual

Fluciclovine PET/CT	Description

Imaging protocol	• Patient preparation
	  ◦ Avoid significant exercise for ≥1 d before PET imaging.
	  ◦ Nothing to eat or drink for ≥4 h (other than small amounts of water for taking medications) before radiotracer administration.
	  ◦ Avoid voiding before starting the scanning procedure to decrease occasional variant bladder excretion.
	• Dose and injection
	  ◦ 10 mCi/370 MBq as an IV bolus injection while the patient is positioned in the PET/CT scanner with arms down.
	  ◦ Injection into the right arm is suggested to avoid misinterpretation of stasis in left axillary vein as Virchow node.
	  ◦ Subsequently, administer an intravenous flush of sterile sodium chloride injection, 0.9%, to ensure full delivery of the dose.
	• Image acquisition
	  ◦ Position the patient supine with arms above the head if possible.
	  ◦ High-quality CT acquisition for anatomic correlation and attenuation correction.
	  ◦ Begin PET 3–5 min after injection (goal of 4 min).
	  ◦ Image from the mid thighs to base of skull.
	  ◦ Imaging guidelines recommend 5 min per bed position acquisition in the pelvis and 3 min per bed position in the remainder of the body, but these suggestions are scanner dependent.
	• Image reconstruction
	  ◦ The highest quality scanner at an institution should be used.
	  ◦ If a scanner has time of flight, iterative reconstruction and/or a reconstruction algorithm using recovery resolution should be used.
	  ◦ Gaussian smoothing filter (if applicable) should not exceed 5 mm.

Diagnostic criteria	• Generally defined as
	  ◦ Localization of prostate cancer recurrence in sites typical for prostate cancer recurrence in comparison with tissue background.
	• Prostate/bed
	  ◦ Prostatectomy. Typical sites for local recurrence: Urethral anastomosis and seminal vesicle bed/remnants.
	    ■ Focal uptake, visually equal to or greater than bone marrow, in sites typical for prostate cancer recurrence suspicious for cancer.
	    However, if a focus of uptake is small (<1 cm), it may be considered suspicious if the if uptake is at or approaching marrow and significantly greater than blood pool
	• Nonprostatectomy.
	  ◦ Moderate focal asymmetric uptake, visually equal to or greater than bone marrow, is suspicious for cancer recurrence.
	    1. However, if a focus of uptake is small (<1 cm) and in a site typical for recurrence, it may still be considered suspicious if the uptake is visually greater than blood pool.
	• Lymph nodes
	  ◦ Typical sites for prostate cancer recurrence: external iliac (obturator), common iliac, aortocaval, paraaortic, retroperitoneal, and internal iliac/presacral lymph nodes.
	    ■ Uptake, visually equal to or greater than bone marrow, is considered suspicious for cancer.
	    However, if a node is small (<1 cm) and in a site typical for recurrence, it may still be considered suspicious if uptake is at or approaching marrow and significantly greater than blood pool.
	  ◦ Atypical sites for recurrence (inguinal, hilar, and axillary nodes).
	    ■ Mild, symmetric uptake is typically considered physiologic uptake, but if uptake is present within the context of other clear malignant disease, it may be considered suspicious for cancer recurrence.

(continued on next page)

Fluciclovine PET/CT	Description

	• Bone
	  ○ Focal uptake clearly visualized on MIP or PET-only images is considered suspicious for cancer.
	    1. A bone abnormality visualized on CT (eg, dense sclerosis without uptake) does not exclude the presence of metastasis. Alternative imaging, for example, MRI, NaF PET-CT, or SPECT-CT bone scan, should be considered.

Differential diagnosis	• Prostate
	  ○ Cancer, inflammatory changes, benign prostatic hypertrophy.
	• Extraprostate
	  ○ Typical locations for nodal spread of prostate cancer: metastatic prostate cancer.
	  ○ Uptake may occur in other cancers.
	  ○ Nodal inflammation, especially if mild and symmetric and in atypical locations for prostate cancer spread such as inguinal or distal external iliac.
	  ○ Uptake may also occur from benign processes such as infection, and metabolically active benign bone lesions such as osteoid osteoma.

Pearls, pitfalls, variants	• Performance affected by PSA levels. Positivity rate increases with increasing PSA.
	• Read from the "inside out." That is, be aware of typical locations for prostate cancer spread (eg, deep pelvic vs peripheral inguinal or distal external iliac nodes).
	  1. Mild benign symmetric uptake within the inguinal lymph nodes may be seen and should not be called positive unless "disease pattern marching out of pelvis."
	• Higher false-positive rate within intact or treated prostate.
	• Abnormal activity in postprostatectomy bed is more specific.
	  1. Sagittal images helpful with identification of disease at urethral anastomosis.
	• Uptake in lytic skeletal lesions is typically intense, moderate in mixed lesions, but may be absent in densely sclerotic lesions.
	  1. If skeletal lesion is seen on CT, consider skeletal-specific imaging.
	• Degenerative uptake in bone is not a common variant in fluciclovine as it is with FDG and should be further evaluated for the presence of metastatic bone lesions. Skeletal metastases that resemble Schmorl nodes but with fluciclovine uptake within them have been described.
	• Fluciclovine may be taken up by other cancer cells with upregulated amino acid transport. Be familiar with normal physiologic patterns of activity. In these instances, further correlation with clinical presentation and/or other imaging may be helpful.
	• In a small percentage of patients, fluciclovine may demonstrate moderate early bladder activity, interfering with evaluation of the prostate bed.
	• Liver uptake is very intense. SUV_{max} threshold should be increased to evaluate the liver for pathology
	• Bone marrow SUV mean values should be measured from the L3 vertebra, if possible (and likely representative of normal marrow).
	• Blood pool SUV mean should be measured from the same bed position of the suspected lesion (suggested site: aortic bifurcation). Measurements from the mediastinum may result in false low values owing to rapid tracer washout.

What the referring physician needs to know	• Fluciclovine PET/CT demonstrates usefulness in the localization of recurrent prostate cancer disease (FDA-approved indication). • Fluciclovine PET can identify true positive prostate cancer foci even when conventional imaging, such as CT, MRI, and bone scan, is negative. • No absolute PSA threshold is recommended. However, positivity is more likely with PSA >1 ng/mL or if PSA <1 ng/mL with rapid PSA kinetics. • Fluciclovine PET/CT scan should be considered before salvage therapy, for accurate treatment planning.

Abbreviations: CT, computed tomography; FDA, US Food and Drug Administration; FDG, fludeoxyglucose; IV, intravenous; MIP, maximum intensity projection; PSA, prostate-specific antigen; SPECT, single photon emission positron emission tomography; SUV_{max}, maximum standard uptake value.

From Savir-Baruch B, Zanoni L, Schuster DM. Imaging of prostate cancer using fluciclovine. PET Clin 2017;12(2):152–3; with permission.

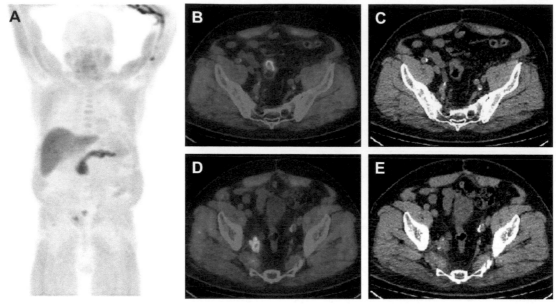

Fig. 6. In biochemically recurrent prostate cancer and incidental sigmoid cancer, 18F fluciclovine PET/computed tomography (CT) detects nodal metastasis. A patient with prostate cancer treated with radical surgery, salvage radiation, and hormonal therapy, now presents with low but rapidly increasing prostate-specific antigen (PSA) (PSA trigger, 0.94 ng/mL; PSA doubling time, 5.9 months; PSA velocity, 1.1 ng/mL/y) and negative transrectal ultrasound examination. The 18F fluciclovine image showed 2 focal lesions in maximum intensity projection images (A) corresponding with right internal iliac tissue (D, E transaxial fused and low-dose CT), causing grade II hydro-ureteronephrosis, and sigmoid wall thickening (B, C). Urologic contrast-enhanced CT scanning and bowel endoscopy confirmed the findings, in keeping with secondary nodal lesions from prostate cancer and new sigmoid cancer. The patient was treated with ureteral stenting, hormonal therapy, and bowel resection, achieving PSA response. (*Courtesy of* Dr Cristina Nanni, Programma di ricerca Regione-Università 2010–2012 Regione Emilia Romagna-Bando giovani Ricercatori, Bologna, Italy.)

cancer is essential to minimize false positive interpretation.[20,24,37,61] Uptake visually equal to or greater than that of lumbar marrow should be considered abnormal, although with nodes less than 1 cm, uptake may be suspicious if in a typical pattern of spread and greater than blood pool. Nevertheless, for example, inguinal lymph nodes may demonstrate nonspecific moderate symmetric inflammatory uptake. For bone lesions to be considered positive, focal uptake should be clearly seen on maximum intensity projection images. Densely sclerotic lesions may not be fluciclovine avid. In contradistinction to FDG-PET, degenerative uptake is not a common variant. Skeletal metastases resembling Schmorl nodes but with fluciclovine uptake have been described. **Table 1** provides more detailed interpretative guidelines as well as pearls, pitfalls, and variants.

GUIDELINES FOR THE USE OF FLUCICLOVINE IMAGING IN PATIENTS WITH RECURRENT PROSTATE CANCER

Fluciclovine PET is highly useful in the detection of recurrent prostate cancer even in the presence of negative or equivocal conventional imaging. The current FDA-approved indication is for men with suspected prostate cancer recurrence based on elevated blood PSA levels after prior treatment. There is no absolute threshold for PSA level in the recommendation of when to obtain fluciclovine PET, yet clearly, diagnostic performance varies with PSA level and kinetics. The fluciclovine PET positivity rate will increase with increasing PSA and with more rapid doubling times.[20,21,66] Based on logistic regression analysis in 1 study, a PSA of 1 ng/mL equated to a 71.8% probability of a positive fluciclovine scan.[37] One group has reported that functional imaging with choline or fluciclovine PET/CT together with MP-MRI to be the most valuable imaging techniques in the detection of prostate cancer relapse and should be highly considered before treatment planning.[67] The group acknowledged the limitation of these PET radiotracers with underlying low PSA levels of less than 1 ng/mL. They suggested that functional images may be cost effective when PSA velocity is high and PSA doubling time is short. Therefore, until more data are available, an elevated PSA or a concerning PSA velocity or doubling time, which

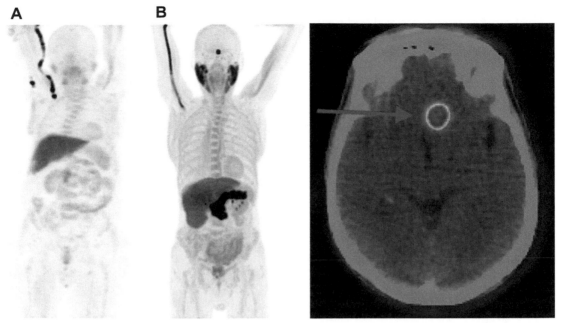

Fig. 7. Variants and pitfalls. (*A*) Uptake of 18F fluciclovine along the vessel of intravenous administration. (*B*) An 18F fluciclovine–avid meningioma. It is well-established that physiologic tracer biodistribution in normal brain is very low or absent. In this case, PET/computed tomography images showed intense and focal brain uptake (maximum standard uptake value, 17; maximum intensity projection and transaxial fused; *red arrow*) in keeping with known meningioma. (*Courtesy of* [*A*] Dr Cristina Nanni, Programma di ricerca Regione-Università 2010 to 2012 Regione Emilia Romagna-Bando Giovani Ricercatori, Bologna, Italy; and [*B*] Dr Lucia Zanoni, Programma di ricerca Regione-Università Area 1-Bando Giovani ricercatori "Alessandro Liberati" 2013, Bologna, Italy.)

clinically triggers salvage therapy in patients, may be a useful reference as to when a fluciclovine PET study should be obtained in suspected recurrent prostate cancer.

SUMMARY

Fluciclovine is currently FDA approved for the localization of recurrent prostate cancer in a patient with elevated PSA. Based on comprehensive clinical data, fluciclovine is beneficial in the identification of disease even when other conventional imaging is negative. Knowledge of normal physiologic distribution and variants as well as typical patterns of prostate cancer spread is important for proper interpretation of fluciclovine PET.

REFERENCES

1. Huang C, McConathy J. Radiolabeled amino acids for oncologic imaging. J Nucl Med 2013;54(7): 1007–10.
2. Jager PL, Vaalburg W, Pruim J, et al. Radiolabeled amino acids: basic aspects and clinical applications in oncology. J Nucl Med 2001;42(3):432–45.
3. Morgan TM, Koreckij TD, Corey E. Targeted therapy for advanced prostate cancer: inhibition of the PI3K/ Akt/mTOR pathway. Curr Cancer Drug Targets 2009; 9(2):237–49.
4. Wibmer AG, Burger IA, Sala E, et al. Molecular imaging of prostate cancer. Radiographics 2016; 36(1):142–59.
5. Chuaqui RF, Englert CR, Strup SE, et al. Identification of a novel transcript up-regulated in a clinically aggressive prostate carcinoma. Urology 1997; 50(2):302–7.
6. Cole KA, Chuaqui RF, Katz K, et al. cDNA sequencing and analysis of POV1 (PB39): a novel gene up-regulated in prostate cancer. Genomics 1998;51(2):282–7.
7. Fuchs BC, Bode BP. Amino acid transporters ASCT2 and LAT1 in cancer: partners in crime? Semin Cancer Biol 2005;15(4):254–66.
8. Heublein S, Kazi S, Ogmundsdottir MH, et al. Proton-assisted amino-acid transporters are conserved regulators of proliferation and amino-acid-dependent mTORC1 activation. Oncogene 2010; 29(28):4068–79.
9. Muller A, Chiotellis A, Keller C, et al. Imaging tumour ATB0,+ transport activity by PET with the cationic amino acid O-2((2-[18F]fluoroethyl)methyl-amino) ethyltyrosine. Mol Imaging Biol 2014;16(3):412–20.
10. Okudaira H, Shikano N, Nishii R, et al. Putative transport mechanism and intracellular fate of

trans-1-amino-3-18F-fluorocyclobutanecarboxylic acid in human prostate cancer. J Nucl Med 2011; 52(5):822–9.

11. Sakata T, Ferdous G, Tsuruta T, et al. L-type amino-acid transporter 1 as a novel biomarker for high-grade malignancy in prostate cancer. Pathol Int 2009;59(1):7–18.

12. Segawa A, Nagamori S, Kanai Y, et al. L-type amino acid transporter 1 expression is highly correlated with Gleason score in prostate cancer. Mol Clin Oncol 2013;1(2):274–80.

13. Smolarz K, Krause BJ, Graner FP, et al. (S)-4-(3-18F-fluoropropyl)-L-glutamic acid: an 18F-labeled tumor-specific probe for PET/CT imaging–dosimetry. J Nucl Med 2013;54(6):861–6.

14. Wang Q, Tiffen J, Bailey CG, et al. Targeting amino acid transport in metastatic castration-resistant prostate cancer: effects on cell cycle, cell growth, and tumor development. J Natl Cancer Inst 2013; 105(19):1463–73.

15. McConathy J, Yu W, Jarkas N, et al. Radiohalogen-ated nonnatural amino acids as PET and SPECT tumor imaging agents. Med Res Rev 2012;32(4): 868–905.

16. Oka S, Okudaira H, Yoshida Y, et al. Transport mechanisms of trans-1-amino-3-fluoro[1-(14)C] cyclobutanecarboxylic acid in prostate cancer cells. Nucl Med Biol 2012;39(1):109–19.

17. Okudaira H, Oka S, Ono M, et al. Accumulation of trans-1-amino-3-[(18)F]fluorocyclobutanecarboxylic acid in prostate cancer due to androgen-induced expression of amino acid transporters. Mol Imaging Biol 2014;16(6):756–64.

18. Ono M, Oka S, Okudaira H, et al. [(14)C]Fluciclovine (alias anti-[(14)C]FACBC) uptake and ASCT2 expression in castration-resistant prostate cancer cells. Nucl Med Biol 2015;42(11):887–92.

19. Nanni C, Schiavina R, Boschi S, et al. Comparison of 18F-FACBC and 11C-choline PET/CT in patients with radically treated prostate cancer and biochemical relapse: preliminary results. Eur J Nucl Med Mol Imaging 2013;40(Suppl 1):S11–7.

20. Nanni C, Zanoni L, Pultrone C, et al. (18)F-FACBC (anti1-amino-3-(18)F-fluorocyclobutane-1-carboxylic acid) versus (11)C-choline PET/CT in prostate cancer relapse: results of a prospective trial. Eur J Nucl Med Mol Imaging 2016;43(9):1601–10.

21. Odewole OA, Tade FI, Nieh PT, et al. Recurrent prostate cancer detection with anti-3-[18F]FACBC PET/CT: comparison with CT. Eur J Nucl Med Mol Imaging 2016;43(10):1773–83.

22. Schuster DM, Votaw JR, Nieh PT, et al. Initial experience with the radiotracer anti-1-amino-3-F-18-fluorocyclobutane-1-carboxylic acid with PET/CT in prostate carcinoma. J Nucl Med 2007;48(1):56–63.

23. Schuster DM, Nanni C, Fanti S, et al. Anti-1-amino-3-18F-fluorocyclobutane-1-carboxylic acid: physiologic uptake patterns, incidental findings, and variants that may simulate disease. J Nucl Med 2014;55(12): 1986–92.

24. Schuster DM, Savir-Baruch B, Nieh PT, et al. Detection of recurrent prostate carcinoma with anti-1-amino-3-18F-fluorocyclobutane-1-carboxylic acid PET/CT and 111In-capromab pendetide SPECT/CT. Radiology 2011;259(3):852–61.

25. Schuster DM, Taleghani PA, Nieh PT, et al. Characterization of primary prostate carcinoma by anti-1-amino-2-[(18)F]-fluorocyclobutane-1-carboxylic acid (anti-3-[(18)F] FACBC) uptake. Am J Nucl Med Mol Imaging 2013;3(1):85–96.

26. Sorensen J, Owenius R, Lax M, et al. Regional distribution and kinetics of [18F]fluciclovine (anti-[18F] FACBC), a tracer of amino acid transport, in subjects with primary prostate cancer. Eur J Nucl Med Mol Imaging 2013;40(3):394–402.

27. Nye JA, Schuster DM, Yu W, et al. Biodistribution and radiation dosimetry of the synthetic nonmeta-bolized amino acid analogue anti-18F-FACBC in humans. J Nucl Med 2007;48(6):1017–20.

28. Washburn LC, Sun TT, Anon JB, et al. Effect of structure on tumor specificity of alicyclic alpha-amino acids. Cancer Res 1978;38(8):2271–3.

29. Washburn LC, Sun TT, Byrd B, et al. 1-aminocyclo-butane[11C]carboxylic acid, a potential tumor-seeking agent. J Nucl Med 1979;20(10):1055–61.

30. Shoup TM, Olson J, Hoffman JM, et al. Synthesis and evaluation of [18F]1-amino-3-fluorocyclobutane-1-carboxylic acid to image brain tumors. J Nucl Med 1999;40(2):331–8.

31. Martarello L, McConathy J, Camp VM, et al. Synthesis of syn- and anti-1-amino-3-[18F]fluoromethyl-cyclobutane-1-carboxylic acid (FMACBC), potential PET ligands for tumor detection. J Med Chem 2002;45(11):2250–9.

32. McConathy J, Voll RJ, Yu W, et al. Improved synthesis of anti-[18F]FACBC: improved preparation of labeling precursor and automated radiosynthesis. Appl Radiat Isot 2003;58(6):657–66.

33. Oka S, Hattori R, Kurosaki F, et al. A preliminary study of anti-1-amino-3-18F-fluorocyclobutyl-1-carboxylic acid for the detection of prostate cancer. J Nucl Med 2007;48(1):46–55.

34. Okudaira H, Nakanishi T, Oka S, et al. Kinetic analyses of trans-1-amino-3-[18F]fluorocyclobutanecarboxylic acid transport in Xenopus laevis oocytes expressing human ASCT2 and SNAT2. Nucl Med Biol 2013; 40(5):670–5.

35. Schuster DM, Nye JA, Nieh PT, et al. Initial experience with the radiotracer anti-1-amino-3-[18F] Fluorocyclobutane-1-carboxylic acid (anti-[18F] FACBC) with PET in renal carcinoma. Mol Imaging Biol 2009;11(6):434–8.

36. Available at: http://www.blueearthdiagnostics.com/u-s-fda-approves-blue-earth-diagnostics-axumintm-

fluciclovine-f-18-injection-priority-review-pet-imaging-recurrent-prostate-cancer. Accessed July 29, 2016.

37. Schuster DM, Nieh PT, Jani AB, et al. Anti-3-[(18)F] FACBC positron emission tomography-computerized tomography and (111)In-capromab pendetide single photon emission computerized tomography-computerized tomography for recurrent prostate carcinoma: results of a prospective clinical trial. J Urol 2014;191(5):1446–53.

38. Cookson MS, Aus G, Burnett AL, et al. Variation in the definition of biochemical recurrence in patients treated for localized prostate cancer: the American Urological Association Prostate guidelines for localized prostate cancer update panel report and recommendations for a standard in the reporting of surgical outcomes. J Urol 2007;177(2):540–5.

39. Savir-Baruch B, Odewole O, Alaei Taleghani P, et al. Anti-3-[F18] FACBC uptake pattern in the prostate affects positive predictive value and is associated with the presence of brachytherapy seeds. J Nucl Med 2013;54(2_MeetingAbstracts):346.

40. Fanti S, Minozzi S, Castellucci P, et al. PET/CT with (11)C-choline for evaluation of prostate cancer patients with biochemical recurrence: meta-analysis and critical review of available data. Eur J Nucl Med Mol Imaging 2016;43(1):55–69.

41. Inoue Y, Asano Y, Satoh T, et al. Phase IIa clinical trial of trans-1-amino-3-18F-fluoro-cyclobutyl-carboxylic acid in metastatic prostate cancer. Asia Ocean J Nucl Med Biol 2014;2(2):87–94.

42. Gill H, Iclal E, Toslak E, Solanki AA, et al. Initial experience with commercial 18F-fluciclovin. Sunday November 26, 2017. SSA16-02 RSNA 2017. Chicago, 2017.

43. Sandblom G, Sorensen J, Lundin N, et al. Positron emission tomography with C11-acetate for tumor detection and localization in patients with prostate-specific antigen relapse after radical prostatectomy. Urology 2006;67(5):996–1000.

44. Mena E, Turkbey B, Mani H, et al. 11C-Acetate PET/CT in localized prostate cancer: a study with MRI and histopathologic correlation. J Nucl Med 2012; 53(4):538–45.

45. Brogsitter C, Zophel K, Kotzerke J. 18F-Choline, 11C-choline and 11C-acetate PET/CT: comparative analysis for imaging prostate cancer patients. Eur J Nucl Med Mol Imaging 2013;40(Suppl 1): S18–27.

46. Afshar-Oromieh A, Zechmann CM, Malcher A, et al. Comparison of PET imaging with a (68)Ga-labelled PSMA ligand and (18)F-choline-based PET/CT for the diagnosis of recurrent prostate cancer. Eur J Nucl Med Mol Imaging 2014;41(1):11–20.

47. Afshar-Oromieh A, Hetzheim H, Kubler W, et al. Radiation dosimetry of (68)Ga-PSMA-11 (HBED-CC) and preliminary evaluation of optimal imaging timing. Eur J Nucl Med Mol Imaging 2016;43(9):1611–20.

48. Afshar-Oromieh A, Haberkorn U, Schlemmer HP, et al. Comparison of PET/CT and PET/MRI hybrid systems using a 68Ga-labelled PSMA ligand for the diagnosis of recurrent prostate cancer: initial experience. Eur J Nucl Med Mol Imaging 2014;41(5):887–97.

49. Afshar-Oromieh A, Avtzi E, Giesel FL, et al. The diagnostic value of PET/CT imaging with the (68)Ga-labelled PSMA ligand HBED-CC in the diagnosis of recurrent prostate cancer. Eur J Nucl Med Mol Imaging 2015;42(2):197–209.

50. Ackerstaff E, Pflug BR, Nelson JB, et al. Detection of increased choline compounds with proton nuclear magnetic resonance spectroscopy subsequent to malignant transformation of human prostatic epithelial cells. Cancer Res 2001;61(9):3599–603.

51. Cimitan M, Evangelista L, Hodolic M, et al. Gleason score at diagnosis predicts the rate of detection of 18F-choline PET/CT performed when biochemical evidence indicates recurrence of prostate cancer: experience with 1,000 patients. J Nucl Med 2015;56:209–15.

52. Freitag MT, Radtke JP, Hadaschik BA, et al. Comparison of hybrid (68)Ga-PSMA PET/MRI and (68)Ga-PSMA PET/CT in the evaluation of lymph node and bone metastases of prostate cancer. Eur J Nucl Med Mol Imaging 2016;43(1):70–83.

53. Lutje S, Heskamp S, Cornelissen AS, et al. PSMA ligands for radionuclide imaging and therapy of prostate cancer: clinical status. Theranostics 2015;5(12): 1388–401.

54. Lutje S, Rijpkema M, Franssen GM, et al. Dual-modality image-guided surgery of prostate cancer with a radiolabeled fluorescent anti-PSMA monoclonal antibody. J Nucl Med 2014;55(6):995–1001.

55. Schwenck J, Rempp H, Reischl G, et al. Comparison of (68)Ga-labelled PSMA-11 and (11)C-choline in the detection of prostate cancer metastases by PET/CT. Eur J Nucl Med Mol Imaging 2017;44:92–101.

56. Bluemel C, Krebs M, Polat B, et al. 68Ga-PSMA-PET/CT in patients with biochemical prostate cancer recurrence and negative 18F-Choline-PET/CT. Clin Nucl Med 2016;41:515–21.

57. Dietlein M, Kobe C, Kuhnert G, et al. Comparison of [(18)F]DCFPyL and [(68)Ga]Ga-PSMA-HBED-CC for PSMA-PET imaging in patients with relapsed prostate cancer. Mol Imaging Biol 2015;17:575–84.

58. Giesel FL, Hadaschik B, Cardinale J, et al. F-18 labelled PSMA-1007: biodistribution, radiation dosimetry and histopathological validation of tumor lesions in prostate cancer patients. Eur J Nucl Med Mol Imaging 2017;44:678–88.

59. Turkbey B, Albert PS, Kurdziel K, et al. Imaging localized prostate cancer: current approaches and new developments. AJR Am J Roentgenol 2009;192(6):1471–80.

60. Turkbey B, Mena E, Shih J, et al. Localized prostate cancer detection with 18F FACBC PET/CT: comparison with MR imaging and histopathologic analysis. Radiology 2014;270(3):849–56.

61. Nanni C, Schiavina R, Brunocilla E, et al. 18F-fluci-clovine PET/CT for the detection of prostate cancer relapse: a comparison to 11C-choline PET/CT. Clin Nucl Med 2015;40(8):e386–91.

62. Savir-Baruch B, Odewole O, Master V, et al. Diagnostic performance of synthetic amino acid anti-3-[18F] FACBC PET in recurrent prostate carcinoma utilizing single-time versus dual-time point criteria. J Nucl Med 2014;55(Suppl 1):21.

63. Available at: http://www.axumin.com/. Accessed July 30, 2016.

64. Gill HS, Tade F, Greenwald DT, et al. Metastatic male breast cancer with increased uptake on 18F-Fluci-clovine PET/CT scan. Clin Nucl Med 2018;43:23–4.

65. Fei B, Nieh PT, Schuster DM, et al. PET-directed, 3D Ultrasound-guided prostate biopsy. Diagn Imaging Eur 2013;29(1):12–5.

66. Kairemo K, Rasulova N, Partanen K, et al. Preliminary clinical experience of trans-1-amino-3-(18)F-fluorocyclobutanecarboxylic acid (anti-(18) F-FACBC) PET/CT imaging in prostate cancer patients. Biomed Res Int 2014;2014:305182.

67. Schiavina R, Brunocilla E, Borghesi M, et al. Diagnostic imaging work-up for disease relapse after radical treatment for prostate cancer: how to differentiate local from systemic disease? The urologist point of view. Rev Esp Med Nucl Imagen Mol 2013;32(5):310–3.

Advances in Urologic Imaging
Prostate-Specific Membrane Antigen Ligand PET Imaging

Michael S. Hofman, MBBS, FRACP, FAANMS[a,b],
Amir Iravani, MD, FRACP[a,*],
Tatenda Nzenza, BMedSci, MBBS, PGDipAnat[c],
Declan G. Murphy, MBBS, FRACS[d]

KEYWORDS

- Prostate cancer • Prostate-specific membrane antigen • PET • PSMA PET/CT • PSMA PET

KEY POINTS

- Prostate-specific membrane antigen PET (PSMA PET) imaging is a valuable diagnostic tool with promising performance for detection of prostate cancer and its metastases.
- PSMA PET imaging has the advantage of high specificity, independence of PSA-level, and low nonspecific tracer uptake in surrounding tissue.
- Although PSMA imaging has been most commonly investigated in the biochemical recurrence of prostate cancer, an increasing number of studies are exploring its utility in the different aspects of prostate cancer management.
- Multiple studies have consistently shown high clinical impact of PSMA imaging in guiding the management of prostate cancer.
- PSMA may prove an important imaging biomarker in prostate cancer, paving the way for precision medicine.

INTRODUCTION

Prostate cancer (PCa) is one of the most common malignancies in men worldwide and leads to substantial morbidity and mortality. Imaging is indicated in multiple aspects of PCa management, including primary diagnosis, staging, localization of recurrent disease, and response assessment in metastatic disease. Currently, conventional imaging modalities, including, bone scintigraphy, computed tomography (CT), and MRI, are used to detect primary and metastatic PCa for staging and risk stratification.

The main limitation of conventional imaging modalities is their low sensitivity in detecting metastases in primary diagnosis or in recurrent PCa,

Portions of this article were previously published in *PET Clinics* 12:2, April 2017.
Disclosure Statement: The authors have nothing to disclose.
[a] Department of Cancer Imaging, Centre for Molecular Imaging, Peter MacCallum Cancer Centre, 305 Grattan Street, Melbourne, Victoria 3000, Australia; [b] Sir Peter MacCallum Department of Oncology, University of Melbourne, 305 Grattan Street, Melbourne, Victoria 3000, Australia; [c] Sir Peter MacCallum Department of Surgical Oncology, University of Melbourne and Austin Hospital, 305 Grattan Street, Melbourne, Victoria 3000, Australia; [d] Sir Peter MacCallum Department of Surgical Oncology, University of Melbourne, 305 Grattan Street, Melbourne, Victoria 3000, Australia
* Corresponding author.
E-mail address: Amir.iravani@petermac.org

Urol Clin N Am 45 (2018) 503–524
https://doi.org/10.1016/j.ucl.2018.03.016

especially with low prostatic-specific antigen (PSA) levels when disease is often small in volume. In a meta-analysis of 24 studies the pooled sensitivity and specificity of CT for lymph node (LN) diagnosis was 42% and 82% respectively. For MRI, this review reported the pooled sensitivity and specificity of 39% and 82%, respectively.[1]

Molecular imaging with PET using an increasing list of biologically relevant radiotracers is facilitating precision and personalized medicine in PCa.[2] Prostate-specific membrane antigen (PSMA) has received a resurgence of attention over the last few years as a useful biomarker in the imaging of PCa. Among the available tracers and ligands available to image PSMA-expressing tumors, 68Ga-PSMA HBED-CC or 68Ga-PSMA-11, developed by the Heidelberg group in Germany, has become a successful radiotracer for PET/CT imaging with rapid adoption across many countries.[3–5] Subsequently, second-generation fluorinated PSMA agents (fluorine 18 [18F]-DCFPyL and 18F-PSMA-1007) offered several advantages, especially the possibility of large-scale batch production; but published experience with these agents remains limited. In this article, the current position of the literature in the role of advanced molecular imaging in different aspects of PCa management is presented.

RADIOLABELED PROSTATE-SPECIFIC MEMBRANE ANTIGEN LIGANDS

PSMA is a type II integral membrane glycoprotein that was first detected on the human prostatic carcinoma cell line LN cancer of prostate (LNCaP).[6] It consists of 750 amino acid integral membrane glycoprotein (100–120 kDa), with a 19 amino acid intracellular component, a 24 amino acid intramembrane segment, and a large 707 amino acid extracellular domain.[7] It has several enzymatic functions and is known to be upregulated in castrate-resistant and metastatic PCa.[8] PSMA is not specific to the prostate gland and is expressed in other normal tissues, including salivary glands, duodenal mucosa, proximal renal tubular cells, and subpopulation of neuroendocrine cells in the colonic crypts. In PCa, PSMA is overexpressed in the order of 100 to 1000 times compared with normal prostate tissue.[9] Overexpression occurs in greater than 90% of local PCa lesions as well as in metastatic LNs and bone metastases.[10–12] There is no known natural ligand for PSMA, and the reasons for its upregulation in PCa remain unclear. PSMA undergoes constitutive internalization and, therefore, can serve not only as an imaging biomarker but is also suitable for theranostic agents by attaching to radioactive molecules enabling targeted delivery of radiation to the sites of tumors.[13–17]

PSMA expression seems to increase with higher tumor grade and pathologic stage. Of clinical importance is that PSMA expression is upregulated when tumors become androgen independent and also following antiandrogen therapy (ADT).[18] This characteristic makes PSMA particularly valuable because it has potential as an early indicator of tumor progression after ADT and could play a role as a prognostic factor for disease recurrence.[19]

One of the first imaging probes specifically targeting PSMA was indium 111 (111In)–capromab pendetide, an 111In-labeled anti-PSMA antibody.[20] A significant limitation of capromab pendetide is binding to the intracellular epitope of the transmembrane PSMA glycoprotein. Therefore, capromab pendetide either binds to viable tumor cells following internalization or to dying cells with disrupted cellular membranes. Furthermore, slow plasma clearance of the antibody results in relatively poor tumor-to-background contrast; the application of 111In-capromab pendetide for imaging prostatic malignancies remained limited.[21,22]

Subsequently, high affinity antibodies directed against extracellular epitopes of PSMA have been developed, such as J415, J533, and J591.[23] It was shown that 111In-J591 accurately targets bone and soft tissue metastatic PCa lesions[24] and that lutetium 177 (177Lu)–labeled J591 can be used safely in radioimmunotherapy directed against micrometastatic PCa.[25] Major disadvantages limiting the use of radiolabeled monoclonal antibodies as theranostic radiopharmaceuticals are their relatively long circulatory half-life (3–4 days), poor tumor penetration, and low tumor-to-normal tissue ratios, especially at early time points. Small molecules, in contrast, exhibit rapid extravasation, rapid diffusion in the extravascular space, and faster blood clearance which results in high tumor-normal tissue contrast early after injection of the tracer.

In search for PSMA tracers with such favorable characteristics, modified forms of N-acetyl-L-aspartyl-L-glutamate peptidase (NAALAdase) inhibitors, which were originally developed for possible neuroprotective effects in neurologic disorders, such as amyotrophic lateral sclerosis,[26] have been evaluated for their potential to diagnose and treat PCa. A series of preclinical studies evaluated the role of radiolabeled small-molecule PSMA-inhibiting ligands for imaging of human PCa using various radionuclides, such as carbon 11 (11C),[27] 18F,[28] iodine 123 (123I),[29] technetium-99m (99mTc),[30,31] and 68Ga.[32,33] Overall, the

PSMAs tested in these preclinical studies showed high tumor uptake peaking at 0.5 to 1.0 hour in mice with PSMA-expressing tumors. For imaging purposes, this time frame matches best with radio-nuclides with half-lives of 1 to 2 hours, such as ^{68}Ga or ^{18}F. In some of these preclinical studies, remarkable changes in affinity and tumor uptake were observed on changes in the radiolabel, chelator, and linker. First, it has been suggested that a spacer is required between the PSMA binding motif and the chelator. Chen and colleagues[34] compared PSMAs with different linker lengths and showed that an increased linker length enhanced the affinity for PSMA and increased tumor uptake.

Since 2012, numerous clinical studies using a variety of urea-based PSMAs have been undertaken, including $^{123/124/131}$IMIP-1072/-1095,[35] ^{99m}Tc-MIP-1404/-1405,[36] ^{68}Ga-HBED-PSMA, ^{18}F-DCFBC,[37] ^{18}F-DCFPyl,[38] and ^{68}Ga-THP-PSMA.[39] Among these agents, the ^{68}Ga- and ^{18}F-labeled compounds have attracted the most attention, as these compounds can be used for PET/CT imaging. However, the availability of ^{123}I or ^{99m}Tc allows single-photon emission CT/CT imaging in centers without facilities for PET.

PET/COMPUTED TOMOGRAPHY IMAGING WITH GALLIUM 68 RADIOLABELED PROSTATE-SPECIFIC MEMBRANE ANTIGEN

During the past few years, the application of ^{68}Ga-labeled peptides has attracted considerable interest for cancer imaging because of the physical characteristics of ^{68}Ga[40] and the availability of reliable germanium 68 (^{68}Ge)/^{68}Ga generators. This development enabled ^{68}Ga-dodecanetetraacetic acid (Tyr3)-octreotate (DOTATATE) PET/CT imaging of neuroendocrine tumors[41,42] owing to the rapid binding and cellular uptake of DOTATATE, and this is now widely recognized as the new gold standard for imaging these tumors. Moreover, the half-life of ^{68}Ga is suitable for the pharmacokinetics of the small PSMA-inhibiting peptides, which have rapid binding and cellular uptake.

Some of the first PSMA inhibitors available for labeling with ^{68}Ga and PET imaging of PCa were 1,4,7,10-tetraazacyclododecane-1,4,7,10-tetraacetic acid–conjugated urea-based PSMA inhibitors, developed and tested preclinically by Banerjee and colleagues.[32] Eder and colleagues[43] prepared the ^{68}Ga-labeled PSMA inhibitor Glu-NH-CO-NHLys(Ahx)-HBED-CC using the chelator HBED-CC. ^{68}Ga-labeled HBED-CC, also known as ^{68}Ga-PSMA-11, showed fast blood clearance, relatively low liver uptake, and high specific uptake in PSMA-expressing tissues and tumor.

Based on the promising preclinical results, the German Cancer Research Center in Heidelberg performed the first clinical investigation of the ^{68}Ga-PSMA-11 in a cohort of 37 patients. In 84% of the patients, PCa lesions were identified. PCa lesions were found in 60% of the patients with PSA levels less than 2.2 ng/mL, whereas at PSA levels greater than 2.2 ng/mL, PCa lesions were found in all patients. Thus, even at relatively low blood PSA levels, ^{68}Ga-PSMA-11 PET/CT identified lesions with high tumor-to-background ratios. Tumor uptake of ^{68}Ga-PSMA-11 was stable between 1 hour and 3 hours, whereas in normal tissue uptake it slightly decreased between 1 and 3 hours. As a result, late scans exhibited higher tumor-to-background ratios, which might be useful when lesions remain unclear in an early scan.[4] Currently this tracer is the most commonly investigated PSMA agent around the world.

Limitations of ^{68}Ga-PSMA-11 are the synthesis time and the need for on-site radiopharmaceutical expertise or the use of automated synthesis devices, which add additional cost. More recently a new radiopharmaceutical, ^{68}Ga-tris(hydroxypyridinone) (THP)–PSMA, has been developed with a simplified design for one-step kit-based radiolabeling.[44] THP ligand complexes ^{68}Ga3+ rapidly at low concentration, room temperature, and over a wide pH range, enabling direct elution from a ^{68}Ge/^{68}Ga generator into a lyophilized kit in one step without manipulation. Hofman and colleagues,[39] in a first in-human study, evaluated the safety and bio-distribution of this tracer. In this study a head-to-head comparison was performed between ^{68}Ga-PSMA-11 and ^{68}Ga-THP-PSMA in 6 patients. In 5 of 6 patients there was concordance in the number of metastases identified with ^{68}Ga-PSMA-11 and ^{68}Ga-THP-PSMA. In 22 malignant lesions, tumor-to-liver contrast was similar on THP-PSMA compared with PSMA-11, although absolute tumor uptake was significantly higher with PSMA-11 (**Fig. 1**).

PET/COMPUTED TOMOGRAPHY IMAGING WITH FLUORINE 18 RADIOLABELED PROSTATE-SPECIFIC MEMBRANE ANTIGEN

^{18}F-labeled PSMA compounds have several advantages, including large-scale batch production capacity, owing to a higher available amount of the radioisotope ^{18}F produced by a cyclotron compared with ^{68}Ga eluted from a generator.[45] Furthermore, the nuclear decay characteristics of ^{18}F, such as optimal positron energy (0.65 MeV compared with 1.9 MeV ^{68}Ga with shorter tissue penetration and theoretic higher spatial resolution) and a longer half-life (110 minutes compared with 68 minutes for ^{68}Ga enabling delayed PET acquisition), may also translate into refined imaging quality.[45] Unlike

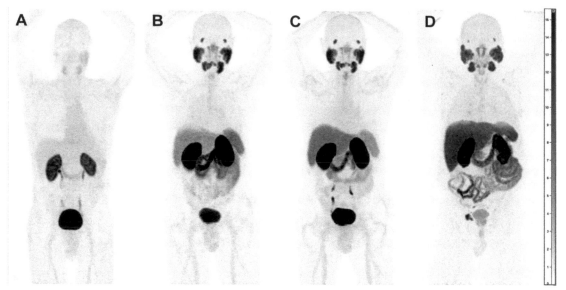

Fig. 1. Physiologic biodistribution of different PSMA PET agents. Maximum intensity projection images of ^{68}Ga-THP-PSMA (*A*), [68]G-PSMA-11 (*B*), ^{18}F-DCFPyL (*C*), and ^{18}F-PSMA-1007 (*D*). Each image is windowed to the same intensity as shown by the intensity scale on the right side demonstrating a fixed upper standardized uptake value threshold. Increasing physiologic hepatic uptake is seen from the left to right PSMA agents. In panel (*D*), PSMA-expressing right pelvic LNs are seen.

^{68}Ga-PSMA-11, the ^{18}F-PSMA compounds are all patented, which may result in higher costs, although commercial development may facilitate the conduct of clinical trials and evidence base required for reimbursement (**Table 1**).

Mease and colleagues[28] described a first-generation ^{18}F-labeled PSMA ligand, ^{18}F-DCFBC. In a clinical study, researchers investigated ^{18}F-DCFBC in 5 patients who had radiological evidence of metastatic disease, and imaging with ^{18}F-DCFBC identified more suspicious lesions than bone scintigraphy or CT.[37] In another preliminary study in 13 patients with PCa, ^{18}F-DCFBC–PET was able to reliably detect clinically significant high-grade (Gleason scores [GS] 8 and 9) and large-volume tumors with relatively low uptake in benign prostatic lesions.[46] However, the major disadvantage of this agent was the considerable blood pool activity, which could potentially interfere with the detection of LN metastases.[37]

Subsequently in 2011, a second-generation ^{18}F-labelled PSMA ligand ^{18}F-DCFPyL was introduced, with favorable results for tissue binding in vitro and in vivo. In the first clinical investigation in 9 patients, ^{18}F-DCFPyL showed very high levels of uptake in sites of metastatic disease as well as in primary tumors.[38] Very low blood pool activity was observed; the conspicuousness of lesions was notably higher with ^{18}F-DCFPyL than with the first-generation radiotracer ^{18}F-DCFBC, making it a promising agent. Data from a first preliminary study

comparing ^{68}Ga-PSMA-11 with ^{18}F-DCFPyL showed that ^{18}F-DCFPyL had a better tumor-to-background ratio, and additional lesions consistent with metastases were detected in 3 of the 14 patients.[45] In a retrospective study, Dietlein and colleagues[47] compared the diagnostic performance of ^{18}F-DCFPyL (62 patients) and ^{68}Ga-PSMA-11 (129 patients) in biochemical recurrence (BCR), which was stratified by PSA levels and matched by GS. ^{18}F-DCFPyL was found noninferior to ^{68}Ga-PSMA-11. In addition, in a subcohort of 25 patients who underwent imaging with both tracers, head-to-head comparison showed noninferiority of the ^{18}F-DCFPyL.

The other promising second-generation ^{18}F-labeled PSMA ligand is ^{18}F-PSMA-1007, which is structurally related to PSMA-617. In an initial study by Giesel and colleagues[48] in 10 patients with primary high-risk PCa with histopathologic validation, ^{18}F-PSMA-1007 correctly detected the primary site and LN metastases in most patients. ^{18}F-PSMA-1007 was reported favorable for primary tumors and local relapse due to low urinary excretion with 1.2% injected dose (ID) over 2 hours, compared with greater than 10% ID over 2 hours in other commonly used PSMA tracers, including ^{18}F-DCFPyL, ^{68}Ga-PSMA-11, and ^{68}Ga-PSMA-617.[49] In an another pilot study by the same group in 12 patients with treatment-naïve PCa, head-to-head comparison was made between ^{18}F-DCFPyL and ^{18}F-PSMA-1007.[50] The investigators reported excellent imaging quality and identical findings for both fluorinated PSMA agents (see **Fig. 1**).

COMPARISON BETWEEN PROSTATE-SPECIFIC MEMBRANE ANTIGEN PET/COMPUTED TOMOGRAPHY AND FLUORINE 18–FLUCICLOVINE PET/COMPUTED TOMOGRAPHY

Upregulation of amino acid transport occurs in some neoplastic processes, such as PCa. Therefore, using an amino acid–based radiotracer can identify the PCa tissues more reliably than conventional imaging techniques. Anti-1-amino-3-F-18-fluorocyclobutane-1-carboxylic acid (fluciclovine) is a synthetic amino acid analogue for which the most comprehensive clinical studies for PCa have been performed to date.[51] Based on multiple studies on 877 subjects, including 797 subjects with PCa, the Food and Drug Administration's approval was granted to ^{18}F-fluciclovine in May 2016 for the clinical indication of suspected PCa recurrence based on elevated PSA levels following prior treatment.[52] Subsequently this led to the Centers for Medicare and Medicaid Services' reimbursement in 2017 for patients with PCa recurrence. Thus, it could serve as a reference standard for evaluating other PET molecular imaging agents under investigation for PCa.

In one of the main retrospective studies, the diagnostic performance of ^{18}F-fluciclovine PET was evaluated in 596 patients with BCR, of whom 143 were assessed against the histologic reference standard.[53] The detection rate in the whole population (mean PSA 5.43 ng/mL) was 67.7%, and it was 41.4% in the lowest quartile of serum PSA levels (<0.79 ng/mL). Although several studies reported higher diagnostic performance of ^{68}Ga-PSMA-11 PET/CT imaging,[54,55] there is only one small case series of head-to-head comparison between these two agents.[56] In this case series including 10 patients with BCR, 7 out of 10 (70%) studies were positive with ^{68}Ga-PSMA-11, whereas 8 out of 10 (80%) ^{18}F-fluciclovine scans were negative; the disease extent was underestimated in both patients with a positive ^{18}F-fluciclovine study. Importantly, 4 ^{18}F-fluciclovine scans were negative despite extensive disease on ^{68}Ga-PSMA-11 scans. It should be noted that the absence of significant tracer excretion in the urine is one of the advantages of ^{18}F-fluciclovine, making detection of the small-volume disease in the prostate bed or pelvic LNs easier; but high uptake in the bone marrow and liver may interfere with the detection of metastases at these sites (**Fig. 2**; see **Table 1**).

COMPARISON BETWEEN PROSTATE-SPECIFIC MEMBRANE ANTIGEN PET/COMPUTED TOMOGRAPHY AND RADIOLABELED CHOLINE PET/COMPUTED TOMOGRAPHY

The use of radiolabeled choline PET/CT for imaging PCa is based on increased phosphorylcholine levels and an elevated phosphatidylcholine turnover in PCa cells. Radiolabeled choline PET/CT is a clinically valuable tool for restaging patients with BCR.[62] ^{68}Ga-PSMA has shown substantially higher detection rates compared with radiolabeled choline PET/CT, including ^{11}C-choline or ^{18}F-fluorocholine.[63] Bluemel and colleagues[64] investigated the value of ^{68}Ga-PSMA-11 PET/CT in patients with biochemically recurring PCa with negative ^{18}F-fluoro-choline PET/CT. With the sequential imaging approach, ^{68}Ga-PSMA-11 identified sites of recurrent disease in 43.8% of the patients with negative ^{18}F-fluoro-choline. Subgroup analysis of ^{68}Ga-PSMA-11 in ^{18}F-fluoro-choline–negative patients revealed detection rates of 28.6%, 45.5%, and 71.4% for PSA levels of 0.2 to 1.0 ng/mL, 1 to 2 ng/mL, and greater than 2 ng/mL, respectively (**Fig. 3**).

POTENTIAL CLINICAL INDICATIONS OF PROSTATE-SPECIFIC MEMBRANE ANTIGEN IMAGING

Since 2012, an increasing number of studies have evaluated the utility of PSMA PET imaging in different aspects of PCa, including screening, active surveillance, primary detection, risk stratification, targeted biopsy, primary staging, persisting raised PSA and BCR following radical treatment (radical prostatectomy [RP], radiotherapy [RT], or brachytherapy), salvage treatment following radical treatment (LN dissection [LND], RT), targeted treatment of oligometastatic disease, and response assessment of systemic and targeted treatment (**Table 2**).

Prostate-Specific Membrane Antigen Imaging in Primary Detection, Risk Stratification, and Systematic Versus Targeted Biopsy

The ability to accurately diagnose clinically significant PCa and risk stratify patients based on cancer aggressiveness is invaluable. This ability is determined by several factors, including PSA level and International Society of Urologic Pathology (ISUP) grade group, which facilitates care decisions, varied from active surveillance to RP or RT. The current standard technique for diagnosis of PCa is transrectal/transperineal ultrasound-guided needle biopsy (TPUS-GB).[65] Despite systematic 10 to 12 core biopsies, in 10% to 25% of cases with initial

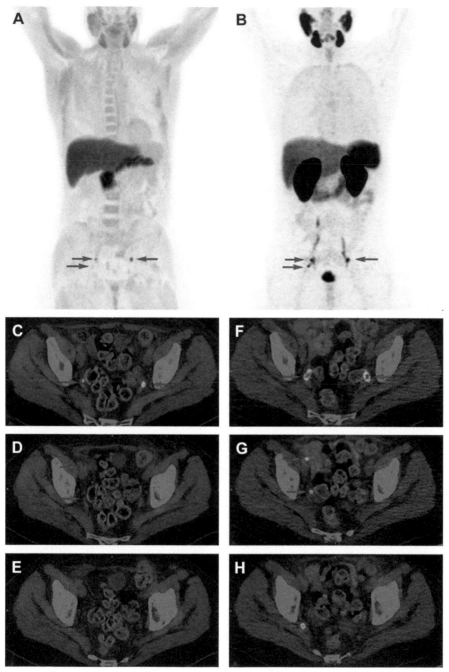

Fig. 2. Comparative ^{18}F-fluciclovine and ^{68}Ga-PSMA-11 PET/CT of a patient with BCR (PSA 12 ng/mL) with 1-week interval between scans. ^{18}F-fluciclovine PET maximum intensity projection (MIP) (*A*) and PET/CT (*C–E*) images show physiologic distribution of this tracer and increased uptake in bilateral subcentimeter pelvic LNs (*arrows*). ^{68}Ga-PSMA-11 PET MIP (*B*) and PET/CT (*F–H*) images demonstrate bilateral pelvic LNs (*arrows*) with 2- to 3-fold higher tumor-to-background contrast and maximum standardized uptake value range of 7 to 19 compared with 3 to 9 in ^{18}F-fluciclovine.

negative TRUS-GB, repeat biopsy will yield positive results. Furthermore, in just more than a third of patients, ISUP grade group will be upgraded following prostatectomy.[66,67]

Multi-parametric MRI (mpMRI) has shown promising results in multiple single-center studies for localizing aggressive tumors with a negative predictive value (NPV) and positive predictive

Table 1
Characteristics of the most commonly used prostate-specific membrane antigen PET tracers and fluciclovine

	PSMA-11	DCFPyL	PSMA-1007	Fluciclovine
Target	PSMA	PSMA	PSMA	Amino acid analogue
Radiotracer	^{68}Ga	^{18}F	^{18}F	^{18}F
Production	Generator[a]	Cyclotron	Cyclotron	Cyclotron
Half-life (min)[b]	68	110	110	110
Positron energy (MeV)[c]	1.9	0.65	0.65	0.65
Effective radiation dose (mSv/MBq)	1.6–2.3E-02[57,58]	1.4E-02[38]	2.2E-02[48]	1.6–2.2E-02[59,60]
Urinary excretion[d]	++++	++++	+	−
Hepatic uptake[e]	+	++	+++	+++
Bone marrow uptake[e]	−	−	−	++
Intellectual property	No patent	Patented	Patented	Patented

Abbreviations: +, indicates its presence and number of "+" would indicate relative intensity of excretion or uptake; −, indicates absence of tracer excretion or uptake.

  [a] Cyclotron production of ^{68}Ga is in development.[61] Generator enables on-site on-demand production. Cyclotron enables large-scale production and distribution.

  [b] Longer half-life enables delayed imaging.

  [c] Lower positron energy yields lower radiation burden but may negate with higher half-life.

  [d] Lower urinary excretion has the advantage in the assessment of prostate bed.

  [e] Higher hepatic or bone marrow uptake may interfere with assessment of these sites.

value (PPV) ranging from 63% to 98% and from 34% to 68%.[68,69] The combination of systematic and targeted biopsies (MRI-Tbx) may also better predict the final ISUP grade group.[70] Therefore, some investigators proposed performing mpMRI before a prostate biopsy.[71] However, 2 more recent randomized controlled trials restricted to the initial biopsy yielded contradictory results regarding the added value of MRI-Tbx combined with systematic biopsies.[72,73] Major limitations of mpMRI, however, are its interobserver variability. The Prostate Imaging Reporting and Data System (PI-RADS) scoring system version 1 and more recently version 2 have been designed to

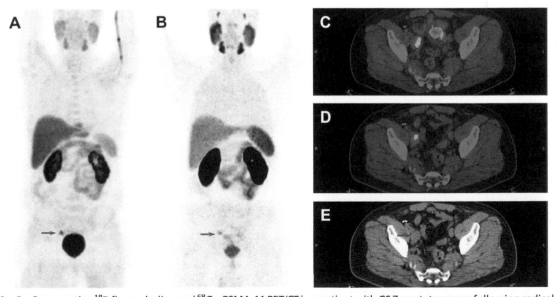

Fig. 3. Comparative ^{18}F-fluorocholine and ^{68}Ga-PSMA-11 PET/CT in a patient with GS 7 prostate cancer following radical prostatectomy and BCR with PSA of 2.38 ng/mL. ^{18}F-fluorocholine PET maximum intensity projection (MIP) (*A*) and PET/CT (*C*), ^{68}Ga-PSMA-11 PET MIP (*B*) and PET/CT (*D*) images show avid right pelvic lymph node (*arrow*). Corresponding CT image (*E*) shows an enlarged lymph node in the right pelvis (*arrow*). Panel A also shows the physiologic distribution of the ^{18}F-fluorocholine with higher bone marrow and liver uptake compared to ^{68}Ga-PSMA-11

Table 2
Potential indications for prostate-specific membrane antigen PET/computed tomography

Benefit of Using PSMA PET/CT	Patient Group
High clinical yield	• Primary staging in intermediate- to high-risk disease (D'Amico risk classification) • BCR with low PSA values (0.2 ng/mL to 10 ng/mL)
Low clinical yield	• Primary staging in low-risk disease (D'Amico risk classification)
Potential application with promising preliminary data	• Biopsy targeting after previous negative biopsy but high suspicion of PCa (especially in combination with multi-parametric MRI using PET/MRI) • Monitoring of systemic treatment in metastatic castration sensitive or resistant PCa
Potential application with current lack of published data	• Active surveillance of the primary (especially in combination with multi-parametric MRI using PET/MRI) • Active surveillance of the low-volume indolent metastatic PCa • Treatment monitoring in metastatic castration-resistant PCa undergoing radioligand therapy targeting PSMA (eg, ^{177}Lu-PSMA-ligand)

Adapted from Rauscher I, Maurer T, Fendler WP, et al. (68) Ga-PSMA ligand PET/CT in patients with prostate cancer: how we review and report. Cancer Imaging 2016;16(1):14; with permission.

standardize image acquisition and reporting of mpMRI.[74]

There is positive correlation between PSMA expression and GS. In immunohistochemistry analysis of 1700 PCa treated by radical prostatectomy, PSMA staining was found in 94% of cancers and was significantly associated with tumor stage and high GS and preoperative PSA. In

this study, tumors with strong PSMA expression had a higher risk of BCR than cancers with weak PSMA expression.[11] In another study on 902 patients with PCa postprostatectomy, high PSMA expression was significantly correlated with higher GS and PSA at diagnosis.[75] Although the understanding of the role of PSMA overexpression in PCa is evolving, it likely captures malignant features, such as GS, tumor angiogenesis, and cell migration, rather than being an independent prognostic factor.

In vivo demonstration of PSMA overexpression of PCa by PSMA imaging has been validated in multiple studies. In correlation with a prostatectomy histopathology sample of patients with intermediate- to high-risk PCa, ^{68}Ga-PSMA PET/CT imaging has yielded promising results. Fendler and colleagues[76] evaluated the accuracy of ^{68}Ga-PSMA-11 PET/CT in localizing PCa at the initial diagnosis in 21 patients. This study demonstrated 67% sensitivity, 92% specificity, and PPV more than 95%. In another study by Woythal and colleagues,[77] 31 patients who underwent prostatectomy and preoperative ^{68}Ga-PSMA-11 PET/CT were analyzed. ^{68}Ga-PSMA-11 PET/CT showed sensitivity and specificity of 87% and 97%, respectively, for the detection of PCa.

Furthermore, multiple studies have assessed the performance of ^{68}Ga-PSMA-11 PET/CT in patients with newly diagnosed PCa in comparison with TRUS-GB or MRI/TRUS-fusion biopsy. In a study by Uprimny and colleagues[78] 90 patients with TRUS-GB–proven PCa underwent ^{68}Ga-PSMA PET/CT. A total of 91% of patients demonstrated pathologic tracer uptake in the primary tumor. Tumors with GS of 6, 7a (3 + 4), and 7b (4 + 3) showed significantly lower PSMA uptake, compared with patients with GS more than 7. Furthermore, patients with PCa with a PSA of 10.0 ng/mL or greater exhibited significantly higher uptake than those with PSA levels less than 10.0 ng/mL. The investigators concluded the GS and PSA level correlated with the intensity of uptake in the primary tumors on ^{68}Ga-PSMA-11 PET/CT. Koerber and colleagues[79] analyzed the ^{68}Ga-PSMA-11 PET/CT of 104 patients with newly diagnosed PCa with approximately half of them had undergone MRI/TRUS-fusion biopsy. It was demonstrated that patients with higher PSA, higher GS, and higher d'Amico risk score had higher intensity of PSMA uptake on PET/CT. In correlation with the mpMRI and ^{68}Ga-PSMA-11 PET/CT findings, there was 89.5% concordance in the detection of PCa with the highest available GS. Similar findings were noted in another study with total or near-total agreement between PSMA PET/CT and mpMRI with regard to PCa detection in patients with a high pretest probability for large tumors.[80]

Notwithstanding less than 10% of PCa may not overexpress PSMA, based on the aforementioned findings PSMA PET/CT may play an important role for localization and risk stratification of most intermediate- to high-risk PCa. By providing additional molecular imaging information to the mpMRI findings, this imaging method may be helpful for identifying target lesions of the highest Gleason pattern before prostate biopsy. In addition, PSMA PET/MRI might be of high potential to improve the current standard TRUS-biopsy in the same way as mpMRI did. Further studies are needed to evaluate the role of PSMA PET/CT or PSMA PET/MRI in challenging situations such as prostatitis or after repeated negative biopsies.

Prostate-Specific Membrane Antigen Imaging in Primary Staging Before Radical Prostatectomy

Current guidelines recommend metastatic screening with at least abdominopelvic cross-sectional imaging (CT or MRI) and a bone scan (BS), only for intermediate- and high-risk PCa.[65,81]

In a meta-analysis consisting of 24 studies, the pooled sensitivity was 42% and 39% and the pooled specificity was 82% and 82%, for CT and MRI, respectively.[1] The investigators concluded reliance on either CT or MRI will potentially misdirect the therapeutic strategies offered to patients. Therefore, clinicians are reliant on preoperative models using PSA levels, ISUP grade group, and T stage to dictate LND protocols.[82]

Extended LND is considered the gold standard for high-risk patients with PCa undergoing RP, which not only determines the LN status but also potentially offers a survival benefit.[83] Nevertheless, this technique is invasive and may underestimate LN involvement; in fact, metastatic LNs can be found outside the standard resection area in approximately 40% to 50% of patients. This situation may be due to the different drainage and dissemination patterns in patients. With the improvement of novel molecular imaging techniques, the identification of patients with PCa with LN involvement has become more accurate.

The evidence favoring PSMA PET/CT imaging for detection of LN metastasis in this cohort of patients is evolving. A meta-analysis of 4 studies included 210 men with intermediate- to high-risk PCa who underwent ^{68}Ga-PSMA-11 PET/CT staging before RP.[84] In these studies, retroperitoneal LND was used as the standard of reference. ^{68}Ga-PSMA-11 PET/CT detected nodal metastases (pN1) in 35% of patients. The pooled sensitivity and specificity

per patient analysis and per LN packet analysis was similar and quoted as 61% and 97%, respectively. The largest cohort of patients in this meta-analysis belonged to a retrospective study including 130 patients by Maurer and colleagues.[85] It was noted that the patients with pN1 that were missed by ^{68}Ga-PSMA-11 PET had either PSMA-negative primary tumors (8.4% of all patients) or micrometastases (3 ± 1 mm) in single LN. In a phase II prospective study by Gorin and colleagues[84] on 25 men with high-risk PCa, ^{18}F-DCFPyL PET/CT performed similarly with sensitivity and specificity of 71% and 88%, respectively, per patient analysis and 66% and 92% per LN packet analysis. In addition, in multiple studies the rate of detection of non-nodal distant metastasis (predominantly bone metastases) was reported between 12% and 18%[78,79,84] (**Fig. 4**).

Prostate-Specific Membrane Antigen Imaging in Biochemical Recurrence After Radical Treatment

BCR following RP or RT occurs in up to half of patients with PCa.[86] According to guidelines, timing and choice of treatment of BCR without clinical recurrence (CR) after RP are still subject to controversy and may include RT, intermittent/ongoing androgen deprivation therapy (ADT), or expectant management.[87] Although only 15% of patients with PCa with BCR after RP will die of this disease, approximately one-third of these patients will develop CR at follow-up.[88] Therefore, detection of the sites of recurrent disease is of paramount importance, as this would avoid futile localized treatment in cases of systemic recurrence and avoid the side effects of systemic treatments in cases of localized recurrence (**Figs. 5** and **6**). This point is particularly important at low serum PSA values, when there are potential curative salvage treatment options. For instance, there is an average 2.6% loss of relapse-free survival for each incremental 0.1 ng/mL PSA at the time of salvage RT; this remains most effective at serum PSA values less than 0.5 ng/mL.[89] Because of the extremely low yield, guidelines do not advocate BS or abdominopelvic CT for asymptomatic patients with BCR after RP who have PSA levels less than 10 ng/mL.[87,90]

PET imaging with choline-based tracers has improved staging and enhanced the detection of recurrent PCa.[63] However, these tracers still lack the ability to identify smaller lesions, especially at low PSA velocity or serum PSA values less than 2 ng/mL.[91] Thus, PET imaging with choline-based tracers is not usually recommended at early stages of recurrence.

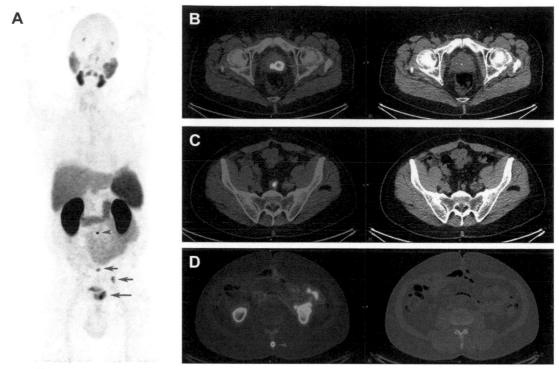

Fig. 4. ^{68}Ga-PSMA-11 PET/CT in primary staging of a patient with GS 9 and PSA 14 ng/mL. PSMA PET maximum intensity projection (*A*) demonstrates PSMA-avid prostate lesion (*arrow*), and further three foci of PSMA activity (*short arrows* and *arrow head*). Corresponding PET/CT and CT images show primary PCa (*B, arrow*), LN metastases (*C, short arrows*) and osseous metastasis (*D, arrow head*).

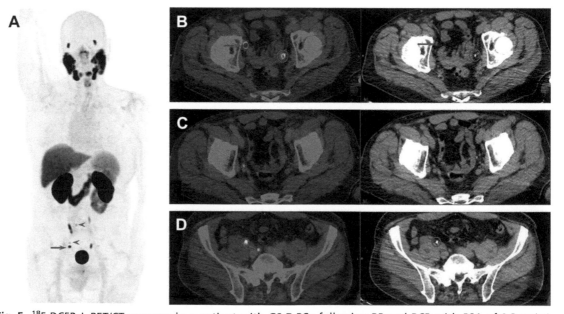

Fig. 5. ^{18}F-DCFPyL PET/CT urogram in a patient with GS 7 PCa following RP and BCR with PSA of 0.3 ng/mL. ^{18}F-DCFPyL PET maximum intensity projection (MIP) (*A*) shows an intensely avid focus in the right pelvis (*arrow*) and two foci of mild activity (*arrowheads*) in this region. Corresponding PET/CT, and CT images demonstrate intensely avid small right pelvic LN (*B, arrow*) and further two small mildly avid LNs in the right pelvis (*C and D, arrowheads*). Foci of trace activity corresponding to contrast opacified urine have been delineated in (*B*) and (*D*) (*circles*).

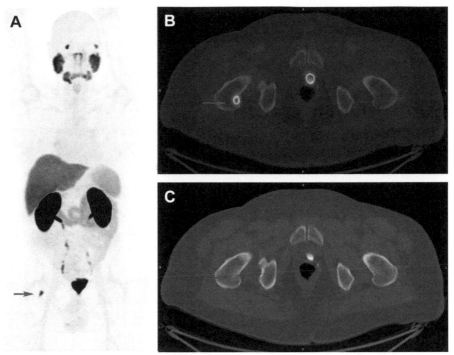

Fig. 6. ^{18}F-DCFPyL PET/CT in 64-year-old patient with BCR after RP with PSA 0.25 ng/mL. PSMA PET maximum intensity projection (*A*), PET/CT (*B*), and CT (*C*) images show intense focal uptake in the right femur with only subtle changes on CT (*arrows*).

In this setting, PSMA PET imaging has shown promising results. In a meta-analysis performed by Perera and colleagues[54] including 16 articles and 1309 patients, the overall percentage of positive ^{68}Ga-PSMA-11 PET was 76% for BCR. PSA values at the time of restaging were positively associated with the detection rate of ^{68}Ga-PSMA-11 PET/CT. The detection rate for the PSA categories 0 to 0.2, 0.2 to 1.0, 1 to 2, and greater than 2 ng/mL were 42%, 58%, 76%, and 95% scans, respectively. On per-patient analysis, the sensitivity and specificity of ^{68}Ga-PSMA-11 PET were both 86%, whereas on per-lesion analysis, the sensitivity and specificity were 80% and 97%, respectively. In another meta-analysis including 9 studies with 983 patients, sites of recurrence were detected in 799 patients (81%) with 50% detection rate for PSA of 0.2 to 0.49 ng/mL and 53% detection rate for PSA of 0.50 to 0.99 ng/mL.[55] All studies reported examinations with PET/CT, and only one study included a subgroup of patients examined with PET/MRI. Seventy-nine (10%) patients had sites in the prostate bed, 164 (22%) patients in pelvic LNs, 100 (13%) patients in distant organs, and 272 (36%) patients in several regions. Two studies undertook patient-based analysis and tested the performance of ^{68}Ga-PSMA PET/CT for restaging of LN metastases versus a histologic reference standard.[92,93] In these two studies, the sensitivities were 87% and 93% and the specificities were 93% and 100%.

Prostate-Specific Membrane Antigen Imaging in Salvage Lymph Nodal Dissection: Preoperative or Intraoperative

Of the patients with BCR, patients with LN metastases, the most common locations of metastatic disease, generally have a better survival outcome compared with patients with bone and/or visceral metastases.[94] Salvage LND (sLND) may be offered to patients with isolated nodal recurrence, which may delay CR, hence, the use of systemic treatments and their associated side effects. However, currently there is no proof that sLND improves the overall survival and may result in adverse events. Imaging techniques with high sensitivity and specificity are essential for precise preoperative staging. Choline-based tracers are the most investigated PET tracer in this setting, with promising results but limited accuracy particularly at low PSA levels.[91,92,95] The role of PSMA imaging in this setting has been the subject of multiple studies.

Hijazi and colleagues[96] reported the first evaluation of ^{68}Ga-PSMA-11 PET/CT-guided pelvic extended LND. In this study including 23 patients with BCR and 12 patients with high-risk PCa, 17 patients with oligometastatic disease underwent LND. At 40 days' postsurgery follow-up, the PSA level was less than 0.2 ng/mL in 82% (14 of 17) of patients.

Pfister and colleagues[92] compared the diagnostic performance of ^{68}Ga-PSMA-11 and ^{18}F-fluoroethylcholine (FEC) PET/CT in series of patients with BCR with postpelvic and/or retroperitoneal LND histopathology sample as the standard. ^{68}Ga-PSMA-11 PET outperformed FEC PET with a significantly higher NPV (96% vs 88%) and accuracy (91% vs 82%) for the detection of locoregional recurrent and/or metastatic lesions before sLND.

In the largest population in this clinical setting, Herlemann and colleagues,[97] performed sLND in 104 patients with isolated nodal recurrence on either FEC or ^{68}Ga-PSMA-11 PET/CT. This study was of importance, as there was a median follow-up of 39.5 months after sLND; apart from the biochemical response (BR), the investigators evaluated the CR and cancer-specific survival (CSS). In this study, 29% of patients developed complete BR (PSA <0.2 ng/mL) and 56% developed partial BR (PSA postoperative < PSA preoperative) after sLND. The rate of complete BR was higher in patients with LN metastases diagnosed on ^{68}Ga-PSMA-11 compared with FEC PET (45% vs 21%). PSA level at sLND and preoperative imaging with ^{68}Ga-PSMA-11 PET seem to be independent predictors of complete

BR. The 5-year BCR-free, CR-free, and CSS rates were 6%, 26%, and 82%, respectively. The investigators concluded that although preoperative staging with ^{68}Ga-PSMA-11 is a superior imaging modality, only a limited number of patients developed complete BR after sLND and most patients experienced BCR and CR during follow-up.

Based on the aforementioned evidence, careful patient selection is critical for individualizing the surgical approach (**Fig. 7**). Future trials are needed to assess whether less extensive surgery with PSMA PET/CT–targeted LND would have similar oncologic outcomes to more extended sLND. In addition, PSMA-derived radio-guided or fluorescence-guided surgery using a probe intraoperatively may facilitate sLND.[98,99]

Management Impact of Prostate-Specific Membrane Antigen Imaging in Primary Staging and Biochemical Recurrence

Multiple retrospective and prospective studies have evaluated the impact of PMSA imaging in intended or actual implemented management of patients with PCa (**Table 3**).

In one of the first studies to evaluate the clinical impact of PSMA PET imaging, Morigi and colleagues[100] prospectively compared ^{68}Ga-PSMA-11 PET/CT and ^{18}F-fluoromethylcholine PET/CT in 37 men with BCR following RP or RT. The

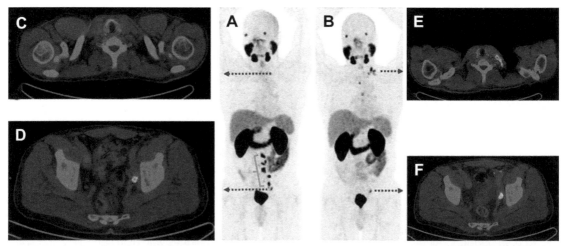

Fig. 7. PSMA PET-informed sLND in a patient with PCa, GS 9, and BCR (PSA 1.8 ng/mL) following RP. PSMA PET maximum intensity projection (MIP) (*A*) and PET/CT (*C, D*) shows multiple left retroperitoneal LNs metastases (*bracket*). The patient underwent sLND, and histopathology showed 23 of 44 involved LNs. Four months following sLND, PSA increased rapidly from 1.4 ng/mL to 3.4 ng/mL in 1 month. PSMA PET MIP (*B*) and PET/CT (*F*) images show resolution of retroperitoneal nodes (except one) and development of new nodal disease above to the sLND field in the retroperitoneum, the mediastinum, the left supraclavicular region, (*E*) as well as multiple osseous metastases. *Arrows* indicate the corresponding trans-axial levels of PET/CT. (*From* Hofman MS, Iravani A. Gallium-68 prostate-specific membrane antigen PET imaging. PET Clin North Am 2017;12(2):219–34; with permission.)

Table 3
Summary of studies investigating management impact of prostate-specific membrane antigen imaging

	Type of Study		Clinical Setting		Management Impact				
	Retrospective	Prospective	PS (N)	BCR (N)	Intended	Implemented	Impact (%) (PS)	Impact (%) (BCR)	Impact (%) (Overall)
Morigi et al,[100] 2015	—	+[a]	—	+ (38)	+	—	—	54	54
Sterzing et al,[102] 2016	+	—	+ (15)	+ (42)	—	+	26	60	51
Bluemel et al,[101] 2016	+	—	—	+ (45)	—	+	—	42	42
Hope et al,[106] 2017	—	+	—	+ (126)	+	—	—	59	59 (53 major)
Roach et al,[105] 2018	—	+	+ (108)	+ (323)	+	—	21	62	51
Afaq et al,[108] 2017	+	—	—	+ (100)	—	+	—	39	39
Albisinni et al,[104] 2017	+	—	—	+ (131)	—	+	—	76	76
Calais et al,[103] 2017	+	—	—	+ (270)	+	—	—	50	50 (19 major)
Calais et al,[107] 2017	—	+	—	+ (101)	+	+	—	53	53
Grubmüller et al,[109] 2018	—	+	—	+ (117)	+	—	—	43	43

Abbreviations: BCR, biochemical recurrence; N, number of patients; PS, primary staging.
[a] + Indicates whether the column's heading applies to the respective study.

investigators reported 54% management impact due to ^{68}Ga-PSMA-11 imaging alone. Bluemel and colleagues[101] assessed the impact of ^{68}Ga-PSMA-11 PET/CT before salvage RT (sRT) in 45 patients with persistence or BCR after radical surgery. Suspicious lesions were detected in 53% of patients; of those, 62% of lesions were only detected by ^{68}Ga-PSMA-11 PET. Accordingly treatment was changed in 42.2% of patients by extending the RT field, dose escalation, or change to systemic therapy. In 21 patients who were treated by sRT and had available clinical follow-up, almost all showed BR (mean PSA decline 78 ±19%). The Heidelberg group assessed the potential role of PSMA PET imaging in individualizing the RT planning in a cohort of 57 patients comprising 15 patients at primary staging and 42 patients at BCR.[102] Stratified by the D'Amico criteria, PSMA PET changed TNM staging in 3 (10.3%) patients with low-risk, 11 (37.9%) with intermediate-risk, and 15 (51.8%) with high-risk cancer. Accordingly, in a primary staging cohort the treatment plan changed in 26% of patients and in 60% patients with BCR.

In a post hoc analysis of an intention-to-treat in homogenous population of 270 patients with BCR and PSA less than 1.0 ng/mL, the impact of PSMA PET on sRT following prostatectomy was assessed.[103] The investigators reported the addition of PMSA PET may potentially impact sRT in half of the patients, of whom 19% with major impact by the extension of the RT field, addition of metastasis-directed stereotactic body RT (SBRT), or RT considered futile because of the presence of poly-metastatic disease. Importantly, the most common PSMA-positive lesion location outside the RT field was bone (44%); the most common nodal regions outside of RT field were the perirectal, distal external iliac, and para-aortic, which are neither assessed by routine LND at prostatectomy nor targeted by routine sRT.

In a retrospective study of 131 patients with BCR, change in treatment plan by a multidisciplinary oncology team was recorded prior and following PSMA PET.[104] In this study, there was an impact on subsequent management in 99 out of 131 patients (76%). A wide range of modifications were noted, including ongoing surveillance, hormonal manipulations, SBRT, sRT, sLND, or salvage local treatment (prostatectomy, high-intensity focused ultrasound).

A prospective Australian multicenter study evaluated PSMA PET imaging impacts on management intent of intermediate- to high-risk PCa at initial diagnosis or following BCR in a cohort of 431 patients.[105] Management intent was recorded by a questioner filled out by the referring physician before and after PSMA PET. Imaging with PSMA PET revealed unsuspected disease in the prostate bed in 27% of patients, locoregional LNs in 39%, and distant metastatic disease in 16% of patients. PSMA PET led to changes in the planned management of 62% of BCR cohort and 21% of primary staging cohort. However, this study did not record whether the change in the planned management was, in fact, implemented. In a similarly designed prospective study by Hope and colleagues[106] on 126 patients with BCR, major management change was reported in 53% of patients, including those with a PSA of less than 0.2 ng/mL. This cohort included patients with a PSA doubling time of less than 12 months, but change in management did not significantly differ by the baseline PSA level.

In a prospective study, referring physicians were surveyed prior, immediately after (intended management), and 3 to 6 months following PSMA PET imaging to ascertain the implemented management change in patients with BCR.[107] Of the 101 of 161 patients who completed all 3 surveys, PSMA PET led to 53% implemented management changes. These changes consisted of conversion to focal treatment/new focal treatment in 29%, conversion to systemic treatment in 13%, change of the systemic treatment approach in 5%, and conversion to active surveillance in 7% patients.

Health care providers and government agencies frequently judge the value of novel diagnostic tests by measuring their impact on patient management and outcomes. Although all of the aforementioned studies demonstrated significant intended or implemented management change, the efficacy of such interventions in terms of progression-free survival, quality of life, cost benefits, and overall survival have not been reported yet. However, the improved performance of such testing offers the opportunity to alter conventional clinical treatment paradigms. Nevertheless, current evidence overwhelmingly supports designing and executing prospective randomized clinical trials in determining whether, in patients with BCR of PCa at very low PSA levels, PSMA PET-informed management would translate into improved patient outcomes and quality of life.

The potential contribution of PSMA PET to more accurate primary staging of patients at the time of initial diagnosis may also change the natural history of the disease and incidence rate of BCR. Currently a prospective randomized multicenter study in Australia is underway to assess the impact of ^{68}Ga-PSMA PET/CT imaging for staging high-risk PCa before curative-intent surgery or RT (ACTRN12617000005358). Another currently running phase II/III prospective trial is evaluating the diagnostic ability of ^{68}Ga-PSMA-11 PET/MRI in patients with intermediate- or high-risk PCa undergoing surgery and LND (NCT02678351).

Molecular Imaging in Response Assessment, Biological Characterization, and Prognostication

PCa is a heterogeneous disease with clonal sub-populations and varied histologic and molecular abnormalities. Intrapatient and interpatient heterogeneity could account for the variability in therapeutic responses[110,111] and poses a significant challenge for imaging response assessment. This point is particularly important in advanced stages of PCa when it becomes castration resistant (metastatic castration-resistant PCa [mCRPC]). Response assessment by conventional imaging in metastatic PCa is often suboptimal because of the limited applicability of Response Evaluation Criteria in Solid Tumors (RECIST 1.1) criteria due to nontarget disease, including nonmeasurable LNs and sclerotic bone metastases. Evaluation with BS also remains a challenge to reliably prove therapy response because of the frequently seen flare phenomenon.

Clinical and translational research in PCa has expanded our understanding of the pathogenesis, different clinicopathologic and molecular subtypes as well as biology of the evolution of CRPC, which has resulted in improving therapeutic armamentarium for the management of mCRPC.[112] These new advances led to the development of the updated Prostate Cancer Clinical Trials Working Group (PCWG3) recommendations.[113] The PCWG3 guidelines stress the importance of biological profiling of the tumor at the initiation of any therapy by biopsies of metastatic sites, liquid biopsies such as circulating tumor cells or circulating DNA analysis, or other blood biomarkers of bone turnover or immune function. There is an ongoing need to better define predictive and prognostic markers, to optimally sequence the approved agents in treatment protocols, and to develop better targeted therapies.[114,115]

Characterization of the disease with different molecular imaging agents, such as ^{18}F fluoro-2-D-deoxyglucose for glycolysis,[116] ^{18}F-fluorodihydrotestosterone for androgen receptor expression,[116] ^{68}Ga-DOTATATE for somatostatin receptor expression in neuroendocrine differentiation,[117] choline-based radiolabeled agents,[118] and PSMA imaging, may play a role as real-time disease biomarkers.

Radiolabeled choline PET imaging has had promising results in predicting the response to treatment modalities, such as ADTs.[119] To date, there is only one published study evaluating the role of PSMA PET in response assessment. In this study by Seitz and colleagues,[120] 6 patients with metastatic castration-sensitive PCa (mCSPC) and 17 patients with mCRPC were treated with docetaxel chemotherapy. The radiological response was evaluated by PSMA PET/CT PET response criteria in solid tumors (PERCIST) and CT (RECIST 1.1) and correlated with BR. The concordance of outcome prediction between PSMA PET/CT and BR was higher than CT and BR in both mCSPC and mCRPC. This preliminary result suggests that PSMA PET/CT may be a promising method for treatment response assessment. However, further larger and prospective studies are needed to confirm the value of PSMA PET/CT as an imaging biomarker for response assessment (**Figs. 8** and **9**).

HARMONIZATION OF INTERPRETATION AND REPORTING

There is an imperative need to standardize interpretation and reporting of any new promising modality for imaging including novel radiopharmaceuticals. The aim of developing consensus guidelines in the interpretation of PSMA imaging would include more consistent reports within clinical practice and clinical trials, more robust assessment of the diagnostic performance, better comparison with other modalities, the ability to accurately guide treatment and subsequently impact on the outcome, as well as providing prognostic stratification. To this end, the Joint European Association of Nuclear Medicine/Society of Nuclear Medicine and Molecular Imaging published the first procedure guideline for ^{68}Ga-PSMA PET/CT in PCa in 2017.[121] Several other groups have proposed criteria in harmonization of PSMA imaging interpretation and reporting.

Fanti and colleagues[122] performed a study evaluating the interobserver agreement among nuclear physicians in 7 international centers with extensive prior experience in ^{68}Ga-PSMA PET/CT, in the setting of BCR. They found that the interobserver agreement for the presence of an abnormality by 7 expert readers was only moderate. However, following multiple Delphi rounds the consensus reading improved and interpretation criteria were devised. It was also suggested that most cases of disagreement between observers related either to extremely subtle abnormalities of uncertain significance or differing interpretation of the nomenclature appropriate for describing the abnormalities. In another multicenter international study, Fendler and colleagues[123] assessed the interobserver agreement between imaging specialists with different levels of experience in

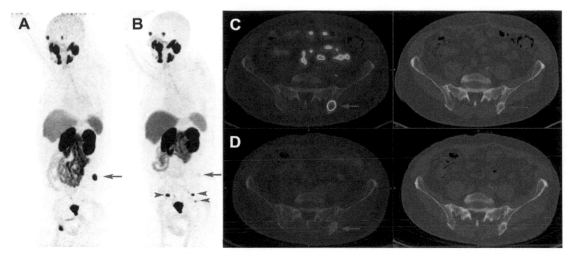

Fig. 8. Response assessment by PSMA PET/CT following SBRT for a solitary osseous metastasis in a patient with BCR and PSA 36 ng/mL. PSMA PET maximum intensity projection (MIP) (*A*), PET/CT, and CT (*C*) show solitary left pelvic osseous metastasis (*arrow*). Following SBRT, PSA nadir of 2.3 ng/mL at 6 months' follow-up was achieved. PSA increased to 8.4 ng/mL at 12 months' follow-up and PSMA MIP (*B*), PET/CT, and CT (*D*) showed complete response in the treated left pelvic osseous metastasis on PSMA imaging (*arrows*); but new LNs and osseous metastases were detected (*arrowheads*).

PSMA PET imaging. The interobserver agreement among highly experienced observers was either substantial or almost perfect in the primary staging and BCR in all regions (the local disease, nodal or distant metastases). It was, however, noted that the level of experience positively correlated with agreement between observers. The investigators concluded initial training on at least 30 cases are needed to achieve acceptable consistency. As the availability of PSMA imaging is rapidly increasing, the necessity of a standardized framework for consistent reporting among centers with different levels of expertise is underscored by the aforementioned findings.

Two reporting criteria for PSMA imaging have been proposed recently. The RADS provides a standardized framework for conveying findings and recommendations to clinicians and has been

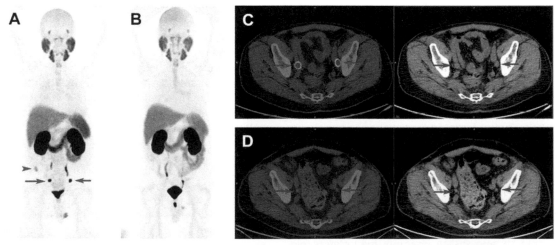

Fig. 9. Response assessment by PSMA PET/CT in a patient with BCR and PSA 0.4 ng/mL. PSMA PET maximum intensity projection (MIP) (*A*), PET/CT, and CT (*C*) show pelvic LNs (*arrows*) and right pelvic osseous (*arrowhead*) metastases. The patient was commenced on androgen deprivation therapy; at 24 months' follow-up PSMA PET MIP (*B*), PET/CT, and CT (*D*) demonstrate decline in the size of LNs (*arrows*) and complete response on PSMA imaging in LNs and bone. Contemporaneous PSA level at the time of follow-up PSMA PET was less than 0.1 ng/mL.

adopted in multiple solid organ malignancies, such as PCa (PI-RADS).[124] Based on this concept, Rowe and colleagues[125] proposed the first version of PSMA-RADS. The investigators used their clinical experience and published literature in interpreting PSMA imaging for guiding clinical management to develop PSMA-RADS. The goal of the PSMA-RADS reporting system is to convey the imaging specialist's level of confidence for the presence of PCa as well as the potential need for any additional workup. PSMA-RADS differs from systems such as PI-RADS, as it is whole-body based rather than organ based and is most useful in the lesions outside of the prostate. Using a 5-point scale, the reader's level of confidence is classified as benign (PSMA-RADS-1), likely benign (PSMA-RADS-2), equivocal (PSMA-RADS-3), PCa highly likely (PSMA-RADS-4), and PCa almost certainly present (PSMA-RADS-5). Subgroup classifications are also defined within each category. The impression of the report is proposed to include a patient-based as well as lesion-based PSMA-RADS score for up to 5 lesions. The latter is on the basis that oligometastatic disease would qualify patients to be considered for targeted treatment. An important consideration has been given to incorporate the clinical history in the report, including indication for the study, history of treatments (type, duration, and date of last treatment), current PSA level, any important imaging findings on other modalities, and any other relevant clinical history. A strength of this proposed method is the incorporation of clearly defined levels of confidence in imaging findings with actionable recommendations, ranging from benign, equivocal (requiring confirmatory workup or follow-up imaging), or positive disease not requiring confirmatory biopsy.

The American Joint Committee on Cancer's clinicopathologic TNM system is the most widely used PCa staging system.[126] Based on this, the Prostate Cancer Molecular Imaging Standardized Evaluation criteria proposed a molecular imaging TNM system (miTNM version 1.0) as the standardized reporting framework for PSMA PET/CT or PET/MRI.[127] The aim of the miTNM is to serve as standardized reporting for the presence, location, and extent of local PCa; presence, location, extent, and distribution pattern of extrapelvic metastases; PSMA expression level of tumor lesions; and diagnostic confidence of reported findings. Local tumor described as absence of local recurrence in the pelvis both after RP or RT (miT0), tumor extent with prostate in place (miT2–miT4), confined organ unifocal (miT2u), and confined organ multifocal (miT2m). Pelvic LN metastases will be categorized into single (miN1a) and multiple (miN1b) involved nodal regions. Distant metastases are separated into 3 categories, extrapelvic LNs (miM1a), bone metastases (miM1b), and organ metastases (miM1c). The visual level of PSMA uptake (miPSMA) scored from 0 to 3 relative to the organs of reference (blood pool, liver, and parotid glands), with score 2 and 3 typical for PCa lesions. The final diagnostic certainty is based on a 5-point scale, which will substantially vary depending on uptake, location, and conventional imaging findings. One of the strengths of this criteria is the 6-segment (sextant) schema for PSMA PET/MRI reporting of the primary PCa. However, using proposed visual scoring for miPSMA would need further refinement and verification, especially using different PSMA PET radiotracers with varying biodistribution.

Although the abovementioned proposed criteria are necessary preliminary steps toward the standardization of PSMA PET reporting, prospective outcome-oriented clinical trials are essential for progressive refinement and validation of these guidelines.

SUMMARY

Experience with PSMA PET/CT imaging has rapidly evolved, with an increasing number of studies showing promising results. Although it was first used for detection of BCR and low PSA where conventional imaging is known to have low utility, PSMA PET seems to have a broader role in diagnosis, primary staging, assessment of response to systemic therapies, and selection of patients for ^{177}Lu-PSMA radionuclide therapy. Newer-generation PSMA ligands, including ^{18}F derivatives, will further improve the availability of PSMA PET/CT. Prospective studies are needed to directly compare PSMA PET with existing standards of care, including CT, bone scintigraphy, and MRI, in order for health care providers to reimburse this novel modality and for it to be incorporated into clinical guidelines. Research is also required to demonstrate improved patient-related outcomes and health economic benefits of PSMA PET.

REFERENCES

1. Hovels AM, Heesakkers RA, Adang EM, et al. The diagnostic accuracy of CT and MRI in the staging of pelvic lymph nodes in patients with prostate cancer: a meta-analysis. Clin Radiol 2008;63(4):387–95.
2. Jadvar H. Molecular imaging of prostate cancer with PET. J Nucl Med 2013;54(10):1685–8.
3. Afshar-Oromieh A, Haberkorn U, Hadaschik B, et al. PET/MRI with a 68Ga-PSMA ligand for the

detection of prostate cancer. Eur J Nucl Med Mol Imaging 2013;40(10):1629–30.

4. Afshar-Oromieh A, Malcher A, Eder M, et al. PET imaging with a [68Ga]gallium-labelled PSMA ligand for the diagnosis of prostate cancer: biodistribution in humans and first evaluation of tumour lesions. Eur J Nucl Med Mol Imaging 2013;40(4):486–95.

5. Roethke MC, Kuru TH, Afshar-Oromieh A, et al. Hybrid positron emission tomography-magnetic resonance imaging with gallium 68 prostate-specific membrane antigen tracer: a next step for imaging of recurrent prostate cancer-preliminary results. Eur Urol 2013;64(5):862–4.

6. Israeli RS, Powell CT, Fair WR, et al. Molecular cloning of a complementary DNA encoding a prostate-specific membrane antigen. Cancer Res 1993; 53(2):227–30.

7. Mease RC, Foss CA, Pomper MG. PET imaging in prostate cancer: focus on prostate-specific membrane antigen. Curr Top Med Chem 2013;13(8): 951–62.

8. Demirkol MO, Acar O, Ucar B, et al. Prostate-specific membrane antigen-based imaging in prostate cancer: impact on clinical decision making process. Prostate 2015;75(7):748–57.

9. Sokoloff RL, Norton KC, Gasior CL, et al. A dual-monoclonal sandwich assay for prostate-specific membrane antigen: levels in tissues, seminal fluid and urine. Prostate 2000;43(2):150–7.

10. Ananias HJ, van den Heuvel MC, Helfrich W, et al. Expression of the gastrin-releasing peptide receptor, the prostate stem cell antigen and the prostate-specific membrane antigen in lymph node and bone metastases of prostate cancer. Prostate 2009;69(10):1101–8.

11. Minner S, Wittmer C, Graefen M, et al. High level PSMA expression is associated with early PSA recurrence in surgically treated prostate cancer. Prostate 2011;71(3):281–8.

12. Rybalov M, Ananias HJ, Hoving HD, et al. PSMA, EpCAM, VEGF and GRPR as imaging targets in locally recurrent prostate cancer after radiotherapy. Int J Mol Sci 2014;15(4):6046–61.

13. Bostwick DG, Pacelli A, Blute M, et al. Prostate specific membrane antigen expression in prostatic intraepithelial neoplasia and adenocarcinoma: a study of 184 cases. Cancer 1998;82(11):2256–61.

14. Graham K, Lesche R, Gromov AV, et al. Radiofluorinated derivatives of 2-(phosphonomethyl) pentanedioic acid as inhibitors of prostate specific membrane antigen (PSMA) for the imaging of prostate cancer. J Med Chem 2012;55(22):9510–20.

15. Kawakami M, Nakayama J. Enhanced expression of prostate-specific membrane antigen gene in prostate cancer as revealed by in situ hybridization. Cancer Res 1997;57(12):2321–4.

16. Troyer JK, Beckett ML, Wright GL Jr. Detection and characterization of the prostate-specific membrane antigen (PSMA) in tissue extracts and body fluids. Int J Cancer 1995;62(5):552–8.

17. Bouchelouche K, Choyke PL, Capala J. Prostate specific membrane antigen- a target for imaging and therapy with radionuclides. Discov Med 2010;9(44):55–61.

18. Wright GL Jr, Grob BM, Haley C, et al. Upregulation of prostate-specific membrane antigen after androgen-deprivation therapy. Urology 1996; 48(2):326–34.

19. Ross JS, Sheehan CE, Fisher HA, et al. Correlation of primary tumor prostate-specific membrane antigen expression with disease recurrence in prostate cancer. Clin Cancer Res 2003;9(17):6357–62.

20. Horoszewicz JS, Kawinski E, Murphy GP. Monoclonal antibodies to a new antigenic marker in epithelial prostatic cells and serum of prostatic cancer patients. Anticancer Res 1987;7(5B): 927–35.

21. Franc BL, Cho SY, Rosenthal SA, et al. Detection and localization of carcinoma within the prostate using high resolution transrectal gamma imaging (TRGI) of monoclonal antibody directed at prostate specific membrane antigen (PSMA)–proof of concept and initial imaging results. Eur J Radiol 2013;82(11):1877–84.

22. Ponsky LE, Cherullo EE, Starkey R, et al. Evaluation of preoperative ProstaScint scans in the prediction of nodal disease. Prostate Cancer prostatic Dis 2002;5(2):132–5.

23. Liu H, Rajasekaran AK, Moy P, et al. Constitutive and antibody-induced internalization of prostate-specific membrane antigen. Cancer Res 1998; 58(18):4055–60.

24. Bander NH, Trabulsi EJ, Kostakoglu L, et al. Targeting metastatic prostate cancer with radiolabeled monoclonal antibody J591 to the extracellular domain of prostate specific membrane antigen. J Urol 2003;170(5):1717–21.

25. Tagawa ST, Milowsky MI, Morris M, et al. Phase II study of lutetium-177-labeled anti-prostate-specific membrane antigen monoclonal antibody J591 for metastatic castration-resistant prostate cancer. Clin Cancer Res 2013;19(18):5182–91.

26. Tsukamoto T, Wozniak KM, Slusher BS. Progress in the discovery and development of glutamate carboxypeptidase II inhibitors. Drug Discov Today 2007;12(17–18):767–76.

27. Foss CA, Mease RC, Fan H, et al. Radiolabeled small-molecule ligands for prostate-specific membrane antigen: in vivo imaging in experimental models of prostate cancer. Clin Cancer Res 2005; 11(11):4022–8.

28. Mease RC, Dusich CL, Foss CA, et al. N-[N-[(S)-1,3-dicarboxypropyl]carbamoyl]-4-[18F]

fluorobenzyl-L-cysteine, [18F]DCFBC: a new imaging probe for prostate cancer. Clin Cancer Res 2008;14(10):3036–43.

29. Maresca KP, Hillier SM, Femia FJ, et al. A series of halogenated heterodimeric inhibitors of prostate specific membrane antigen (PSMA) as radiolabeled probes for targeting prostate cancer. J Med Chem 2009;52(2):347–57.

30. Banerjee SR, Foss CA, Castanares M, et al. Synthesis and evaluation of technetium-99m- and rhenium-labeled inhibitors of the prostate-specific membrane antigen (PSMA). J Med Chem 2008;51(15):4504–17.

31. Hillier SM, Maresca KP, Lu G, et al. 99mTc-labeled small-molecule inhibitors of prostate-specific membrane antigen for molecular imaging of prostate cancer. J Nucl Med 2013;54(8):1369–76.

32. Banerjee SR, Pullambhatla M, Byun Y, et al. 68Ga-labeled inhibitors of prostate-specific membrane antigen (PSMA) for imaging prostate cancer. J Med Chem 2010;53(14):5333–41.

33. Schafer M, Bauder-Wust U, Leotta K, et al. A dimerized urea-based inhibitor of the prostate-specific membrane antigen for 68Ga-PET imaging of prostate cancer. EJNMMI Res 2012;2(1):23.

34. Chen Y, Pullambhatla M, Banerjee SR, et al. Synthesis and biological evaluation of low molecular weight fluorescent imaging agents for the prostate-specific membrane antigen. Bioconjug Chem 2012;23(12):2377–85.

35. Barrett JA, Coleman RE, Goldsmith SJ, et al. First-in-man evaluation of 2 high-affinity PSMA-avid small molecules for imaging prostate cancer. J Nucl Med 2013;54(3):380–7.

36. Vallabhajosula S, Nikolopoulou A, Babich JW, et al. 99mTc-labeled small-molecule inhibitors of prostate-specific membrane antigen: pharmacokinetics and biodistribution studies in healthy subjects and patients with metastatic prostate cancer. J Nucl Med 2014;55(11):1791–8.

37. Cho SY, Gage KL, Mease RC, et al. Biodistribution, tumor detection, and radiation dosimetry of 18F-DCFBC, a low-molecular-weight inhibitor of prostate-specific membrane antigen, in patients with metastatic prostate cancer. J Nucl Med 2012;53(12):1883–91.

38. Szabo Z, Mena E, Rowe SP, et al. Initial evaluation of [(18)F]DCFPyL for prostate-specific membrane antigen (PSMA)-targeted PET imaging of prostate cancer. Mol Imaging Biol 2015;17(4):565–74.

39. Hofman MS, Eu P, Jackson P, et al. Cold Kit PSMA PET imaging: phase I study of (68)Ga-THP-PSMA PET/CT in patients with prostate cancer. J Nucl Med 2018 Apr;59(4):625–31.

40. Reubi JC, Maecke HR. Peptide-based probes for cancer imaging. J Nucl Med 2008;49(11):1735–8.

41. Hofman MS, Kong G, Neels OC, et al. High management impact of Ga-68 DOTATATE (GaTate) PET/CT for imaging neuroendocrine and other somatostatin expressing tumours. J Med Imaging Radiat Oncol 2012;56(1):40–7.

42. Hofman MS, Lau WF, Hicks RJ. Somatostatin receptor imaging with 68Ga DOTATATE PET/CT: clinical utility, normal patterns, pearls, and pitfalls in interpretation. Radiographics 2015;35(2):500–16.

43. Eder M, Schafer M, Bauder-Wust U, et al. 68Ga-complex lipophilicity and the targeting property of a urea-based PSMA inhibitor for PET imaging. Bioconjug Chem 2012;23(4):688–97.

44. Young JD, Abbate V, Imberti C, et al. (68)Ga-THP-PSMA: a PET imaging agent for prostate cancer offering rapid, room-temperature, 1-step kit-based radiolabeling. J Nucl Med 2017;58(8):1270–7.

45. Dietlein M, Kobe C, Kuhnert G, et al. Comparison of [(18)F]DCFPyL and [(68)Ga]Ga-PSMA-HBED-CC for PSMA-PET imaging in patients with relapsed prostate cancer. Mol Imaging Biol 2015;17(4):575–84.

46. Rowe SP, Gage KL, Faraj SF, et al. (1)(8)F-DCFBC PET/CT for PSMA-based detection and characterization of primary prostate cancer. J Nucl Med 2015;56(7):1003–10.

47. Dietlein F, Kobe C, Neubauer S, et al. PSA-stratified performance of (18)F- and (68)Ga-PSMA PET in patients with biochemical recurrence of prostate cancer. J Nucl Med 2017;58(6):947–52.

48. Giesel FL, Hadaschik B, Cardinale J, et al. F-18 labelled PSMA-1007: biodistribution, radiation dosimetry and histopathological validation of tumor lesions in prostate cancer patients. Eur J Nucl Med Mol Imaging 2017;44(6):678–88.

49. Kesch C, Kratochwil C, Mier W, et al. (68)Ga or (18)F for prostate cancer imaging? J Nucl Med 2017;58(5):687–8.

50. Giesel F, Will L, Lawal I, et al. Intra-individual comparison of (18)F-PSMA-1007 and (18)F-DCFPyL PET/CT in the prospective evaluation of patients with newly diagnosed prostate carcinoma: a pilot study. J Nucl Med 2017 [pii:jnumed.117.204669] [Epub ahead of print].

51. Savir-Baruch B, Zanoni L, Schuster DM. Imaging of prostate cancer using fluciclovine. PET Clinics 2017;12(2):145–57.

52. FDA approves 18F-Fluciclovine and 68Ga-DOTATATE products. J Nucl Med 2016;57(8):9N.

53. Bach-Gansmo T, Nanni C, Nieh PT, et al. Multisite experience of the safety, detection rate and diagnostic performance of fluciclovine ((18)F) positron emission tomography/computerized tomography imaging in the staging of biochemically recurrent prostate cancer. J Urol 2017;197(3 Pt 1):676–83.

54. Perera M, Papa N, Christidis D, et al. Sensitivity, specificity, and predictors of positive 68Ga-prostate-specific membrane antigen positron emission tomography in advanced prostate cancer: a

systematic review and meta-analysis. Eur Urol 2016;70(6):926–37.

55. von Eyben FE, Picchio M, von Eyben R, et al. (68) Ga-labeled prostate-specific membrane antigen ligand positron emission tomography/computed tomography for prostate cancer: a systematic review and meta-analysis. Eur Urol Focus 2016 [pii:S2405-4569(16)30160-2]. [Epub ahead of print].

56. Calais J, Fendler WP, Herrmann K, et al. Head-to-head comparison of 68Ga-PSMA-11 PET/CT and 18F-fluciclovine PET/CT in a case series of 10 patients with prostate cancer recurrence. J Nucl Med 2017.

57. Afshar-Oromieh A, Hetzheim H, Kubler W, et al. Radiation dosimetry of (68)Ga-PSMA-11 (HBED-CC) and preliminary evaluation of optimal imaging timing. Eur J Nucl Med Mol Imaging 2016;43(9):1611–20.

58. Pfob CH, Ziegler S, Graner FP, et al. Biodistribution and radiation dosimetry of (68)Ga-PSMA HBED CC-a PSMA specific probe for PET imaging of prostate cancer. Eur J Nucl Med Mol Imaging 2016;43(11):1962–70.

59. McParland BJ, Wall A, Johansson S, et al. The clinical safety, biodistribution and internal radiation dosimetry of [(1)(8)F]fluciclovine in healthy adult volunteers. Eur J Nucl Med Mol Imaging 2013;40(8):1256–64.

60. Nye JA, Schuster DM, Yu W, et al. Biodistribution and radiation dosimetry of the synthetic nonmetabolized amino acid analogue anti-18F-FACBC in humans. J Nucl Med 2007;48(6):1017–20.

61. Pandey MK, Byrne JF, Jiang H, et al. Cyclotron production of (68)Ga via the (68)Zn(p,n)(68)Ga reaction in aqueous solution. Am J Nucl Med Mol Imaging 2014;4(4):303–10.

62. Picchio M, Briganti A, Fanti S, et al. The role of choline positron emission tomography/computed tomography in the management of patients with prostate-specific antigen progression after radical treatment of prostate cancer. Eur Urol 2011;59(1):51–60.

63. Brogsitter C, Zophel K, Kotzerke J. 18F-choline, 11C-choline and 11C-acetate PET/CT: comparative analysis for imaging prostate cancer patients. Eur J Nucl Med Mol Imaging 2013;40(Suppl 1):S18–27.

64. Bluemel C, Krebs M, Polat B, et al. 68Ga-PSMA-PET/CT in patients with biochemical prostate cancer recurrence and negative 18F-choline-PET/CT. Clin Nucl Med 2016;41(7):515–21.

65. Mottet N, Bellmunt J, Bolla M, et al. EAU-ESTRO-SIOG guidelines on prostate cancer. Part 1: screening, diagnosis, and local treatment with curative intent. Eur Urol 2017;71(4):618–29.

66. Welch HG, Fisher ES, Gottlieb DJ, et al. Detection of prostate cancer via biopsy in the Medicare-SEER population during the PSA era. J Natl Cancer Inst 2007;99(18):1395–400.

67. Epstein JI, Feng Z, Trock BJ, et al. Upgrading and downgrading of prostate cancer from biopsy to radical prostatectomy: incidence and predictive factors using the modified Gleason grading system and factoring in tertiary grades. Eur Urol 2012;61(5):1019–24.

68. Futterer JJ, Briganti A, De Visschere P, et al. Can clinically significant prostate cancer be detected with multiparametric magnetic resonance imaging? A systematic review of the literature. Eur Urol 2015;68(6):1045–53.

69. Ahmed HU, El-Shater Bosaily A, Brown LC, et al. Diagnostic accuracy of multi-parametric MRI and TRUS biopsy in prostate cancer (PROMIS): a paired validating confirmatory study. Lancet 2017;389(10071):815–22.

70. Le JD, Stephenson S, Brugger M, et al. Magnetic resonance imaging-ultrasound fusion biopsy for prediction of final prostate pathology. J Urol 2014;192(5):1367–73.

71. Moore CM, Robertson NL, Arsanious N, et al. Image-guided prostate biopsy using magnetic resonance imaging-derived targets: a systematic review. Eur Urol 2013;63(1):125–40.

72. Panebianco V, Barchetti F, Sciarra A, et al. Multiparametric magnetic resonance imaging vs. standard care in men being evaluated for prostate cancer: a randomized study. Urol Oncol 2015;33(1):17.e1-7.

73. Baco E, Rud E, Eri LM, et al. A randomized controlled trial to assess and compare the outcomes of two-core prostate biopsy guided by fused magnetic resonance and transrectal ultrasound images and traditional 12-core systematic biopsy. Eur Urol 2016;69(1):149–56.

74. Barentsz JO, Weinreb JC, Verma S, et al. Synopsis of the PI-RADS v2 guidelines for multiparametric prostate magnetic resonance imaging and recommendations for use. Eur Urol 2016;69(1):41–9.

75. Kasperzyk JL, Finn SP, Flavin R, et al. Prostate-specific membrane antigen protein expression in tumor tissue and risk of lethal prostate cancer. Cancer Epidemiol Biomarkers Prev 2013;22(12):2354–63.

76. Fendler WP, Schmidt DF, Wenter V, et al. 68Ga-PSMA PET/CT detects the location and extent of primary prostate cancer. J Nucl Med 2016;57(11):1720–5.

77. Woythal N, Arsenic R, Kempkensteffen C, et al. Immunohistochemical validation of PSMA expression measured by 68Ga-PSMA PET/CT in primary prostate cancer. J Nucl Med 2018;59(2):238–43.

78. Uprimny C, Kroiss AS, Decristoforo C, et al. (68) Ga-PSMA-11 PET/CT in primary staging of prostate cancer: PSA and Gleason score predict the intensity of tracer accumulation in the primary tumour. Eur J Nucl Med Mol Imaging 2017;44(6):941–9.

79. Koerber SA, Utzinger MT, Kratochwil C, et al. (68) Ga-PSMA-11 PET/CT in newly diagnosed

carcinoma of the prostate: correlation of intraprostatic PSMA uptake with several clinical parameters. J Nucl Med 2017;58(12):1943–8.

80. Giesel FL, Sterzing F, Schlemmer HP, et al. Intra-individual comparison of (68)Ga-PSMA-11-PET/CT and multi-parametric MR for imaging of primary prostate cancer. Eur J Nucl Med Mol Imaging 2016;43(8):1400–6.

81. Sanda MG, Cadeddu JA, Kirkby E, et al. Clinically Localized Prostate Cancer: AUA/ASTRO/SUO Guideline. Part I: Risk Stratification, Shared Decision Making, and Care Options. J Urol 2017 Dec 15. pii: S0022-5347(17)78003-2. [Epub ahead of print].

82. Briganti A, Blute ML, Eastham JH, et al. Pelvic lymph node dissection in prostate cancer. Eur Urol 2009;55(6):1251–65.

83. Barentsz JO, Thoeny HC. Prostate cancer: can imaging accurately diagnose lymph node involvement? Nature reviews. Urology 2015;12(6):313–5.

84. Gorin MA, Rowe SP, Patel HD, et al. Prostate specific membrane antigen targeted 18F-DCFPyL positron emission tomography/computerized tomography for the preoperative staging of high risk prostate cancer: results of a prospective, phase ii, single center study. J Urol 2018;199(1):126–32.

85. Maurer T, Gschwend JE, Rauscher I, et al. Diagnostic efficacy of (68)gallium-PSMA positron emission tomography compared to conventional imaging for lymph node staging of 130 consecutive patients with intermediate to high risk prostate cancer. J Urol 2016;195(5):1436–43.

86. Heidenreich A, Bastian PJ, Bellmunt J, et al. EAU guidelines on prostate cancer. Part II: treatment of advanced, relapsing, and castration-resistant prostate cancer. Eur Urol 2014;65(2):467–79.

87. Cornford P, Bellmunt J, Bolla M, et al. EAU-ESTRO-SIOG guidelines on prostate cancer. Part II: treatment of relapsing, metastatic, and castration-resistant prostate cancer. Eur Urol 2017;71(4): 630–42.

88. Pound CR, Partin AW, Eisenberger MA, et al. Natural history of progression after PSA elevation following radical prostatectomy. JAMA 1999; 281(17):1591–7.

89. King CR. The timing of salvage radiotherapy after radical prostatectomy: a systematic review. Int J Radiat Oncol Biol Phys 2012;84(1):104–11.

90. Beresford MJ, Gillatt D, Benson RJ, et al. A systematic review of the role of imaging before salvage radiotherapy for post-prostatectomy biochemical recurrence. Clin Oncol 2010;22(1):46–55.

91. Krause BJ, Souvatzoglou M, Tuncel M, et al. The detection rate of [11C]choline-PET/CT depends on the serum PSA-value in patients with biochemical recurrence of prostate cancer. Eur J Nucl Med Mol Imaging 2008;35(1):18–23.

92. Pfister D, Porres D, Heidenreich A, et al. Detection of recurrent prostate cancer lesions before salvage lymphadenectomy is more accurate with (68)Ga-PSMA-HBED-CC than with (18)F-fluoroethylcholine PET/CT. Eur J Nucl Med Mol Imaging 2016;43(8): 1410–7.

93. Rauscher I, Maurer T, Beer AJ, et al. Value of 68Ga-PSMA HBED-CC PET for the assessment of lymph node metastases in prostate cancer patients with biochemical recurrence: comparison with histopathology after salvage lymphadenectomy. J Nucl Med 2016;57(11):1713–9.

94. Gandaglia G, Karakiewicz PI, Briganti A, et al. Impact of the site of metastases on survival in patients with metastatic prostate cancer. Eur Urol 2015;68(2):325–34.

95. Cimitan M, Bortolus R, Morassut S, et al. [18F]fluorocholine PET/CT imaging for the detection of recurrent prostate cancer at PSA relapse: experience in 100 consecutive patients. Eur J Nucl Med Mol Imaging 2006;33(12):1387–98.

96. Hijazi S, Meller B, Leitsmann C, et al. Pelvic lymph node dissection for nodal oligometastatic prostate cancer detected by 68Ga-PSMA-positron emission tomography/computerized tomography. Prostate 2015;75(16):1934–40.

97. Herlemann A, Kretschmer A, Buchner A, et al. Salvage lymph node dissection after (68)Ga-PSMA or (18)F-FEC PET/CT for nodal recurrence in prostate cancer patients. Oncotarget 2017; 8(48):84180–92.

98. Maurer T, Weirich G, Schottelius M, et al. Prostate-specific membrane antigen-radioguided surgery for metastatic lymph nodes in prostate cancer. Eur Urol 2015;68(3):530–4.

99. Baranski AC, Schafer M, Bauder-Wust U, et al. PSMA-11 derived dual-labeled PSMA-inhibitors for preoperative PET imaging and precise fluorescence-guided surgery of prostate cancer. J Nucl Med 2018 Apr;59(4):639–45.

100. Morigi JJ, Stricker PD, van Leeuwen PJ, et al. Prospective comparison of 18F-fluoromethyl-choline versus 68Ga-PSMA PET/CT in prostate cancer patients who have rising PSA after curative treatment and are being considered for targeted therapy. J Nucl Med 2015;56(8): 1185–90.

101. Bluemel C, Linke F, Herrmann K, et al. Impact of 68Ga-PSMA PET/CT on salvage radiotherapy planning in patients with prostate cancer and persisting PSA values or biochemical relapse after prostatectomy. EJNMMI Res 2016;6(1):78.

102. Sterzing F, Kratochwil C, Fiedler H, et al. (68)Ga-PSMA-11 PET/CT: a new technique with high potential for the radiotherapeutic management of prostate cancer patients. Eur J Nucl Med Mol Imaging 2016;43(1):34–41.

103. Calais J, Czernin J, Cao M, et al. (68)Ga-PSMA PET/CT mapping of prostate cancer biochemical recurrence following radical prostatectomy in 270 patients with PSA<1.0ng/ml: impact on salvage radiotherapy planning. J Nucl Med 2018;59(2):230–7.

104. Albisinni S, Artigas C, Aoun F, et al. Clinical impact of (68) Ga-prostate-specific membrane antigen (PSMA) positron emission tomography/computed tomography (PET/CT) in patients with prostate cancer with rising prostate-specific antigen after treatment with curative intent: preliminary analysis of a multidisciplinary approach. BJU Int 2017;120(2):197–203.

105. Roach PJ, Francis R, Emmett L, et al. The impact of 68Ga-PSMA PET/CT on management intent in prostate cancer: results of an Australian prospective multicenter study. J Nucl Med 2018;59(1):82–8.

106. Hope TA, Aggarwal R, Chee B, et al. Impact of (68)Ga-PSMA-11 PET on management in patients with biochemically recurrent prostate cancer. J Nucl Med 2017;58(12):1956–61.

107. Calais J, Fendler WP, Eiber M, et al. Impact of (68)Ga-PSMA-11 PET/CT on the management of prostate cancer patients with biochemical recurrence. J Nucl Med 2018;59(3):434–41.

108. Afaq A, Alahmed S, Chen SH, et al. (68)Ga-PSMA PET/CT impact on prostate cancer management. J Nucl Med 2018 Jan;59(1):89–92.

109. Grubmüller B, Baltzer P, D'Andrea D, et al. (68)Ga-PSMA 11 ligand PET imaging in patients with biochemical recurrence after radical prostatectomy - diagnostic performance and impact on therapeutic decision-making. Eur J Nucl Med Mol Imaging 2018;45(2):235–42.

110. Katsogiannou M, Ziouziou H, Karaki S, et al. The hallmarks of castration-resistant prostate cancers. Cancer Treat Rev 2015;41(7):588–97.

111. Lian F, Sharma NV, Moran JD, et al. The biology of castration-resistant prostate cancer. Curr Probl Cancer 2015;39(1):17–28.

112. Geethakumari PR, Cookson MS, Kelly WK, Prostate Cancer Clinical Trials Working Group 3. The evolving biology of castration-resistant prostate cancer: review of recommendations from the prostate cancer clinical trials working group 3. Oncology 2016;30(2):187–95, 199.

113. Scher HI, Morris MJ, Stadler WM, et al. Trial design and objectives for castration-resistant prostate cancer: updated recommendations from the prostate cancer clinical trials working group 3. J Clin Oncol 2016;34(12):1402–18.

114. Lorente D, Mateo J, Perez-Lopez R, et al. Sequencing of agents in castration-resistant prostate cancer. Lancet Oncol 2015;16(6):e279–92.

115. Valenca LB, Sweeney CJ, Pomerantz MM. Sequencing current therapies in the treatment of metastatic prostate cancer. Cancer Treat Rev 2015;41(4):332–40.

116. Fox JJ, Gavane SC, Blanc-Autran E, et al. Positron emission tomography/computed tomography-based assessments of androgen receptor expression and glycolytic activity as a prognostic biomarker for metastatic castration-resistant prostate cancer. JAMA Oncol 2018;4(2):217–24.

117. Gofrit ON, Frank S, Meirovitz A, et al. PET/CT with 68Ga-DOTA-TATE for diagnosis of neuroendocrine: differentiation in patients with castrate-resistant prostate cancer. Clin Nucl Med 2017;42(1):1–6.

118. Giovacchini G, Picchio M, Garcia-Parra R, et al. 11C-choline PET/CT predicts prostate cancer-specific survival in patients with biochemical failure during androgen-deprivation therapy. J Nucl Med 2014;55(2):233–41.

119. De Giorgi U, Caroli P, Scarpi E, et al. (18)F-Fluorocholine PET/CT for early response assessment in patients with metastatic castration-resistant prostate cancer treated with enzalutamide. Eur J Nucl Med Mol Imaging 2015;42(8):1276–83.

120. Seitz AK, Rauscher I, Haller B, et al. Preliminary results on response assessment using 68Ga-HBED-CC-PSMA PET/CT in patients with metastatic prostate cancer undergoing docetaxel chemotherapy. Eur J Nucl Med Mol Imaging 2018;45(4):602–12.

121. Fendler WP, Eiber M, Beheshti M, et al. (68)Ga-PSMA PET/CT: joint EANM and SNMMI procedure guideline for prostate cancer imaging: version 1.0. Eur J Nucl Med Mol Imaging 2017;44(6):1014–24.

122. Fanti S, Minozzi S, Morigi JJ, et al. Development of standardized image interpretation for 68Ga-PSMA PET/CT to detect prostate cancer recurrent lesions. Eur J Nucl Med Mol Imaging 2017;44(10):1622–35.

123. Fendler WP, Calais J, Allen-Auerbach M, et al. (68)Ga-PSMA-11 PET/CT interobserver agreement for prostate cancer assessments: an international multicenter prospective study. J Nucl Med 2017;58(10):1617–23.

124. Weinreb JC, Barentsz JO, Choyke PL, et al. PI-RADS prostate imaging - reporting and data system: 2015, version 2. Eur Urol 2016;69(1):16–40.

125. Rowe SP, Pienta KJ, Pomper MG, et al. Proposal of a structured reporting system for prostate-specific membrane antigen (PSMA)-targeted PET imaging: PSMA-RADS version 1.0. J Nucl Med 2018;59(3):479–85.

126. Cheng L, Montironi R, Bostwick DG, et al. Staging of prostate cancer. Histopathology 2012;60(1):87–117.

127. Eiber M, Herrmann K, Calais J, et al. PROstate cancer molecular imaging standardized evaluation (PROMISE): proposed miTNM classification for the interpretation of PSMA-ligand PET/CT. J Nucl Med 2018;59(3):469–78.

Moving?

Make sure your subscription moves with you!

To notify us of your new address, find your **Clinics Account Number** (located on your mailing label above your name), and contact customer service at:

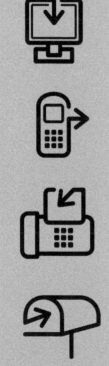

Email: journalscustomerservice-usa@elsevier.com

800-654-2452 (subscribers in the U.S. & Canada)
314-447-8871 (subscribers outside of the U.S. & Canada)

Fax number: 314-447-8029

Elsevier Health Sciences Division
Subscription Customer Service
3251 Riverport Lane
Maryland Heights, MO 63043

*To ensure uninterrupted delivery of your subscription, please notify us at least 4 weeks in advance of move.

ELSEVIER